The Source® Dysphagia

Fourth Edition

Nancy B. Swigert

pro·ed
An International Publisher

800-897-3202   Fax 800-397-7633
www.proedinc.com

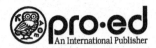

© 2019, 2007, 2000, 1996 by PRO-ED, Inc.

1301 W. 25th St., Suite 300

Austin, TX 78705-4248

800-897-3202   Fax 800-397-7633

www.proedinc.com

Limited Photocopy License

Library of Congress Cataloging-in-Publication Data

Names: Swigert, Nancy B., author.
Title: The source : dysphagia / Nancy B. Swigert.
Other titles: Source for dysphagia
Description: Fourth edition. | Austin, Texas : PRO-ED, Inc. [2019] |
    Preceded by Source for dysphagia / by Nancy B. Swigert. 3rd ed. 2007. |
    Includes bibliographical references.
Identifiers: LCCN 2018035433 (print) | LCCN 2018036194 (ebook) | ISBN
    9781416411628 (ebook) | ISBN 9781416411611
Subjects: | MESH: Deglutition Disorders—therapy | Deglutition
    Disorders—diagnosis | Patient Care Planning
Classification: LCC RC815.2 (ebook) | LCC RC815.2 (print) | NLM WI 258 |
DDC
    616.3/23—dc23
LC record available at https://lccn.loc.gov/2018035433

Art Director: Jason Crosier
Designer: Tom de Lorenzo

Printed in the United States of America

3 4 5 6 7 8 9 10 11   31 30 29 28 27 26 25 24 23 22

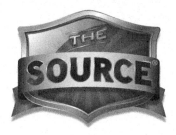

Disorder	Ages
Dysphagia	Adults

Evidence-Based Practice

Evidence-based practice (EBP) has been defined as "the conscientious, explicit, and judicious use of current best evidence in making decisions about the care of individual patients . . . [by] integrating individual clinical expertise with the best available external clinical evidence from systematic research" (Sackett et al., 1996). Guyatt et al. (2000) and Sackett et al. (2000) have emphasized the need to integrate patient values and preferences along with best current research evidence and clinical expertise in making clinical decisions. To the extent possible, this book provides the evidence available on techniques and methods for dysphagia evaluation and treatment.

ASHA practice documents on dysphagia support the following guidelines, which are incorporated in this book:

Speech–language pathologists (SLPs) should have a basic understanding of the following areas:

- Normal and abnormal anatomy and physiology related to swallowing function
- Signs and symptoms of dysphagia
- Indications for instrumental evaluations
- Analyzing clinical and instrumental information to establish a diagnosis and prepare appropriate documentation
- Determining candidacy for intervention
- Implementing compensations and therapy techniques
- Educating and counseling individuals with swallowing problems and their care providers
- Quality-of-life issues related to the individual and the individual's family
- Identifying and using appropriate functional outcome measures
- Related medical issues

SLPs are the primary providers of evaluation and treatment for feeding and swallowing disorders. SLPs should not train individuals or groups of individuals from other professions in the delivery of evaluation and treatment for infants, children, and adults with swallowing and feeding disorders.

The Source: Dysphagia–Fourth Edition incorporates these principles and is also based on expert professional practice.

About the Author

Nancy B. Swigert, MA, CCC-SLP, BCS-S (retired), is the president of Swigert & Associates Inc., providing consulting and education services on dysphagia, documentation, coding, and reimbursement. She recently retired from Baptist Health Lexington (KY) as the process excellence coordinator, with a Green Belt in Lean/Six Sigma. Prior to that she was the director of Speech-Language Pathology and Respiratory Care for 10 years. Before joining Baptist staff, for 26 years Nancy's private practice provided speech–language pathology services in the Central Kentucky area. She is a board-certified specialist in swallowing and swallowing disorders (retired).

Nancy received her master's degree from the University of Tennessee–Knoxville. She is a former president of the Kentucky Speech-Language-Hearing Association (KSHA), the Council of State Association Presidents, the American Speech-Language-Hearing Association, and the American Speech-Language-Hearing Foundation Board of Trustees. She was on the Steering Committee for ASHA Special Interest (Group) Division 13, Swallowing and Swallowing Disorders, for 6 years and coordinator for 3 of those 6 years. She chaired the American Board of Swallowing and Swallowing Disorders for 3 years and currently serves on the Medical Advisory Board for the National Foundation on Swallowing Disorders. Nancy is a fellow of ASHA and was awarded Honors of ASHA in 2015.

Nancy's main interests are in the areas of pediatric and adult dysphagia and other neurogenic disorders. She has authored these publications with LinguiSystems/PRO-ED: *The Source for Dysphagia, The Source for Dysarthria, The Source for Pediatric Dysphagia, The Source for Reading Fluency, The Early Intervention Kit*, and *The Source for Children's Voice Disorders*. She has also published *Documentation and Reimbursement for SLPs: Principles and Practice*. She lectures extensively in the areas of pediatric and adult dysphagia, documentation, and reimbursement. She and her husband recently retired to the mountains of North Carolina.

Dedication

This edition is dedicated to my best friend and husband of 43 years, Keith, who patiently entertains himself while I am at the desk working on projects like this book. Now that the fourth edition is finished, let the true retirement begin!

Acknowledgments

I am indebted to the following individuals for their contributions to this book:

- Fellow board-certified specialists in swallowing at Baptist Health who served as an informal review panel during the revision:
    - Stefanie Moynahan, MS, CCC-SLP, BCS-S
    - Ashley Wright, MS, CCC-SLP, BCS-S
    - Sarah Groppo-Lawless, MS, CCC-SLP, BCS-S
    - Amber Valentine, MS, CCC-SLP, BCS-S
- Curt Hohenecker, AAS, RRT, RPFT, respiratory care manager at Baptist, for reviewing information on all matters respiratory and for providing some of the artwork
- Nicole Wells, BS, RRT, respiratory care supervisor at Baptist, for reviewing information on critical care
- Carla Townsend, MLIS, librarian at Baptist, for finding each and every resource article requested

Illustrated by Margaret Warner and Cindy Maxwell.

Contents

Supplemental Materials

SLP Resources	Referenced in chapter(s)
Case Examples: Choosing the Appropriate Exam	2, 3
Case Examples: Treatment Planning	4
Chart Review Information	1
Clinical Swallow Evaluation Form A	2
Clinical Swallow Evaluation Form B	2
Clinical Swallow Evaluation Summary Sheet	2
Cranial Nerve Assessment During Instrumental Exam	3
Cranial Nerve Exam	2
Discharge Summary Example	5
FEES® Examination Protocol	3
FEES Interpretation	3
FEES Report Form	3
FEES Report Sample	3
Frazier Free Water Protocol Guidelines	4
Goals and Treatment Objectives	4, 5
MBS/VFSS Interpretation	3
MBS/VFSS Report Form	3
MBS/VFSS Report Samples	3
Nerves and Muscles Involved in Swallowing	2
Outpatient Instrumental Exam Referral Form	3
Progress Report Examples	5
Recertification Example	5
Swallowing Questionnaire: Additional History	1
Treatment Notes Examples	5
Treatment Plan Examples	5
Education Materials Patient/Family	
Clinical or Bedside Swallowing Evaluation Information	2, 8
Dementia: Stages and Eating	8
Endoscopic Evaluation of Swallowing Q&A	3
Fiberoptic Endoscopic Evaluation of Swallowing (FEES) Information	3, 8
Lifestyle Modifications for Patients with Gastroesophageal Reflux Disease (GERD)	1, 8

Education Materials Patient/Family	Referenced in chapter(s)
Modified Barium Swallow/VFSS Q&A	3, 8
Modified Barium Swallow/VFSS Information	3, 8
Oral Care Guidelines for Patients Who Cannot Have Thin Liquids	8
Oral Care Handout	2, 8
Phases of Swallow	1, 3
Safe Feeding Goals for Family	8
Safe Feeding Instructions for Family	8
Swallowing Exercises List	4, 8
Swallowing Exercises Instructions	4, 8
Education Materials Staff	
Suctioning Competency Validation Tool	6
Swallowing Screen for Training Nurses Validation Tool	2
Education Materials Staff/Physician	
Aspiration and Aspiration Pneumonia FAQs	8
Dysphagia Q&A	8
Instrumental Examination of Swallowing	7, 8
Letter to Physician Samples	8
Training Materials	
Dysphagia and Palliative Care (PowerPoint)	8
Dysphagia In-Service (PowerPoint)	8
Dysphagia In-Service Pre- and Posttest	8
Dysphagia In-Service (Supplemental Materials)	8
Helping the Patient with Dementia Eat (PowerPoint)	8
Managing Dysphagia: Role of Food Service Staff (PowerPoint)	8
Oral Hygiene Importance (PowerPoint)	8
Oral Care Validation Tool	8
Swallowing Guidelines Signs	8
References	
Efficacy References for Treatment Techniques	4

Introduction

Working with adults with dysphagia is a challenging and rewarding part of the practice of speech–language pathology. I am fortunate to have had the opportunity to evaluate and treat patients in a variety of settings, and this book is a compilation of what I have learned and how I have applied that information to different practice settings. It is meant to be a practical resource for you to use on a day-to-day basis but also has reference information that will help you when you encounter a challenging patient. It should be just one of many resources you use to build your knowledge and skills in dysphagia management.

The Source for Dysphagia was first published in 1996 and then updated in 2000 and again in 2007. Because it is crucial to practice from an evidence base in dysphagia, and research in the area provides new information on an almost monthly basis, it was time again for a comprehensive review and update. This fourth edition provides information that is current in evaluation and treatment, with particular attention paid to updating evidence for treatment techniques.

Most chapters contain significant revisions, such as the following:

- Additional information about what to know before you evaluate a patient, including information on oral hygiene, staging of disease, and standardized questionnaires

- Validated screening tools and the use of screening with different populations

- A streamlined clinical swallow evaluation tool in two formats, each including cranial nerve assessment

- A helpful chart for interpreting findings on VFSS and a new chart for FEES

- Information on the ICF and the importance of keeping a focus on function in treatment planning

- A helpful chart on matching treatment techniques to the impaired physiology

- Revised long- and short-term goals and treatment objectives based on current evidence

- Background information on the principles of neuroplasticity and motor learning

- Updated educational materials with new handouts on the SLP's role in palliative care and end-of-life decision making and the ethical challenges encountered with the end of life

- Information about the International Dysphagia Diet Standardisation Initiative (IDDSI)

- An updated reference list and a list organized by treatment technique

As in the third edition, because of the expanded information, many of the pages are included in the Supplemental Materials (available online) either in addition to the hard copy in the book or instead of a hard copy. You will find a complete listing of the Supplemental Materials immediately following the Table of Contents. Pages you might want to reproduce (e.g., education materials, forms) are included in the Supplemental Materials for ease of use. For example, you can print patient handouts or signs, or forms such as the Clinical Swallow Exam, for use with clients.

Speech–language pathologists are the preferred providers of services to patients with dysphagia. To remain in this position, we must continually update our knowledge and skills. I hope

Dysphagia–Fourth Edition is one of the ways you will keep your skills on the cutting edge of dysphagia services. I also hope you'll take advantage of ASHA's Special Interest Group 13, Swallowing and Swallowing Disorders, which is a great value and an easy way to stay current in our area of practice. In addition, I challenge you to consider seeking Board Certification in Swallowing. Visit the website of the American Board of Swallowing and Swallowing Disorders (http://www.swallowingdisorders.org) for more information.

Nancy

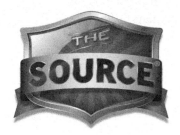

Chapter 1
Preparing for a Patient Assessment

Preparing for assessing a patient with dysphagia starts long before you open the inpatient's chart for review or read the case history the outpatient has completed. The clinician must have a solid understanding of the anatomy and physiology of the normal swallow and abnormal swallow. In-depth knowledge about different causes of dysphagia is required, including structural and neurological causes, and the ways dysphagia symptoms and management can change over the course of a disease. Armed with that base of information, the speech–language pathologist (SLP) is ready to prepare for the evaluation of a particular patient.

There are many reasons to take the time to collect a patient's history before beginning the assessment:

- To get a general idea of the probable etiology of the dysphagia. This allows the clinician time to review any related material (e.g., pull a textbook off your shelf, do a quick internet search).

- To learn whether the patient has family support.

- To determine which food consistencies, if any, to present in the clinical swallow exam. Perhaps the patient has already been on an altered diet before admission, and this information might indicate that you should exclude certain textures or consistencies.

- To learn whether the patient's physical or cognitive condition will preclude full participation in the evaluation.

The information on the following pages is important to obtain *before* you evaluate a patient's swallowing abilities.

The Patient's Chart

At inpatient facilities the clinician should review the medical chart. If the chart is fully electronic, the review can be completed in an expeditious manner once the SLP learns the charting system and knows where to look for necessary information. Paper charts can be more cumbersome to navigate, and some facilities use both electronic and paper charting. In that case, the clinician should review both. The following information can usually be found in the patient's chart. Clinicians may find the form Chart Review Information, found in the Supplemental Materials (SLP Resources), helpful when reviewing a chart.

Medical History

ADMIT DIAGNOSIS
Determine whether the patient has a diagnosis that might account for the dysphagia. For instance, the patient may have had a recent stroke or may have a progressive disorder, such as Parkinson's disease or multiple sclerosis, and has been admitted for an exacerbation.

The admit diagnosis might not seem related to the dysphagia. For example, a patient may have been admitted for a broken hip or cardiac problems. In this case, it would be necessary to delve more deeply into the patient's medical record to determine whether a complication occurred after admission that would have caused the dysphagia. In an acute-care setting, the patient might have undergone surgery or have delirium. However, it may be that the dysphagia is related to a decrease in the patient's functional reserve. Consider this analogy: A healthy individual is able to push a heavy desk across the room. That same person then experiences an illness and has been bedridden for several days and is very weak. That person would likely not be able to push the desk upon getting out of bed because her reserve was depleted. The same thing happens with swallowing skills. An otherwise healthy elderly person may start to display symptoms of dysphagia after an acute event that seems unrelated to neurological status, such as an exacerbation of congestive heart failure or surgery for a broken hip. The acute event has depleted the patient's reserve and revealed a new dysphagia.

Check the chart to be sure that an appropriate medical diagnosis is listed. Medicare can deny reimbursement if the diagnostic code (ICD-10) does not make sense with the procedure code (CPT). For example, if the only medical diagnosis listed is hip fracture, a CPT code for clinical dysphagia evaluation (92610) would be illogical. If a related medical diagnosis does not make sense with the procedure code(s) for dysphagia, consult with the physician to ensure that the diagnosis of dysphagia is added to the medical record as a medical diagnosis.

LEVEL OF ALERTNESS
The more alert a patient is, the better a candidate he or she is for therapeutic intervention. If a patient is not alert and has an alternative source of nutrition, it may be better to delay the intervention until later.

PREVIOUS DIAGNOSES AND TREATMENT
Note any other diagnoses the patient has had. The patient may have had several strokes that resulted in oral motor problems affecting swallowing. A patient may have had radiation treatment for a head and neck cancer years before, with symptoms of dysphagia just beginning to appear. Also note whether the patient has had any previous treatment for dysphagia or related disorders.

PREMORBID STATUS
Find out what the patient's status was before the most recent event that caused the dysphagia. It may be that the patient has eaten pureed foods for some time, and therefore, it may not be reasonable to expect the patient to return to a regular diet at this time.

Advance Directive/Code Status

Check to see whether the patient has filled out an advance directive indicating his or her wishes for resuscitation. Code status indicates which efforts the health-care team will take if the patient's heart stops or the patient stops breathing. Full code status typically means that if the patient's heart stops, the team will use chest compressions, medications, and electric shocks. If the patient stops breathing they will intubate the patient. The abbreviations DNR (do not resuscitate) and DNI (do not intubate) may be used. However, the term most commonly used today, particularly with patients in palliative care or hospice, is *allow natural death* (AND).

An order to allow natural death is meant to ensure that only comfort measures are provided to the patient. The term acknowledges that the person is dying and that everything that is being done for the patient will allow for the dying process to occur as comfortably as possible. This includes withdrawal of artificial nutrition and hydration. To compare the terms *DNR* and *AND*, consider this example. While a DNR patient in intensive care might be put on a ventilator, given artificial hydration, or have a feeding tube inserted, a patient with an AND order would have all those things withdrawn, discontinued, or not even started (see Meyer, n.d., for more information).

Because the recommendations for management of dysphagia will differ in a patient who is acutely ill versus a patient with AND status, the SLP must be fully aware of the patient's and family's wishes. See Chapter 7 for further discussion of managing dysphagia in patients in palliative and hospice care.

Referral/Order

REASON FOR REFERRAL

Your evaluation should state the reason the patient was referred to you. If you do not have the information, look through the patient's records to find out why he or she was referred. The reasons for referral can be many. The patient may have been referred to you because of functional problems, to rule out silent aspiration as a possible cause for pneumonia, or to determine whether dysphagia is related to a recent weight loss, for example.

SIGNED PHYSICIAN'S ORDER

Most settings and payers require that you have a signed physician's order or have obtained a verbal order before you assess the patient. In electronic health records (EHRs) there will be not a physical signature but rather wording that indicates the physician has entered the order. This might say something like "authenticated by" or "order entered by." Familiarize yourself with the charting system in use. Verbal orders also have to be entered or written in a specific way, and they likely require that you document that you "read back" and "verified" the order you took.

FUNCTIONAL PROBLEMS OBSERVED

Information on functional problems observed can often be obtained from nursing notes. Look for terminology such as *coughing or choking when drinking, refusing to take certain foods,* or *drooling.* This information can be obtained in more depth from the patient and caregiver interview.

Signs of Dysphagia

Signs are something that the clinician or another provider has observed. Although the terms *signs* and *symptoms* are sometimes used interchangeably, symptoms are things the patient reports and will be discussed in the section Interpreting the Symptoms the Patient Reports.

DROOLING/INCREASED SECRETIONS

A patient showing drooling or complaining of "excess saliva" (usually means the patient is not swallowing secretions as well as previously) may indicate dysphagia.

WEIGHT LOSS

If a patient has experienced an unintentional weight loss, dysphagia is a possible cause. A patient may have trouble swallowing certain food consistencies and avoid eating them. He or she then experiences weight loss.

COUGHING OR CHOKING

Coughing and choking are very obvious signs of dysphagia.

POCKETING

If the patient has poor oral skills, you may find information indicating that the nurses have to clean food out of the patient's mouth long after a meal.

PNEUMONIA

Aspiration pneumonia is an infection in the lungs. If a patient has aspirated, he or she may develop symptoms of pneumonia, such as cough and fever. Some patients who aspirate may not develop pneumonia. It is very difficult for a physician to determine whether pneumonia is due to aspiration unless the pneumonia developed soon after an observable episode of aspiration. It is just as difficult for a radiologist to look at a chest X-ray and identify aspiration pneumonia versus pneumonia due to another infectious process. Therefore, question any mention of pneumonia in a patient's chart. For more information, see the section below on respiratory status.

CHANGES IN DIET
Recent changes in eating or drinking habits may be an unconscious reaction to difficulty handling certain textures or types of foods.

PATIENT COMPLAINT
A patient's complaint about difficulty swallowing will often trigger a referral.

DEHYDRATION
Patients who have developed dysphagia may begin to avoid liquids and become dehydrated. The dehydration may not be mentioned specifically in the chart. If not, some signs that the patient may be dehydrated include confusion, constipation, poor skin turgor or skin breakdown, and renal insufficiency. Dehydration can contribute to patient falls, stroke, and renal failure.

Patients may also become dehydrated as a result of conditions that cause water loss (e.g., fever or infection, high environmental temperature or low environmental humidity, diuretic therapies) and/or conditions that cause both water and electrolyte loss (e.g., vomiting, diarrhea, food or fluid malabsorption, losses through a fistula or an ostomy).

REFLUX
Look for any mention of the patient's complaints of heartburn, reflux, or tightness in the chest. For more information on reflux and other esophageal disorders, see the section Esophageal Dysphagia in this chapter.

Nutrition and Hydration Status

CURRENT DIET
Document the patient's current diet. If a patient is in an acute-care setting and recently had surgery, he or she may initially be placed on a clear-liquid or full-liquid diet to reduce the risk of an upset stomach and vomiting. However, the clear-liquid diet may be the most difficult for the patient with dysphagia to handle.

The patient may have been on a modified diet for some time. For instance, patients who have had all their teeth removed may have already altered the kinds of food they are eating. Patients with dementia may have been placed on a pureed diet for ease of feeding. It is important to know what the baseline is before evaluating the patient.

DIETARY RESTRICTIONS
There may be restrictions other than the texture of a patient's diet that need to be considered. For instance, patients may be on the American Heart Association diet or a diabetic, carbohydrate-controlled diet. Collaborate with the dietitian at the facility to learn more about the specific diets used there.

ALTERNATE METHOD OF FEEDING
Determine whether the patient is on a nasogastric/nasojejunal (NG/NJ) or percutaneous endoscopic gastrostomy (PEG) tube or is receiving parenteral nutrition. Feeding that uses the gut is enteral feeding (e.g., NG, NJ, PEG, PEJ), whereas parenteral bypasses the intestinal system (Table 1.1). Total parenteral nutrition (TPN) delivers nutrients directly to the bloodstream and is often used when the gut is not working properly. For more information on TPN, see Chapter 6.

Table 1.1
Comparison of Feeding Tubes

Types of tubes	Description	Indications	Advantages	Disadvantages
Nasogastric (NG tube)	• Available in a variety of sizes • Placed into the nare through the nasopharynx, down the esophagus, into the stomach • Radiopaque (shows up on X-ray to verify placement)	• Usually used short term (less than 6 weeks) • Patient's GI tract has to be functioning • Often used for patients with swallowing disorders secondary to neurological impairment, tumors of the head and neck or esophagus	• Putting tube into stomach is more natural than directly into intestine • Stomach acid helps destroy microorganisms and may reduce risk of infection • Intermittent feedings may be better tolerated in the stomach	• Some patients find the tube uncomfortable • Sometimes difficult for the patient to self-feed around a feeding tube • Sometimes patients pull at the tube and have to have hands restrained • May be contraindicated for patients at high risk for aspiration, as it keeps the LES slightly open and may permit reflux • Easily dislodged by the patient, can coil in the hypopharynx or be placed incorrectly into trachea
Nasoduodenal or nasojejunal	• Very similar to NG tube, but tip goes through stomach into the duodenum or jejunum • May be used postoperatively if the patient has had gastric surgery	• Same as NG tube	• May be less risk for aspiration than NG tube	• Same as NG tube
Gastrostomy (G-tube)	• Surgically placed directly into the stomach (very few tubes are surgically placed unless patient is already undergoing abdominal surgery)	• Used for long-term feedings • Patient's GI tract has to be functioning • Often used for patients with swallowing disorders secondary to neurological impairment, tumors of the head and neck or esophagus	• Same as NG tube but more comfortable and aesthetic	• Requires surgery to place
Percutaneous endoscopic gastrostomy (PEG tube)	• Same as G-tube but placed under local anesthesia or conscious sedation at bedside	• Same as G-tube	• Same as G-tube	• Contraindicated for patients with peritonitis, esophageal obstruction, morbid obesity, or severe gastroesophageal reflux

(continues)

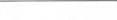

Table 1.1. *(continued)*

Types of tubes	Description	Indications	Advantages	Disadvantages
Jejunostomy (J-tube)	• Tube surgically placed directly into the jejunum	• For long-term feeding • Also used for short-term feeding after GI tract surgery • When severe reflux and emesis are present	• Little to no aspiration risk because of negative pressure below pyloric sphincter • Tube cannot be misplaced • More comfortable and aesthetic	• Contraindicated for patients with peritonitis or morbid obesity
Percutaneous endoscopic jejunostomy (PEJ)	• Same as J-tube but placed under local anesthesia or conscious sedation at bedside	• Same as J-tube	• Same as J-tube	• Contraindicated for patients with peritonitis, esophageal obstruction, or morbid obesity

Medications

Almost any patient you will evaluate for dysphagia will be taking some kind of medication. Some medications have no impact on the dysphagia or its symptoms, whereas others might have a significant role in causing the symptoms or addressing the cause of the dysphagia (Table 1.2). A common problem in the elderly is polypharmacy, a term that refers to multiple, excessive, or unnecessary drug consumption. Factors that contribute to polypharmacy are low health literacy (not understanding what a medication is intended to do) and the availability of many over-the-counter drugs. The speech–language pathologist should consult with the pharmacist concerning any questions about the medications the patient is taking and how the interaction of the medications may affect the patient's symptoms (Evans & McLeod, 2003; Mintzer & Burns, 2000; Mortazavi et al., 2016).

MENTAL STATUS CHANGE, CONFUSION, AND SEDATION RELATED TO MEDICATIONS

Elderly patients are at risk of confusion caused by drugs, especially if they already have some cognitive impairments. Drugs that may cause confusion include anticholinergics, analgesics, psychotropics, and antiepileptics. Many of these drugs can also cause drowsiness. If a patient is on sedatives, it is important to time your evaluation so the patient is alert. Be aware that if you evaluate the patient when he or she is alert and make recommendations, the patient still may be sedated for a large part of the day and not able to do as well at mealtimes as during your evaluation.

MEDICATIONS TO TREAT DISEASES THAT MAY AFFECT SWALLOW

If the patient is taking a medication to treat a specific neurological disorder, it is important to find out whether that medicine has any effect on enhancing or interfering with the swallow function. For example, one systematic review reported conflicting results on whether levodopa (L-DOPA), typically used to treat Parkinson's disease, causes a decline or an improvement in swallowing skills. One study found that more than half of patients experienced improvement of the swallowing function, possibly due to the reduction of bradykinesia and rigidity of the tongue (Mancopes et al., 2013). Another pilot study found that swallowing efficiency was reduced (Lim, Leow, Huckabee, Frampton, & Anderson, 2008).

Another consideration is that a side effect of levodopa is xerostomia, which often negatively affects the oral phases of the swallow. Because there are conflicting findings, it might be beneficial to see what the effects are on your patient. Levodopa is typically at its peak in the bloodstream 1 hour after administration. The speech–language pathologist can assess the patient at that time compared

Table 1.2
Types of Medications: Intended Use and Side Effects

Type of medication	Examples: Intended use	Side effects (examples)
ACE inhibitors (angiotensin converting enzyme) and ARB (angiotensin receptor blockers)	Hypertension Heart failure	Dry cough Loss of taste
Antibiotics	Infections	GI symptoms, allergic reaction
Anticoagulants	Prophylactic for DVT	Bleeding, bruising
Anticholinergics • Anti-Parkinson • Bronchodilators • Antispasmodics	 • Parkinson's • COPD • GI and bladder conditions	Dry mouth Memory impairment
Antidepressants	Depression	Dry mouth, nausea, constipation
Antidiabetic	Type 2 diabetes	GI symptoms
Analgesics	Acute pain	Dry mouth, drowsiness
Benzodiazepines	Anxiety Seizure disorder	Weakness, confusion, slurred speech
Beta blockers	Hypertension	Drowsiness, GI symptoms, GERD
Calcium channel blockers	Hypertension	Drowsiness, GI symptoms, GERD
Corticosteroids	Diseases of immunity, inflammation, rashes	Increased risk of infections, thinning bones
Diuretics	Edema associated with heart failure, high blood pressure, liver disease	Headache, dizziness, thirst
H2 receptor antagonists	Ulcers, GERD, esophagitis	Headache
Nitrates	Chest pain, angina	Headache, dizziness
Nonsteroidal anti-inflammatories (NSAIDs)	Inflammatory conditions like arthritis	Stomach pain, headaches and dizziness
Opioid analgesic	Pain control	Constipation, respiratory depression, sedation
Phosphate binding agents	Chronic kidney disease	GI symptoms, myopathy
Proton pump inhibitors	GERD, erosive esophagitis	Headache, GI symptoms
Psychotropics, including antipsychotics	Anxiety, depression, schizophrenia	Mouth, eating and digestion problems
Respiratory agents such as bronchodilators	COPD	Nausea, tachycardia, problems sleeping
SSRI (selective serotonin reuptake inhibitor) and SNRI (serotonin norepinephrine reuptake inhibitor)	Depression	Anorexia, constipation, xerostomia
Statins	High cholesterol	Muscle pain and weakness (and some have been known to weaken muscles of swallowing)

Note. Adapted from Muldoon et al. (2002); PDR Network (2011); Stockley (2002).

to at a nonpeak time. If the patient's swallowing skills are better at peak time after administration of the drug, then having the patient arrange meals around peak effects of medication could be beneficial (National Parkinson Foundation, 2017).

Patients with myasthenia gravis are typically treated with Mestinon, which has its peak effect at an hour postadministration. Therefore, having a discussion with the physician about changing the timing of medication may significantly improve the patient's ability to swallow (see the website www.myasthenia.org for specific information).

MEDICATIONS THAT CAN CAUSE SYMPTOMS OF DYSPHAGIA

Many medications can have a side effect causing symptoms of dysphagia. Some may affect the smooth muscles of the esophagus, whereas others can cause xerostomia. Others have side effects on the central nervous system (e.g., antiepileptics, benzodiazepines), causing muscle weakness or incoordination. Some even cause movement disorders (e.g., antipsychotic drugs) like tardive dyskinesia, which usually involves the muscles in the face and tongue. If the dysphagia is severe, the patient may not be able to chew or swallow. Still other medications (e.g., aspirin, nonsteroidal anti-inflammatory drugs, potassium chloride) can cause injury to the esophagus if the pill gets stuck, called pill-induced esophagitis.

GASTROESOPHAGEAL REFLUX DISEASE (GERD) MEDICATIONS

Gastroesophageal reflux disease (GERD) is often treated with medications, so it is important to note whether the patient is currently taking any of the following: antacids, such as over-the-counter calcium carbonate to neutralize stomach acid (e.g., Tums, Rolaids); histamine-2 receptor antagonists (e.g., ranitidine, cimetidine, famotidine, or nizatidine, with brand names like Zantac, Pepcid, Axid, and Tagamet), which help reduce stomach acids; or proton pump inhibitors (e.g., omeprazole, pantoprazole, and so on, with brand names like Nexium, Prevacid, Protonix, and Prilosec) to block the formation of acid. In addition, many medications may make reflux worse, such as antidepressants, anticholinergics, asthma medications, and sedatives (Galmiche, Barthelemy, & Hamelin, 1997; Tytgat et al., 2008).

ROUTE OF ADMINISTRATION

Determine how medications are being given to the patient. If the patient is NPO (nothing by mouth) with an NG tube, is he or she still getting his medications by mouth? Are any of the medications liquid (e.g., potassium chloride), and can the patient safely take liquids? Do the pills need to be crushed and mixed with a thickened liquid?

Oral Hygiene

Is the patient edentulous? If so, does the patient have dentures, and are the dentures present for the evaluation? If the patient has teeth, is there any information about caries and dental health?

Respiratory Status

LUNG DISEASES

Chronic obstructive pulmonary disease (COPD) is a blanket term with features of chronic bronchitis (inflammation of the airways) and emphysema (destruction of the alveoli). The result is significant trapping of air and impaired oxygen and carbon dioxide exchange. In a small study of outpatients with COPD referred for videofluoroscopic swallowing evaluation, nearly 85% had some degree of dysphagia, and there was a high percentage of silent penetration and aspiration (Good-Fratturelli, Curlee, & Holle, 2000). Upper-airway protections may be impaired as a result of incoordination between breathing and swallowing (Cvejic et al., 2011).

LUNG SOUNDS

Respiratory therapists, nurses, and physicians may make comments about the patient's lung sounds. Look for terms such as the following:

rhonchi   coarse, dry rale in the bronchial tubes

rale   abnormal respiratory sound heard on inspiration

wheeze   a whistling respiratory sound

There is no one-to-one correspondence between the sound heard on auscultation and underlying pulmonary issues. There are numerous websites on which one can listen to different adventitious breath sounds.

CHEST X-RAYS

Look at recent reports from chest X-rays to determine whether any infiltrates have been observed. Remember that something may not be reported as aspiration related when it actually is. In addition, if the patient has actually aspirated, the area of infiltrate in the lung will be the area of the lung that was dependent at the time of the aspiration event, not necessarily the right lower lobe. This means that if the patient lies down a lot, then both lower lobes may be affected, or even the middle lobes. If the patient aspirated when he or she was lying on the left side, the aspiration may be in the left lobe. See Table 1.3 for common terms used in radiology reports (Maron, 2003; Potchen et al., 2000; Van Ginneken, Stegmann, & Loog, 2006).

OXYGEN THERAPY AND MODE OF DELIVERY

If the patient is on oxygen therapy, it will give you some indication of his respiratory status. Oxygen is provided for several reasons, including hypoxemia, increased working of breathing, and hemodynamic insufficiency. The goal of oxygen therapy is to provide optimal oxygenation of tissue while reducing the work of the heart and lungs. Oxygen administration can be delivered via low-flow or high-flow systems, with humidity or not, and with a reservoir or not (Table 1.4). Humidity helps prevent the nasal passages from drying out. Reservoir systems incorporate a mechanism for gathering and storing oxygen during inspiration and exhalation. Patients draw from the oxygen reservoir anytime their minute ventilation flow exceeds the device delivery flow.

It is helpful to understand two factors about how the oxygen is provided, as different oxygen-delivery devices can provide oxygen at only certain concentrations and flow (liters per minute, or lpm).

Concentration of oxygen. Concentration of oxygen describes the fraction of oxygen in the air being breathed (FiO_2). Room air is 21% oxygen. The percentage of oxygen delivered can be inconsistent or precise, depending on the delivery device. Regarding the FiO_2 range, oxygen systems can be divided into those indicated for low oxygen (<35%), moderate delivery (35%–60%), or high delivery (>60%).

Liters per minute. Liters per minute describes the rate of flow at which the oxygen is delivered. As the flow increases, so does the percentage of oxygen delivered (Miller, 2015).

Determine whether the patient is receiving oxygen through a nasal cannula or a face mask (Figure 1.1). If the patient is using a face mask, find out if it can be changed to a nasal cannula so you can present food during your assessment. If patients cannot maintain a stable SpO_2 with a change in oxygen-delivery device, then perhaps they are not stable enough for an evaluation of their swallowing skills.

RECENT INTUBATIONS

If the patient has recently been orally intubated, he may have some edema of the vocal folds. This condition alone may be enough to cause some decreased laryngeal closure and possible aspiration during swallowing.

Table 1.3
Radiology Terms Used to Describe Chest Radiographs

Term	What is it describing?
Atelectasis	Complete or partial collapse of the alveoli in the lung; complication of surgery. This occurs when compressed from the outside (e.g., pleural effusion, pneumothorax) or when airway is obstructed (e.g., lung cancer, cystic fibrosis, inhaled foreign objects, tumors, respiratory weakness).
Infiltrates	Substance denser than air, such as pus, blood, or protein, which lingers within the parenchyma of the lungs. Associated with pneumonia but does not necessarily mean there is a pneumonia. Somewhat controversial term as it is vague. Preferred term is *pulmonary opacification*.
Pulmonary opacification	Caused by air space or interstitial disease.
Pleural effusion	Abnormal collection of fluid that lines the pleura of the lungs, between the lungs and the rib cage. Most common cause is congestive heart failure. On chest X-ray appears as blunted angles. Effusion causes shortness of air.
Consolidation/density	When alveoli, usually filled with air, instead are filled with fluid, cells, or tissue. Can be caused by pneumonia, edema, atelectasis.
Mass	Well-defined area of opacification.
Opacities	More solid matter has infiltrated an air-filled space.
Edema	Fluid saturating an area.
Cardiomegaly	Congestive heart failure (CHF), commonly called "enlarged heart." The heart then takes up space in the chest cavity and the lungs cannot fully expand.
Density	The term *density* is often used interchangeably with opacity. Density means an area on the X-ray is brighter than expected because the X-rays are being blocked by something.
Lucency	Opposite of density. More X-rays are passing through less dense regions. Too much lucency can be seen in emphysema.
Pneumothorax	Air occupying the pleural space between the lungs and the rib cage.
Cardiomyopathy	Disease of the heart muscle that results in enlargement of the heart.
Nodule	Rounded and defined tissue surrounded by air. Can be benign or malignant.
Pulmonary edema	Occurs when too much fluid accumulates in the lungs. The fluid leaks out of the blood vessels, usually when it is backed up from the heart.
Parenchymal/ interstitial lung disease	Can be caused by long-term exposure to hazardous materials like asbestos or autoimmune diseases like rheumatoid arthritis. Results in progressive scarring of the lungs.
Fibrosis	The condition of having scar tissue.
Pulmonary or vascular congestion	Increased pressure in the blood vessels in the lungs without leakage. Caused by heart failure.

Note. Adapted from Dorland (2011); Venes (2017).

VENTILATOR, TRACHEOSTOMY TUBES, AND SPEAKING VALVE

For more information on intubation and ventilators and tracheostomy, see Chapter 6.

Nursing Assessment

In inpatient settings, the nursing database and daily assessments provide helpful information to prepare you for the dysphagia evaluation. A conversation with the nurse before entering the patient's room is essential. Look for information in the nursing notes about the following.

Table 1.4
Oxygen-Delivery Devices, Concentration, and Flow

Type of device	Low flow	High flow	Humidity possible?	Concentration range	Flow rate range (liters per minute, lpm)
Nasal cannula	Yes		Yes	22%–44%	1–6 lpm
Nasal cannula with reservoir	Yes		No; because these conserve oxygen, the device can give a higher percentage at lower flow rates because flow is with each breath instead of continuous.	22%–40%	Up to 8 lpm
Simple face mask	Yes		No; short term use because FIO$_2$ is not exact	44%	6–8 lpm
Non-rebreather		Yes	No due to back pressure from humidifier and flow	60%–90% Varies due to patients' inspiratory flow, respiratory rate, and depth of breath	12–15 lpm
Venturi mask		Yes	No, does not work well with humidity	25%–55%	4–8 lpm
HFNC		Yes	Required	35%–98%	20–65 lpm

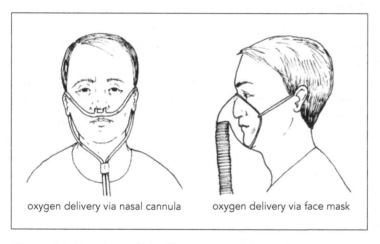

oxygen delivery via nasal cannula   oxygen delivery via face mask

Figure 1.1 Examples of low-flow oxygen-delivery device.

COGNITIVE ASSESSMENT

Nursing notes usually make some statement about the patient's cognitive skills. This is important information when you are going to assess a patient.

SIGNS OF DYSPHAGIA

Nursing notes may also provide some information about signs or symptoms of dysphagia. Key words to look for include *coughing, choking, throat clearing, pocketing of food, inability to finish meals*, and *refusal of certain foods*.

SETTING BEFORE ADMISSION

You may want to note the patient's living situation before admission to the facility to help determine whether he or she was cooking for himself and to determine the type of meals the patient previously ate. If the patient came to your facility from another facility (e.g., admit to inpatient rehab from acute care, admit to skilled nursing from inpatient rehab), look for the discharge records from that facility, particularly any notes from the SLP there.

FAMILY SUPPORT AND INVOLVEMENT

Find out whether there are family members or others who can be taught safe techniques for feeding the patient. If the patient is discharged from your facility, what kind of support will he or she have for following the techniques at home?

SENSORY IMPAIRMENTS

It is also important to consider whether the patient can see the food in front of him, listen to your directions, and smell and taste the food. Check for hearing aids and glasses.

ORAL HEALTH

Nursing documentation will likely include statements about the patient's oral health. Does the patient have his or her own teeth? Or is the patient partially or completely edentulous? Does the patient have a partial plate or full dentures, and does the patient usually eat with those in her mouth? If the patient has at least some teeth, what is the health of those teeth and the overall oral health? Recent epidemiological research provides evidence of possible associations between oral infections—particularly periodontal disease—and diabetes and cardiovascular disease. Also, if the patient's mouth harbors harmful bacteria and the patient aspirates, the bacteria may be carried into the lungs.

A healthy mouth contains helpful oral flora. Certain medications can have a negative impact on the health of the oral cavity. As shown in Table 1.2, many medications cause dry mouth.

Inhalers for asthma can also cause problems, specifically oral thrush, which causes white patches of fungus in the mouth that can be irritating or painful. Some medications, such as cardiovascular agents, central nervous system stimulants, nonsteroidal anti-inflammatory drugs, and smoking-cessation products, can leave a bitter or metallic taste in the mouth, or even interfere with overall sense of taste (Evans & McLeod, 2003).

Other Evaluations

Examinations by other health-care professionals can yield important background information for the SLP. Here are examples of other evaluation reports that should be reviewed.

GI SERIES

The patient may have had an upper or lower GI evaluation because of initial complaints of dysphagia. Helpful information can be found in these reports. Some physicians do not carefully delineate between a barium swallow and a modified barium swallow when ordering diagnostic tests. Therefore, a patient who complains of dysphagia or "choking" may have had a barium swallow ordered and performed. The patient may also have had an upper gastrointestinal tract series (UGI), which includes a barium swallow and a follow-through of the contrast materials. It is not likely that these reports will include any information about the oral or pharyngeal phases, but it is worth checking.

There are several important differences between a modified barium swallow study and a barium swallow and UGI study. A modified barium swallow study is designed to assess the oral and pharyngeal phases of the swallow. A barium swallow study assesses the esophageal phase and the function of the stomach. The UGI includes assessment of the esophageal phase but also provides information about movement of the barium through the intestines. During a modified barium swallow study, the patient sits upright in the lateral, and often anterior–posterior (AP), view and is presented with small amounts of various liquid consistencies and solids. The barium swallow study and UGI series are performed with the patient lying down, drinking a whole bottle of liquid barium sulfate.

The purpose of the modified barium swallow is only partially to diagnose the problem. In large part, the modified barium swallow (MBS) or videofluoroscopic swallowing study (VFSS) is conducted to identify the physiological causes of the symptoms and to select appropriate treatment techniques based on the physiology. Modifications to texture, different postures, and compensatory techniques may be tried to study their effect on swallowing. The barium swallow and UGI are strictly diagnostic procedures, designed to identify problems and possible causes. No trial treatment techniques are used.

ESOPHAGOGASTRODUODONOSCOPY (EGD)

The EGD is an endoscopic procedure that is typically used to assess structural deficits (e.g., inflammation, ulcers, tumors) in the esophagus, stomach, and first part of the small intestine. Because the patient does not swallow anything during this test (as doing so would obscure the view), it is not a good assessment of motility.

NEUROLOGICAL CONSULT

If a patient has had a recent neurological consult, read it carefully for any information about etiology of the dysphagia. The most common neurological causes of dysphagia are stroke, Parkinson's disease, and dementia, but almost any neurological disease can cause dysphagia (e.g., multiple sclerosis, myasthenia gravis, amyotrophic lateral sclerosis, traumatic brain injury).

DIETARY CONSULT

The dietary consult may have important information about the patient's nutritional status. A dietitian's note may include target levels for calorie and protein intake and diet modifications that are required on the basis of the patient's diagnosis. It may also include laboratory values indicative of both nutritional status and treatment progress. The dietitian should clearly state when lab values can and cannot be used as nutrition indicators. For example, a serum albumin is seldom a valid indicator of nutritional status during an illness, as the value is affected by most disease conditions, including simple stress. A patient may present with protein calorie malnutrition such that his or her physical condition is significantly weakened. Malnutrition can be the sole cause of a patient's dysphagia.

SURGERY

There are several ways a recent surgery can have an impact on swallowing. Patients may be debilitated and weak as a result of the surgery and have short-term swallowing problems as a result. If the surgery was to the chest or neck, there may have been some compromise of the laryngeal nerve or one of its branches that contributes to swallowing. If the surgery was to the oral or pharyngeal region (as with cancer), the structures for swallowing may have changed along with the physiology. If the surgery was to the brain, control of swallowing may be affected.

RADIATION TREATMENT

Radiation treatment to the head or neck will almost certainly have an effect on swallowing. Chemoradiation is now the standard of care for organ preservation, but preserving the organ does not mean preserving function. Cancers of the oropharynx are on the rise, particularly those caused by the human papillomavirus (HPV). The effects of radiation differ in the acute, chronic, and late stages because the effects are cumulative. Sometimes the dysphagia does not appear until years after the treatment was completed. The changes in swallowing typically happen gradually; often, the patient is not aware of the subtle changes until the compounded effects present a significant problem

(Chaturvedi et al., 2011). Evaluating and treating patients with dysphagia as a result of head and neck cancer necessitates a different bank of knowledge from that for treating dysphagia resulting from a neurological cause. Clinicians are encouraged to seek out information from other sources.

Interviewing the Patient

You may glean critical information by asking the patient or caregivers for a description of the problem. It may be necessary to reword your question to get the information. For example, you might ask a patient if he ever chokes when eating, and he might answer no. If you reword your question and ask whether food or liquid ever goes down the wrong way, the patient may reply yes.

Involving the patient and caregivers in the identification of swallowing problems also helps keep the focus on function, as in the ICF model (see Chapter 4).

The Supplemental Materials contain a questionnaire that provides several different ways to ask questions. (See Supplemental Materials, SLP Resources, Swallowing Questionnaire: Additional History.)

Standardized Patient Questionnaires

Some standardized questionnaires have been developed to help capture information from the patient's perspective. These can be considered Patient-Reported Outcome Tools (PROs). Several examples of PROs in dysphagia are SWAL-QOL, SWAL-CARE, MDADI, and EAT10. Initially the SWAL-QOL was a 93-item quality-of-life and quality-of-care outcomes tool for dysphagia researchers and clinicians. Because its length made it impractical for clinical use, the researchers used psychometric techniques to reduce the 93-item instrument into two patient-centered outcomes tools: the SWAL-QOL, a 44-item tool that assesses 10 quality-of-life concepts, and the SWAL-CARE, a 15-item tool that assesses quality of care and patient satisfaction. The scales have been shown to have good internal consistency reliability and short-term reproducibility. The scales differentiate normal swallowers from patients with oropharyngeal dysphagia and are sensitive to differences in the severity of dysphagia as clinically defined (McHorney et al., 2000).

The Eating Assessment Tool is a self-administered, symptom-specific outcome instrument for dysphagia. The researchers concluded that the EAT-10 has good internal consistency, test–retest reproducibility, and criterion-based validity. The normative data suggest that an EAT-10 score of 3 or higher is abnormal. The instrument may be utilized to document the initial dysphagia severity and monitor progress in treatment (Belafsky et al., 2008).

The MDADI, MD Anderson Dysphagia Inventory, was the first validated and reliable self-administered questionnaire designed specifically for evaluating the impact of dysphagia on the quality of life of patients with head and neck cancer. The MDADI is a 20-item, 5-point Likert questionnaire that assesses dysphagia in three domains (functional, emotional, physical) (Chen et al., 2001).

Tools like this can be used to provide a baseline for comparison at a later point in time. This can help the clinician measure functional gains in the patient's swallowing status. The use of patient-reported tools also helps the clinician keep a focus on function, measuring change that is important to the patient.

Interpreting the Symptoms the Patient Reports

QUALITY OF LIFE

How is the dysphagia affecting the patient's quality of life? Has the patient changed the types of foods eaten? Limited the places and situations in which he or she will eat? Restricted the people with whom he or she will eat?

OBSTRUCTION OR PAIN
The medical term for the condition of obstruction or pain is *odynophagia*. Ask the patient to point to the area where this occurs. A sharp pain could indicate an ulcerative lesion of the pharynx or esophagus. If the patient describes a dull or squeezing pain, it could be an esophageal spasm.

GLOBUS
This is a descriptive term for the sensation of a lump or fullness in the throat, sometimes caused by a mass but frequently due to gastroesophageal reflux (GER). Some patients may be more sensitive to esophageal distention and describe the sensation. Globus may be a better symptom of GER than heartburn is. Eighty percent of patients complaining of globus have a functional cause, and it is often related to GER and, more specifically, laryngopharyngeal reflux.

Patients are usually fairly accurate when identifying where the problem is in the pharynx, but a patient who is having problems with the esophagus will often tell you that he or she feels the sensation much higher in his throat. This is called *symptom referral* and is often caused by food remaining in the esophagus that is then jetted up against a closed upper esophageal sphincter (UES). Globus is often momentarily relieved by a second, dry swallow.

HEARTBURN
Heartburn is a very common symptom of esophageal reflux disease; however, the severity reported does not correlate with the severity of the reflux-induced damage to the esophagus. Ask whether the patient's heartburn is more common after meals or at night.

WHEN THE PROBLEM OCCURS
Are the symptoms observed at the start of the meal or not until the patient is part way through eating? If the latter, it may be related to reflux.

PARTICULAR FOODS
Which foods seem to cause the most trouble? Are liquids or solids more challenging? Trouble with solids usually points toward esophageal problems.

TEMPERATURE OF FOODS
If the problem occurs only with very cold foods, the patient may be experiencing a cricopharyngeal spasm. A cricopharyngeal spasm is usually described by the patient as a pain in the chest or a feeling of being unable to swallow a solid. However, spasms can occur with hot foods as well. Cricopharyngeal spasm may be related to reflux (Veenker, Andersen, & Cohen, 2003).

TIME OF DAY
Does the patient experience the symptoms at every meal, or are the symptoms more severe later in the day? In the latter case, the symptoms might be more related to fatigue, and the etiology of the dysphagia might be a disease in which motor function is worse with fatigue.

TERRIBLE TASTE IN MOUTH
Ask whether the patient often has a bad taste in his or her mouth upon awakening. Also determine whether the patient has excessive burping. These symptoms are frequently caused by esophageal reflux.

NASAL BURNING AND DRIPPING
A patient who reports burning in the nose, sniffs frequently, or wipes his or her nose excessively during a meal may be experiencing reflux of food or liquid into the nasal cavity. Stimulation to the trigeminal nerve can also cause this reaction. Nasal burning or dripping has no relationship to aspiration.

CHOKING AND COUGHING

Patients often answer in the negative when asked if they feel like they are choking when they swallow. You may want to reword your question. You might ask patients if they ever feel like the food goes down the wrong way, or if they are unable to breathe when food gets caught.

LATE REGURGITATION

If the patient is vomiting hours after a meal, it probably indicates an esophageal disorder such as GER or achalasia, an esophageal disorder in which food is retained in the esophagus.

APPETITE

Ask whether the patient has noticed a decrease in appetite. Poor appetite might be caused by a fear of choking or by early muscle fatigue while eating. The patient may be so fatigued by eating that he or she stops eating and does not finish the meal.

LENGTH OF TIME TO FINISH A MEAL

Some people eat more slowly than others, but dysphagia can also cause a person to take longer to eat. If there is an oral dysphagia, the person may take longer to prepare each bolus. If the patient is aware of difficulties in the pharyngeal phase, he or she may eat slowly to try to avoid problems.

TASTE

Taste deficits, especially if accompanied by olfactory disturbances, may interfere with the sensory component of swallowing and the desire to eat. It would be rare to have isolated damage to cranial nerves VII and IX, which would reduce or eliminate the ability to taste.

CHANGES IN SPEECH OR VOICE

Ask the patient to be specific when describing any changes to speech or voice. You may need to give examples such as "Is your speech slurred?" "Does your voice sound breathier?" "Are you talking through your nose?" and "Do you need to clear your throat more?" Any problems related to the voice may warrant a referral to otolaryngology (ENT).

Problems Related to Phases of Swallowing

The dysphagia symptoms being described or those found in the medical chart may relate to a particular phase of swallow. A diagram of the phases is provided in the Supplemental Materials (see Education Materials, Patient/Family, Phases of Swallow). The description of separate phases is an artificial distinction because the phases are dynamic and interrelated, but reading about some of the aspects of each one may help you understand the relationships among the phases. There are many possible causes for the various symptoms.

Oral Dysphagia

It is fairly uncommon in adults to have only an oral dysphagia (referring to the oral phases). It could be caused by a neurogenic disorder, decreased salivary flow, or painful lesions in the mouth. It could also be the result of oral surgery or chemoradiation for cancer. Diminished salivary flow makes it extremely difficult to prepare the bolus to swallow. Be aware that more than 400 commonly used drugs can affect salivary flow, including anticholinergics, antihistamines, antidepressants, antihypertensives, and diuretics.

Still, some patients with dementia may show only an oral dysphagia. A patient with dementia often does not recognize food (e.g., agnosia). When food is placed in the patient's mouth, it is as if he or she has forgotten what to do with the bolus of food (e.g., swallowing apraxia). The staff or family may report that the patient will not swallow even when persuaded to take some food into the mouth.

Occasionally, isolated neurogenic oral dysphagia may appear in patients before the onset of other neurological findings. Watch this condition very carefully so you can make a referral to a neurologist if difficulty swallowing is the first symptom to appear. Some oral dysphagia may be psychogenic. Patients may describe a fear of choking, or state that the food just will not go down. They may eat only certain types of foods, which may not always make sense if you analyze the textures (e.g., a patient stating that he can swallow coffee but not water).

Oropharyngeal, Pharyngeal, and Pharyngoesophageal Dysphagia

Dysphagia in the oropharyngeal, pharyngeal, and pharyngoesophageal phases can have many causes, including acute, chronic, or progressive neurological disorders; postsurgery status; chemoradiation to head and neck; overall weakness; history of intubation; placement of tracheostomy tube; and/or surgery to neck or chest with damage to nerves important for swallowing (see Education Materials, Patient/Family, Phases of Swallow). It is important to determine the etiology, as improvement is expected in some cases but not in others. The following is a brief listing of common etiologies of dysphagia. The clinician should explore more in-depth information about any of the disorders prior to assessing the patient.

NEUROLOGICAL CAUSES

Many disorders of the central nervous system (CNS) can cause dysphagia. The neurological etiology does not necessarily indicate the type or severity of dysphagia. As an example, dysphagia after surgery for a brain tumor will differ depending on site, type, and size of tumor. However, there are certain characteristics of dysphagia typically seen with certain diseases or at certain stages of the disease. For example, moderate stages of dementia may result in the patient being distracted or forgetting to eat; in later stages the patient may hold the bolus in the mouth and forget to chew and swallow.

Neurological causes of dysphagia can be divided into degenerative and nondegenerative causes, with different diseases causing the dysphagia. Understanding the nature and course of each disease helps the SLP plan management of the dysphagia (Table 1.5). A few of the more common causes of neurogenic dysphagia are discussed here.

Stroke. Stroke is the leading cause of dysphagia in patients with neurological diseases. Prevalence ranges from 25% to 75 % in patients after stroke. This variability is due to the method of assessing swallowing function, timing of assessment, and number and type of stroke patients studied. The dysphagia improves in most patients following stroke, usually within 14 days, although up to 42% of patients will have dysphagia lasting more than 14 days, and 11% demonstrate persistent problems at 6 months (Mann, Hankey, & Cameron, 2000).

Dysphagia is more common in hemorrhagic than ischemic stroke and may result from

- bilateral hemispheric strokes
- brainstem strokes (especially lateral medullary)
- unilateral strokes of either hemisphere
- cerebellar strokes (Horner, Massey, & Brazer, 1990; Kim, Chung, Lee, & Robbins, 2000; Kumar et al., 2012)

Dysphagia may also result from unilateral strokes of either cerebral hemisphere (Robbins, Levine, Maser, Rosenbek, & Kempster, 1993). There are contradictory findings concerning swallowing lateralization. Some authors indicate that the dismotility pattern and aspiration risk may be related to the hemisphere lesioned (Robbins et al., 1993; Smithard et al., 1996), while others indicate that the hemisphere may not discriminate dismotility pattern or risk of aspiration (Daniels & Foundas, 1999). Robbins et al. (1993) indicate that swallowing behavior differs in left- and right-hemispheric stroke, with left-hemisphere stroke indicative of oral dismotility and

Table 1.5
Neurological Causes of Dysphagia: Examples

Non-degenerative	Degenerative
Vascular	Dementia
• Strokes	• Alzheimer's disease
	• Frontotemporal dementia
	• Lewy body dementia
	• Vascular dementia
Trauma	Movement disorders
• Traumatic brain injury	• Parkinson's disease
	• Progressive supranuclear palsy
	• Huntington's disease
	• Amyotrophic lateral sclerosis (ALS)
Neoplastic	Relapsing-remitting
• Brain tumor	• Multiple sclerosis
Congenital	
• Cerebral palsy	
Iatrogenic	
• Medication induced (tardive dyskinesia)	
• Surgery induced (carotid endarterectomy)	

right-hemisphere stroke more related to pharyngeal dysfunction and aspiration. Daniels and Foundas (1999) found that swallowing behavior did not differ in right- and left-hemisphere strokes. However, evidence is converging to indicate common sites of involvement and to support that there is a distributed neural network involving both cerebral hemispheres and subcortical structures. Involvement of multiple levels is thought to induce more severe or protracted dysphagia.

Traumatic brain injury. Patients who have suffered traumatic brain injuries often have severe dysphagia. The kinds of problems they present may be complicated because of the type of neurological insult (e.g., coup and contra-coup damages result in the areas of damage being more diffuse) and possible structural injuries to the head and neck (e.g., fractures). Management of the patient has to be guided by her level of recovery. For instance, if a patient is in the combative stage, it is not likely that she will allow physical help to achieve a compensatory posture.

Spinal cord injury. Patients with traumatic brain injury may also have spinal cord injuries that compound their swallowing problems. Patients with spinal cord injuries alone can also present with dysphagia, including problems such as a delay in the pharyngeal swallow response and impaired movement of the larynx.

Myasthenia gravis. This causes an impairment at the juncture of the muscle and the nerve that diminishes the input to the muscle. The hallmark feature is that performance worsens with fatigue on repetitive trials. Swallowing is usually worse at the end of the meal and at the end of the day.

Guillain-Barré. This is a viral disease with rapid onset of paresis. It may progress to the point that the patient requires ventilator support. One of the first signs of this disease may be swallowing difficulty. As the disease progresses, it is not unusual for the patient to require tube feeding.

Dementia. Dementia has various etiologies, and the etiology, as well as the stage of the disease, causes different swallowing problems. The prevalence of swallowing difficulties in patients with dementia ranged from 13% to 57%. Dysphagia developed during the late stages of frontotemporal dementia (FTD), but it was seen during the early stage of Alzheimer's dementia (AD) (Alagiakrishnan, Bhanji, & Kurian, 2013; Easterling & Robbins, 2008).

Amyotrophic lateral sclerosis (ALS). Dysphagia will occur with ALS. This progressive disease affects swallowing in both the oral and pharyngeal phases. Impaired swallowing may be one of the first symptoms reported by the patient, particularly when there is bulbar involvement (Kawai et al., 2003).

Parkinson's disease. More than 80% of patients with Parkinson's (PWPs) will develop dysphagia during the course of the disease. More severe dysphagia usually occurs in late stages of the disease.

Patients who have Parkinson's with dementia are more likely to have dysphagia. Although dysphagia is common in PD, it is underreported by patients. No more than 20%–40% are aware of their dysphagia, and less than 10% spontaneously report it (Kalf, De Swart, Bloem, & Munneke, 2012).

This disease may affect oral, pharyngeal, and esophageal phases (Table 1.6). These swallowing problems may be one of the first signs of the disease (Hammer, Murphy, & Abrams, 2013).

Multiple sclerosis. Multiple sclerosis results in plaque-like deposits throughout the neurological system. Patients may present with oral and pharyngeal dysphagia, depending on the location of the lesion. Esophageal symptoms are also reported. Dysphagia symptoms may appear in the early stages of the disease (De Pauw, Dejaeger, D'hooghe, & Carton, 2002; Poorjavad et al., 2010).

STRUCTURAL CAUSES

Structural causes of dysphagia in adults are the result of surgical changes to the oral mechanism, pharynx, larynx, or esophagus, or changes that occur as a result of chemoradiation to these structures. These are treatments for cancers of the head and neck. Radiotherapy can cause changes to the mucosa, such as mucositis, candida, erythema, and edema. Swallowing can be painful (odynophagia), and the patient may experience altered taste (dysgeusia) and smell. Xerostomia, with thick mucous, makes it difficult to swallow. Reduced appetite, fatigue, and nausea often occur during the course of treatment. The late and chronic effects of radiation include fibrosis, or thickening and scarring of connective tissue. Trismus, which is fibrosis of the muscles of mastication, can result in a reduced ability to open the jaw, and lymphedema. Lymphedema, or swelling caused by blockage of the lymphatic system, is seen most in the limbs, but it can also affect the face and neck (and thus swallowing) (Hutcheson et al., 2012; Ohba et al., 2016). Patients can also experience cranial nerve palsies.

IDIOPATHIC FUNCTIONAL DYSPHAGIA

Some patients report symptoms of dysphagia but no specific cause can be determined. That is, there is no apparent neurological or structural deficit causing the swallowing problems. These reports of dysphagia are common in patients who see an otolaryngologist. When no underlying

Table 1.6
Swallowing Deficits in Parkinson's Disease

Oral	Pharyngeal	Esophageal
Repetitive tongue pumping	More residue in valleculae than in pyriform sinuses	Reduced motility
Oral residue	Aspiration	Spasms
Premature loss of bolus posteriorly	Reduced rate of spontaneous swallows	Tertiary contractions
Piecemeal deglutition		

Note. Adapted from Hammer, Murphy, and Abrams (2013).

etiology can be determined, the patient is often labeled as having idiopathic functional dysphagia. However, a recent study found that many of these patients also had laryngeal muscle tension, such as causes muscle tension dysphonia, and laryngeal hyperresponsiveness, such as presents in refractory chronic cough, paradoxical vocal fold motion, and muscle tension dysphonia. The authors propose the use of the term *muscle tension dysphagia* (MTD) (Kang, Hentz, & Lott, 2016).

About the Esophagus

The esophagus is approximately 22–26 cm long and contains both skeletal (striated) and smooth muscle. The top 5% of the esophagus is striated, the middle 35%–40% is a combination, and the bottom 50%–60% is smooth. The striated part starts at the bottom of the cricopharyngeus (CP) muscle. The muscles forming the UES/PES are formed by the horizontal fibers of the CP and muscles of the inferior pharyngeal constrictor. The cricoid cartilage forms the front border of the UES, and the CP muscle is the back and side of the UES. The UES is about 1 cm in length (Kuo & Urma, 2006; Meyer, Austin, Brady, & Castell, 1986)

The UES is naturally in a tonic state (high pressure) to prevent air from entering the esophagus and to prevent contents of the esophagus from retro-flowing into the pharynx. Therefore, the UES has to relax for food to pass into the esophagus. This action is accomplished by the actual relaxation of the sphincter and action of the hyolaryngeal complex pulling up and forward.

At about the sixth cervical vertebra, the actual body of the esophagus starts. At rest, the body of the esophagus is without motor activity. It remains in the state of relaxation until dilated by air or food. The lower esophageal sphincter (LES) also maintains high pressure in a state of constant contraction, serving to keep food in the stomach.

Pressure in the UES and LES is measured manometrically. Manometry assesses motor function of the esophagus and may be needed if barium study or gastroesophageal endoscopy identifies no cause of the problem. A transnasal catheter with multiple electronic pressure probes is passed into the stomach, measuring esophageal contractions and defining upper and lower esophageal responses to swallowing. Manometry detects definitive abnormalities in only 25% of patients with nonobstructive lesions (Feussner, Kauer, & Siewert, 1993; Tutuian & Castell, 2004). High-resolution manometry (HRM) uses up to 36 sensors and produces multicolored spatiotemporal plots for more specific diagnosis of pressure abnormalities in the esophagus (Fox & Bredenoord, 2008). HRM is also being used in some centers to assess pressures in the pharynx (Hoffman et al., 2012; McCulloch, Hoffman, & Ciucci, 2010).

Peristalsis is the wavelike movement that propels the bolus through the esophagus and into the stomach. This squeezing motion can be observed on fluoroscopy. As the contraction travels through the esophagus, the muscular wall just ahead of the squeeze relaxes. This action pushes the contents in the tube toward the stomach. These peristaltic pressures are described as primary, secondary, and tertiary. Primary peristalsis is initiated by a swallow. Secondary peristaltic pressure waves are progressive contractions in the body of the esophagus that can start at any level. They are caused by the bolus (or air) causing distention of the esophagus. This action may clear the esophagus without another swallow. When secondary peristalsis is occurring, inhibition of deglutition occurs. In fact, if the person starts another swallow during secondary peristalsis, there is complete inhibition of the contraction started by the first swallow (Meyer & Castell, 1980). Tertiary contractions are simultaneous contractions in the body of the esophagus in reaction to the distention. These are nonperistaltic contractions that do not clear the esophagus and may occur unrelated to swallowing, such as with GERD or stress (Dent et al., 1980). These tertiary contractions are in-coordinated and may squeeze the remaining bolus up and down in the esophagus.

Esophageal Dysphagia

Patients with esophageal dysphagia often localize their symptoms to the area of the throat. Patients may describe symptoms that sound as if they are occurring in the pharynx when they are actually esopgeal.

Patients with oropharyngeal dysphagia may also have esophageal dysphagia. It is important to understand the relationship between the two. To illustrate that point, for the constrictor muscles in the PES to work well, the hyolaryngeal complex has to be elevated. This constriction is what starts to propel the bolus into the esophagus. In addition, it appears that thicker boluses can increase the stripping wave.

Esophageal dysphagia begins with problems at the level of the upper esophageal sphincter (UES), also called the pharyngoesophageal sphincter or segment (PES), and below as the food travels through the esophagus to the stomach. Remember that the patient will probably not indicate the exact location when reporting problems in the esophagus.

Problems in the esophageal phase are of two basic types. Problems are related to issues with movement of the bolus (motility problems) or are related to structural deficits, as shown in Table 1.7.

COMMON ESOPHAGEAL MOTILITY PROBLEMS

There can be interference in some part of the swallowing sequence with relaxation of the muscle followed by squeezing or peristalsis. These motility abnormalities can occur with liquids and solid boluses, and typically the onset is intermittent. The patient may report that episodes occur when distracted and not paying close attention to swallowing. Oftentimes these episodes may occur when eating out and may be mistakenly attributed to emotional tension.

Esophageal dismotility. Esophageal dismotility is a decrease in the primary contraction wave of the esophagus. This results in slower movement of the bolus into the stomach. In the case of severe dismotility, subsequent boluses may begin "piling up" in the esophagus. The patient may report feeling full or unable to swallow the next bite. There are currently no approved drugs on the market to treat esophageal dismotility. Previously available medications for this purpose had serious side effects. Esophageal spasm is just what the name implies, a tightening of the esophagus that causes a sharp pain. The esophagus may also be affected in collagen vascular diseases, such as dermatomyositis or polymyositis and progressive systemic sclerosis. Effects may range from GERD to reduced UES opening (Shaker, Castell, Schoenfeld, & Spechler, 2003).

Achalasia. Achalasia is an esophageal motility disorder that affects the swallowing of liquids and solids. The patient may complain of a burning sensation or pain behind the sternum. It is chronic and gets worse gradually. When assessed manometrically, it is characterized by lack of esophageal peristalsis and LES relaxation. The view on fluoroscopy is described as a bird's beak because the esophagus is dilated and full of food, no squeezing is occurring, and—because the LES does not relax—the column of food in the esophagus ends in a point that looks like a bird's beak.

Table 1.7
Types of Esophageal Problems

Examples of motility disorders	Examples of structural disorders
Esophageal dismotility	Zenker's diverticulum
Achalasia	Peptic stricture
Esophageal spasm	Esophageal rings
Collagen vascular diseases	Esophageal webs
Cricopharyngeal dysfunction	

Cricopharyngeal dysfunction. In true CP dysfunction, the UES fails to relax. However, what may appear on videofluoroscopy to be a failure of the UES to relax may really be due to limited laryngeal elevation and limited anterior movement of the hyolaryngeal complex, the mechanical actions needed to pull open the UES. If this lifting and forward movement is inadequate, there is insufficient mechanical action to pull open the cricopharyngeus. Before a myotomy is considered, careful assessment of the neuromuscular aspects of the swallow should be completed to determine whether swallowing therapy is indicated rather than surgery. Manometry would determine if increased UES pressures are responsible for failure of the UES to relax.

COMMON ESOPHAGEAL STRUCTURAL PROBLEMS

There can be a narrowing of the opening to the stomach. Often the first symptoms noted will be with solid foods, particularly tough meats. The patient may change his or her diet to pureed food and liquids. If the progression has been very rapid (1–3 months) and the patient has had significant weight loss, it is more likely that the obstruction or narrowing is caused by a malignancy.

Medication-induced esophageal injury. Medication-induced injury occurs if a pill gets stuck and dissolves in the esophagus or stays in the esophagus too long secondary to esophageal dismotility. It may also occur if the medication returns to the esophagus through reflux action. The symptoms are acute substernal pain, odynophagia, and dysphagia. This can cause mucosal injury and possible stricture.

Zenker's diverticulum. A small hernialike pouch that develops on the posterior esophageal wall is called a Zenker's diverticulum. It occurs near the UES. The pouch can be very small or as large as a golf ball. Food and liquid collect in the pouch. Sometimes the food flows out of the pouch and is swallowed, but there is a risk of aspirating the material. Because of this retention of food, patients may report a very bad taste in their mouth and bad breath. They may even state that they cough up pieces of food they have not eaten in days. The diverticulum can be surgically repaired.

Peptic stricture. Peptic stricture is the most common stricture of the esophagus. About 10% of patients with severe reflux disease have such a stricture of the LES; however, the stricture can also occur in proximal esophagus, causing aspiration and choking.

Esophageal rings and webs. Rings and webs can occur proximally (as in Plummer-Vinson or Paterson-Brown-Kelly syndrome) and cause aspiration. These proximal webs may be associated with Zenker's diverticulum. Distal rings are located at the LES and are usually accompanied by a hiatal hernia. Dysphagia is intermittent and usually related to solid foods. These rings are called Schatzki's rings (Shaker et al., 2003).

Gastroesophageal Reflux Disease and Laryngopharyngeal Reflux

One of the most common esophageal disorders is gastroesophageal reflux disease. GERD occurs when gastric contents pass through the LES into the esophagus. This is different from intraesophageal reflux, in which material never empties from the esophagus and moves upward in a retrograde fashion. When evaluating the esophageal phase during a modified barium swallow, note if gastroesophageal reflux or intraesophageal reflux occurs.

Many individuals have some degree of reflux and may never know it because they do not present with any symptoms. Such symptoms include the burning sensation called heartburn, a feeling of tightness or fullness in the chest area (i.e., globus), a bad taste in the mouth, a feeling of being unable to breathe when lying flat, nasal burning or dripping, and/or frequent burping. GERD is more common in the elderly, and older patients are less able to detect the symptoms (DeVault, 2007; Ferguson & DeVault, 2007).

Laryngopharyngeal reflux (LPR) indicates that the reflux material moves through the UES into the pharynx and even into the larynx. LPR typically occurs during the day with the patient in the upright position. The most common symptoms of LPR are hoarseness, globus, dysphagia, chronic throat clearing, coughing, and sore throat (Koufman, Aviv, Casiano, & Shaw, 2002).

Relatively small amounts of acid exposure and intermittent exposure can injure tissues. The acid harms the larynx in several ways. The acid can inflame the posterior structures (e.g., arytenoids, posterior commissure). Pepsin, another digestive juice, can injure the mucosa.

There is also, of course, the risk that gastric contents or acid may be aspirated. This is a risk particularly under anesthesia.

Certain factors may cause or aggravate the symptoms of reflux in individuals prone to the disorder. These include cigarette smoking, obesity, some medications (e.g., anticholinergics), alcohol, clothing that is tight around the waist, lifting heavy objects (especially if leaning over to do so), and eating very large meals. Certain foods can also worsen the symptoms of reflux. These include caffeine, chocolate, mint, spicy foods, foods with high acid content, pepper, pickled items, processed meats (e.g., hot dogs, sausage), and foods with high fat content.

Treatment for GERD depends on the severity of the problem. GERD can be managed through one or a combination of approaches: lifestyle modifications, drugs or surgery. Lifestyle modifications include avoiding foods and activities that aggravate the reflux. (A patient handout is included in the Supplemental Materials, Education Materials, Patient/Family, Lifestyle Modifications for Patients with Gastroesophageal Reflux Disease [GERD].) Drug treatment may be as simple as over-the-counter antacids. If the problem is more severe, other types of medications may be prescribed, including H2 antagonists and proton pump inhibitors (see Table 1.2). Proton pump inhibitors (PPIs) increase the risk of community-acquired pneumonia but not hospital-acquired pneumonia (Thomson, Sauve, Kassam, & Kamitakahara, 2010). PPI therapy is associated with a twofold increase in risk for clostridium-difficile (c-dif) infection (Deshpande et al., 2012).

Surgery may be considered if the GERD does not respond to medication and lifestyle changes, especially if it is contributing to pulmonary disease. Surgery, called Nissen fundoplication, involves surgically reducing the size of the opening into the stomach by wrapping the stomach around the distal esophagus, although several variations are performed (Mayo Clinic, 2017).

Stage of Disease and Underlying Etiology

In addition to understanding the different diseases that can cause dysphagia, the SLP must grasp how management of dysphagia can be impacted by the stage of the disease.

Acute Onset

If the dysphagia is an acute onset, such as with stroke, then some spontaneous recovery is to be expected. In such cases, frequent reassessment may be needed and recommendations adjusted as the patient recovers.

Chronic

Some patients present with chronic dysphagia. This might have initially been caused by a neurological event such as stroke, but recovery has plateaued and no further improvement is expected.

Progressive

Dysphagia caused by progressive neurological diseases (e.g., Parkinson's, ALS, Alzheimer's dementia, myasthenia gravis) will also be progressive in nature. Reevaluations and adjustment of recommendations will be needed periodically over the course of the disease.

Exacerbation of Chronic or Progressive

Patients with both chronic and progressive dysphagia can experience an acute event that exacerbates their dysphagia. This is sometimes described as "acute on chronic." Obtain information from the patient and caregiver concerning what the patient's baseline skills were before the acute event. Make needed adjustments to the recommendations during the acute stage, but as the patient recovers from the exacerbating event, strive to get him back to baseline performance.

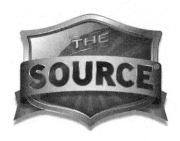

Chapter 2

Screenings and Bedside or Clinical Evaluations

A screening is used with a group of people to identify who does not have the target disorder and who likely does or is at risk to have the disorder. Common medical screening tests include cholesterol screening via blood test, screening mammograms, prostate screening blood tests, and tuberculosis skin tests. Screenings determine who should undergo further diagnostic tests.

Screening for Dysphagia and Aspiration

Swallowing screening refers to a minimally invasive procedure. According to the American Speech-Language-Hearing Association's (ASHA) Preferred Practice Patterns, screening for swallowing is "a pass/fail procedure to identify individuals who require a comprehensive assessment of swallowing function or a referral for other professional and/or medical services" (p. 10). The document indicates that specific to dysphagia, the screening should determine the risk, or likelihood, that the individual has dysphagia or may be aspirating food or liquid. This distinction between screening for dysphagia and screening for aspiration is an important one, because some tools screen for one but not the other.

Swallowing screening identifies persons who are likely to have swallowing impairments related to function, activity, and/or participation, as defined by the World Health Organization (2018). Impairments may cause pulmonary aspiration, airway obstruction, or inadequate nutrition and/or hydration (ASHA, 2004). A screening might include the following components:

- questions about the patient's history (e.g., history of swallowing problems)
- information about specific diagnoses that are associated with dysphagia (e.g., Parkinson's disease, stroke)
- observation of the patient for signs associated with dysphagia (e.g., dysphonia, dysarthria)
- signs of dysphagia that can be determined without presenting any food to the patient (e.g., weak cough, inability to control saliva)
- presentation of food or liquid to the patient to observe for clinical signs of dysphagia or aspiration (e.g., pocketing food, coughing with liquids)

Many of these tools are designed as a flowchart or decision tree so that once a patient fails an item, the screening is terminated and the patient is referred to an SLP for full assessment.

Although speech–language pathologists can perform the screening of swallowing function (as indicated in the Preferred Practice Patterns), in health-care settings it is more typical for the screening to be performed by nursing staff who have been trained by the speech–language pathologist. In some settings, the physician or physician extender performs the screening. Because screenings are administered to patients at risk for dysphagia, it is more efficient to use other personnel to perform the screening and use the speech–language pathologist's time to see patients who fail the screening.

Populations to Screen

Depending on the setting in which services are provided, different populations of patients may be identified to be screened. For example, in an outpatient clinic that sees only patients with amyotrophic lateral sclerosis (ALS), multiple sclerosis, or Parkinson's, all patients might be screened, because the medical diagnosis alone places the patient at high risk for dysphagia. Patients undergoing chemoradiation therapy for head and neck cancer would be another high-risk population that would warrant screening. In contrast to such settings, in a general medical practice, perhaps only patients reporting symptoms or over a certain age might be screened (or the physician might refer such patients directly to the speech–language pathologist for full evaluation on the basis of reported symptoms).

In some inpatient settings, like inpatient rehabilitation facilities or skilled nursing facilities, all new admissions might be screened. There are also questions on patient assessment instruments in these settings that might reveal new signs of dysphagia during periodic reassessments.

In acute-care settings, certain populations of patients are typically identified as high risk and seen for screening. In one hospital in Australia, a small prospective, quasi-experimental study found that twenty-five to 30% of acute hospitalized individuals were identified as having dysphagia. All patients admitted to this facility are screened by nursing (Cichero, Heaton, & Bassett, 2009). However, in many hospitals, it may not be practical to screen all patients admitted to a hospital, as most would not likely present any signs of dysphagia.

STROKE

Historically, the first population in acute-care hospitals to be identified as needing to be screened for dysphagia and aspiration were those patients admitted with stroke. Dysphagia has been reported to occur in 42%–60% of patients with acute stroke (Mann, Hankey, & Cameron, 2000). Dysphagia increases the risk of pneumonia in patients with stroke. Pneumonia increases the cost of care and also mortality. Therefore, a structured screening program for patients with stroke to identify those at risk for aspiration, and for dysphagia, is designed to identify those at risk of developing pneumonia. Several studies have demonstrated that a formal dysphagia screening program can reduce the incidence of pneumonia in patients poststroke (Hinchey et al., 2005; Yeh et al., 2011).

The Joint Commission recognized the importance of screening patients with stroke for dysphagia, and for years this was one of the required core measures on which data had to be collected and reported. In 2010 the Joint Commission removed the reporting requirement, which previously required reporting compliance with administration of dysphagia screening on all patients with stroke before giving any PO intake. The Joint Commission explained that the core measure regarding dysphagia screening allowed the hospital to select its own evidenced-based screening protocol. They stated that because there are several evidenced-based dysphagia screen protocols that can be used, and there is no agreement as to one universal protocol that should be the standard for all hospitals, the dysphagia screen measure was no longer endorsed since it allowed for more than one protocol (i.e., too much variation; Performance Measure FAQs, 2010).

As of this writing, there is still not one universally accepted screening tool for stroke, but there are several standardized measures from which to choose. Therefore in this fourth edition of *The Source: Dysphagia*, the example screening form, which was a facility-designed tool, has been eliminated. Readers are encouraged instead to use a standardized screening form applicable to the population being screened.

An FAQ document developed by ASHA's Special Interest Group 13, Swallowing and Swallowing Disorders, addresses screening specific to the population of patients with stroke. The document stresses the importance of the SLP's involvement in the design of the screening program and in training the other professionals who will perform the screening. It also summarizes the difference between training another profession (e.g., nursing) to screen and cross-training another profession to perform other skilled tasks that the speech–language pathologist performs. That kind of cross-training is not acceptable. It is acceptable, however, to work on a team with other professionals, with others performing tasks such as screening (ASHA, 2009).

POSTEXTUBATION

Another population in acute-care settings at high risk for dysphagia includes patients who have been intubated. Dysphagia is recognized as a complication in patients postextubation and leads to increased morbidity, mortality, and hospital costs (Macht et al., 2011; Skoretz, Flowers, & Martino, 2010; Skoretz, Yau, Ivanov, Granton, & Martino, 2014). The incidence of dysphagia in patients postextubation is reported to be between 3% and 62%, often occurring—up to 25% of the time—without overt signs of aspiration (Ajemian, Nirmul, Anderson, Zirlen, & Kwasnik, 2001) and at times persisting weeks following extubation (Goldsmith, 2000).

EXAMPLES OF OTHER HIGH-RISK POPULATIONS

Depending on the characteristics of the patients served at the facility, there may be other populations at high risk for dysphagia who should be screened.

Admitted with pneumonia. Patients admitted with pneumonia may not be a population typically identified as at high risk for dysphagia. However, many patients who are elderly who are admitted with a diagnosis of community-acquired pneumonia (CAP) may actually have an unidentified dysphagia contributing to or causing the pneumonia. CAP is a major cause of morbidity and mortality in the elderly, and the leading cause of death among residents of nursing homes. Oropharyngeal aspiration is an important factor leading to pneumonia in the elderly, and screening for dysphagia might identify those patients needing intervention (Marik & Kaplan, 2003).

COPD. In a small study of outpatients with COPD referred for videofluoroscopic swallowing evaluation, nearly 85% had some degree of dysphagia and there was a high percentage of silent penetration and aspiration (Good-Fratturelli, Curlee, & Holle, 2000). Upper-airway protections may be impaired as a result of incoordination between breathing and swallowing (Cvejic et al., 2011).

Validation of Swallow Screening Tests

Most screening tests (e.g., Barnes-Jewish) have been standardized on patients with stroke, and clinicians should be cautious in generalizing the validity relative to other populations. Some screening tests have been standardized on more heterogeneous populations (e.g., the Yale Swallow Protocol). Some standardized patient questionnaires are designed for and validated on specific populations (e.g., the MDADI on patients with head and neck cancer), while others are standardized on more diverse groups (e.g., the EAT-10). When selecting a screening tool, the speech–language pathologist should consider the construct and statistical validity of the tool, but also the population on which it was standardized.

Examples of Swallow Screening Tests

WATER-SWALLOW TESTS

Water-swallow tests have been used since the early 1990s, when DePippo, Holas, and Reding (1992) first described a procedure called the 3-oz. water-swallow test for aspiration following stroke (WST). The WST screens for aspiration, not for dysphagia. In the early versions of the 3-ounce water-swallow test, failure criteria were inability to drink the entire amount, interrupted drinking, or coughing during or immediately after drinking. This test has been used increasingly in recent years, and a systematic review and meta-analysis in 2016 provided useful pooled information to clinicians choosing to use this test (Table 2.1).

Table 2.1
Summary of Meta-analysis on Water-Swallow Tests

Presentation	Pooled sensitivity rules out aspiration…	Pooled specificity rules in aspiration…	Conclusions
Single sip	71%	90%	Small volumes with single sips appropriately ruled in aspiration when clinical signs were present.
Consecutive sips of 90–100 ml	91%	53%	Offers the best characteristics to rule out overt aspiration (i.e., a readily observable airway response, voice change associated with swallowing).
Trials of progressively increasing volumes	86%	65%	Combining presentations of both single sips and consecutive sips from a large volume in a stepwise process may boost sensitivity and specificity in the same patient screening session and be the best way to correctly classify patients who are aspirating.

Note. Airway response of cough/choke + voice change improved overall accuracy in identifying aspiration. Adapted from Brodsky et al. (2016).

Airway response (e.g., coughing, choking) with or without voice changes (e.g., wet or gurgly voice quality) was used to identify aspiration during three different bedside WSTs: single sips, consecutive sips large amount, and progressing from small amount to larger amount. The authors concluded that currently used bedside WSTs offer sufficient, though not ideal, utility in screening for aspiration (Brodsky et al., 2016).

YALE SWALLOW PROTOCOL

Leder and Suiter posited that more than a 3-ounce water-swallow test is needed to screen for aspiration. They have combined that test with a brief cognitive assessment and an oral mechanism exam (Leder & Suiter, 2014). Having the patient answer orientation questions and follow commands improved the prediction of odds of aspiration risk for liquid and pureed food consistencies (Leder, Suiter, & Warner, 2009). Facial asymmetry and particularly incomplete lingual range of motion observed on oral mechanism exam potentially increases the odds of aspiration risk (Leder & Suiter, 2014; Leder, Suiter, Murray, & Rademaker, 2013). The Yale Swallow Protocol has been validated on a small population of consecutively referred patients, compared to results of VFSS (Suiter, Sloggy, & Leder, 2014).

BARNES-JEWISH HOSPITAL STROKE DYSPHAGIA SCREEN (BJH-SDS)

The BJH-SDS test combines questions about alertness, oral mechanism examination, and the 3-ounce water-swallow test. It has been validated only on patients with stroke, in one study comparing results to a clinical evaluation of swallowing and in another study, comparing results to VFSS findings. It screens for dysphagia and aspiration. It is designed to be administered by nurses (Edmiaston, Connor, Loehr, & Nassief, 2010; Edmiaston, Connor, Steger-May, & Ford, 2014).

TORONTO BEDSIDE SWALLOWING SCREENING TEST (TOR-BSST)

The TOR-BSST is a two-step test that presents 10 teaspoon amounts of water. The TOR-BSST is a reliable screening tool that does not require lots of preparation. It does require structured, somewhat lengthy training of nurses who will administer the test to patients with neurological deficits (Martino, Maki, & Diamant, 2014; Martino et al., 2009).

OTHER SCREENING TOOLS

Many other screening tools have been developed and described for use with different patient populations. SLPs are encouraged to carefully analyze the information about any tool under consideration. Before embarking on the development of a facility-specific dysphagia screening tool, ascertain that there is not already a valid and reliable tool available.

Standardized Patient Questionnaires as Screening Tools

As described in Chapter 1, patient questionnaires can be used to gather patient report of symptoms of dysphagia. They can also be used as a screening test. Such tools may be particularly helpful in certain outpatient settings. For example, the EAT-10 might be given to all patients being seen at a multiple sclerosis clinic. The EAT-10 has been demonstrated to predict aspiration in outpatients with stable, chronic COPD (Regan, Lawson, & De Aguiar, 2017). As reflected in the previous discussion, such nonswallow information used to screen for dysphagia could be combined with a task like the 3-ounce water-swallow task to more accurately screen for aspiration.

Selecting a Screening Test and Training Nurses to Administer the Tests

When a facility is selecting a dysphagia screening tool, the speech–language pathologist should coordinate that effort. Even though nurses will administer the tool, it is a tool to screen for dysphagia or aspiration, and thus the speech–language pathologist is the most knowledgeable person on staff to guide discussion and decision making. Regardless of the screening tool selected, the speech–language pathologist should also develop and lead the training and competency assessment of the nurses who will administer the screening. Studies have demonstrated that nurses can reliably administer screening tools, but consistent and ongoing training is essential (Anderson, Pathak, Rosenbek, Morgan, & Daniels, 2016; Daniels, Pathak, Rosenbek, Morgan, & Anderson, 2016; Titsworth et al., 2013; Warner, Suiter, Nystrom, Poskus, & Leder, 2014).

Included with the Supplemental Materials is a competency tool designed to check nurses before they began screening patients. This competency tool has been formatted so the facility can customize it to match the screening tool they are using (see Supplemental Materials, Education Materials, Staff, Swallowing Screen for Training Nurses Validation Tool).

Clinical Swallow Evaluation

Patients may be referred for a clinical swallow evaluation after a failed screening or may be referred directly by a physician for this exam. Whereas a screening is designed to determine whether a patient is at risk for having dysphagia or aspirating, the clinical swallow evaluation is a diagnostic test to confirm or rule out oral dysphagia, confirm risk of aspiration and/or pharyngeal dysphagia, but also to determine the nature and extent of the suspected swallowing impairment. The Clinical Swallow Evaluation (CSE) is also an opportunity to assess the patient's swallowing ability (as opposed to the disability) (Carnaby, 2012).

The CSE is often the first step in a complete assessment of a patient with dysphagia. An instrumental procedure (modified barium swallow/videofluoroscopic swallow study [VFSS], or fiberoptic endoscopic evaluation of swallowing [FEES]) is often recommended for more complete assessment of the pharyngeal phase. Unfortunately, there are situations in which only a clinical evaluation can be completed because there is no access to a facility at which an instrumental exam of swallowing can be completed.

Sample cases provide examples of when the CSE might be the only exam needed and when an instrumental exam is needed. (See Supplemental Materials, SLP Resources, Case Examples: Choosing Appropriate Exam.)

Accuracy and Limitations of CSE

A clinical swallow evaluation has definite limitations. Clinicians who treat patients with suspected pharyngeal disorders based solely on results obtained with the CSE place themselves and the patient at risk:

- Aspiration can neither be confirmed nor ruled out with 100% accuracy during a bedside evaluation.
- The function of pharyngeal and laryngeal structures cannot be assessed to determine physiologic deficits.
- Without knowledge of what is wrong in the pharyngeal phase, an accurate treatment plan cannot be developed.

Regarding the pharyngeal phase, the CSE simply allows you to observe for any clinical signs of aspiration and pharyngeal deficits. Many of the same limitations of screening tools, as described earlier, for detecting aspiration are shared by the swallowing portion of a CSE. A systematic review of screening tools and procedures used during clinical exam of swallowing was conducted and found that no bedside screening protocol has been shown to provide adequate predictive value for presence of aspiration. They characterized the study types as subjective clinical exams, questionnaire-based tools, multiple-exam protocols, and individual exam maneuvers. Several individual exam maneuvers demonstrated reasonable sensitivity with ability to exclude aspiration. These include a test for dysphonia through production of a sustained "ah" (McCullough, Wertz, & Rosenbek, 2001) and use of dual-axis accelerometry (Steele et al., 2011) but reproducibility and consistency of these protocols was not established. The authors of the systematic review determined that more research is needed to design an optimal protocol for dysphagia detection (O'Horo, Rogus-Pulia, Garcia-Arguello, Robbins, & Safdar, 2015). Many screening tests use clinical signs of aspiration (e.g., coughing, throat clearing) as part of the pass–fail, and as many as 40%–70% of patients may be silent aspirators, who do not show any clinical signs of aspiration.

Larger volumes of water may accurately identify patients who are silent aspirators on smaller amounts of water (Leder, Suiter, & Green, 2011). Therefore, using a test like a 3-ounce water swallow, as compared to a test using consecutive small sips from a spoon, would likely elicit an airway response in patients who showed no response to aspiration on smaller amounts. The speech–language pathologist must balance the decision to use large volumes of water with the risk this might pose to certain vulnerable patient populations (Daniels, Anderson, & Willson, 2012).

The CSE Is Not a Screening

Some in the SLP community consider a clinical evaluation of swallowing to be a type of screening. However, a thorough CSE can provide much needed information for the management of dysphagia. Although a CSE by a speech–language pathologist might incorporate a screening tool, the CSE is not a screening. Recall that many screening tools screen for presence of or risk for aspiration, not for presence of dysphagia. The CSE can reveal very important information about the oral phases of swallowing that cannot necessarily be obtained during a screening or on an instrumental evaluation. Such information will help you decide which types and textures of food the patient can eat and whether any postural compensations appear to be effective to address oral deficits. The effects of fatigue can be observed and more information about the patient's cognitive and communication skills can be obtained.

Rosenbek, McCullough, and Wertz (2004) are among those who state that the clinical swallowing evaluation is much more than a screening. They emphasize the importance of the clinical exam and the extensive information that can be gained from it. Although their conclusions were based on a small study of 60 patients with stroke, their conclusions should be heeded by all speech–language pathologists: "Perhaps foremost is the need to determine whether the evidence provided by the CSE can define the biomechanical abnormalities responsible for signs of dysphagia, including, but certainly not limited to, aspiration. In the interim it is critical that the CSE not be relegated to the status of a screening tool. It is far too powerful" (Rosenbek, McCullough, & Wertz, 2004, p. 14).

The CSE provides an excellent opportunity to focus on function and obtain information from the patient and caregivers about

- the effects of swallowing impairments on the individual's activities (capacity and performance in everyday contexts) and participation

- contextual factors that serve as barriers to or facilitators of successful swallowing and participation for individuals with swallowing impairments (ASHA, 2004).

ASHA Guidance on Clinical Evaluation

The ASHA Practice Portal and the Preferred Practice Patterns (ASHA, 2004) describe the purposes of the clinical exam. Information from those documents, and additional factors added by this author, indicate that the clinical exam can enable the SLP to do the following:

- Obtain and integrate relevant interview and/or case-history information, including medical status, education, vocation, and socioeconomic, cultural, and linguistic background.

- Collaborate with physicians and other caregivers to obtain necessary background information.

- Review auditory, visual, motor, and cognitive status.

- Observe and assess the integrity of the following structures of the upper airway and digestive tract: face, jaw, lips, oral mucosa, tongue, teeth, hard palate, soft palate.

- Perform a functional assessment of physiological functioning of the muscles and structures used in swallowing, including observations of symmetry, sensation, strength, tone, range and rate of motion, and coordination or timing of movement.

- Obtain information about cranial nerve function related to swallowing.

- Assess saliva management, including frequency and adequacy of spontaneous dry swallowing and ability to swallow voluntarily.

- Perform functional assessment of actual swallowing ability, including observation of mastication, oral containment, and manipulation of the bolus.

- Form impressions about pharyngeal function, such as:
  - briskness of swallow initiation
  - extent of laryngeal elevation during the swallow
  - signs of aspiration such as coughing or wet or gurgly voice quality after the swallow
  - adequacy of airway protection and coordination of respiration and swallowing

- On the basis of clinical signs and symptoms, identify the presence of an oral dysphagia.

- Observe the characteristics that may affect swallowing function, such as bolus size and consistency, fatigue during a meal, posture, positioning, and environmental conditions.

- Identify clinical signs and symptoms of esophageal dysphagia or gastroesophageal reflux in order to make an appropriate referral to another specialty.

- Determine the need for an instrumental evaluation for assessment of the pharyngeal phase of swallowing following the clinical examination.

- Identify and follow up with patients who may require reevaluation, instruction, intervention, or other evaluation procedures prior to instrumental evaluation.

- Determine whether the patient is an appropriate candidate for treatment and/or management from clinical examination findings such as medical stability, cognitive status, nutritional status, and psychological, social, and environmental and behavioral factors.

- Recommend, as appropriate, the route of nutritional management (i.e., oral vs. non-oral).

- Recommend clinical interventions (e.g., positioning, food and liquid consistency modifications, feeding routine alterations) and other clinical strategies to enhance the efficiency and safety of swallowing.

- Provide counseling, education, and training to patients, health-care providers, and caregivers.

Tasks Often Used During CSE

Information is provided in this section about specific procedures often used during clinical swallow exams and whether the use of these procedures is currently supported in the literature (Table 2.2). Research is ongoing on some of these procedures, and SLPs are encouraged to periodically review the new literature.

ORIENTATION

In a large study with a heterogeneous population, the odds of liquid aspiration were 31% greater for patients not oriented to person, place, and time. This was assessed by asking the patient three questions:

1. What is your name?
2. Where are you right now?
3. What year is it? (Leder et al., 2009).

COMMAND FOLLOWING

In that same study, for patients unable to follow single-step verbal commands, the odds of liquid aspiration were 57% higher; for puree aspiration, 47% higher; and for being deemed unsafe for any oral intake, 69% higher. The three commands were the following:

1. Open your mouth.
2. Stick out your tongue.
3. Smile.

COUGH

Daniels, McAdam, Brailey, and Foundas (1997) assessed six clinical features (dysphonia, dysarthria, abnormal volitional cough, abnormal gag reflex, cough after swallow, and voice change after swallow) with a clinical evaluation followed by videofluoroscopic studies. They found that each of the six features was significantly related to aspiration and was a predictor of the subset of patients with silent aspiration. In fact, abnormal volitional cough and cough with swallow together predicted aspiration with 78% accuracy.

McCullough and coauthors investigated the sensitivity and specificity of the bedside/clinical examination for predicting aspiration on videofluoroscopic exam and found that two signs rated on trial swallows predicted aspiration: presence of a spontaneous cough during the swallow and an overall estimate of the presence or absence of aspiration (McCullough, Wertz, Rosenbek, et

Table 2.2
Procedures Sometimes Used During Clinical Swallow Evaluations

Procedure	What it purports to do	Does research currently support its use?	If not supported by research, can anything be gained from using it?
Cough	Indicate that penetration or aspiration has occurred or that patient is at increased risk	Yes	
Wet vocal quality or change in vocal quality on production of "ah"	Indicate that penetration or aspiration has occurred Studies have used pitch, quality, and intensity	Yes Clear postswallow voice should predict that penetration and aspiration did not occur; change in quality or wet vocal quality may indicate that aspiration did occur	
Pitch elevation	Provide information about adequate elevation of larynx	Somewhat	
Digital palpation of larynx during swallowing for hyolaryngeal excursion	Provide information about adequate elevation of larynx during swallow	Somewhat	
Observing for multiple swallows	Indicate extra swallows needed to clear oral and/or pharyngeal residue	Yes	
Delayed or incomplete oral clearance	Clinical predictor of aspiration	Yes	
Gag reflex	Clinical predictor of aspiration in stroke Indication of pharyngeal sensitivity	Yes	
Dysarthria	If present, indicates increased risk for aspiration	Yes	
Oral movements	If impaired, indicate increased risk for aspiration	Yes Particularly for lingual range of motion	
Orientation	If impaired, indicates increased risk of aspiration	Yes What is your name? Where are you right now? What year is it?	
Command following	If impaired, indicates increased risk of aspiration	Yes Open your mouth Stick out your tongue Smile	
Oral health	Poor oral hygiene indicates increased risk of aspiration pneumonia	Yes Oral mucosa, saliva, condition of natural teeth and of dentures	

(continues)

Table 2.2. *(continued)*

Procedure	What it purports to do	Does research currently support its use?	If not supported by research, can anything be gained from using it?
Managing secretions	Inability to manage secretions indicates increased risk of aspirating food or liquid Reduced spontaneous swallowing frequency of saliva may predict severity of dysphagia in stroke	Yes	
Cranial nerve function	Provides information about intact function that can be used to plan rehabilitation	Yes V, VII, IX, X, and XII	
Respiration-swallow coordination	Increased respiratory rate and/or swallow pattern with inhale after swallow can increase risk of aspiration	Yes	
Blue dye test	Used with patients with tracheostomy to show blue secretions indicating aspiration	No	May reveal aspiration of large quantities, but does not show aspiration of small amounts
Watery eyes	Indicate aspiration	No	May indicate irritation of trigeminal nerve
Runny nose or postnasal drip	Indicate aspiration	No	Some individuals with reflux experience this
Sneezing	Indicate aspiration	No	May indicate irritation of trigeminal nerve
Cervical auscultation	Through use of stethoscope, lets the clinician hear different sounds representing different parts of the pharyngeal swallow and predicts aspiration	No, although seems in principle to make sense; research continues	You might "hear" something indicating the patient has swallowed; could be helpful in patients' whose physical position prevents palpating for presence of swallow
Oxygen desaturation or pulse oximetry	Indicate aspiration events	No	Monitor patient stability during exam, noting that a drop in oxygen saturation may indicate stress on patient's respiratory system

al., 2001). Two previous studies (Daniels et al., 1998; Logemann et al., 1999) linked spontaneous cough with predicting aspiration (Daniels et al., 1998; Logemann, Veis, & Colangelo, 1999).

Cough has typically been indicated by the speech–language pathologist as present or absent. That is, did the patient cough or not during or after swallowing? Researchers are looking more closely at cough and measuring it instrumentally. Cough characteristics include duration, volume and peak flow of the inspiration phase, compression phase duration, peak flow and rise time for the expulsive phase, and volume acceleration (expulsive phase peak flow–expulsive phase rise time). In a study of 96 patients with stroke, three objective measures of voluntary cough (expulsive phase rise time, volume acceleration, and expulsive phase peak flow) were each associated with an aspiration risk. Clinicians should stay abreast of research on cough, as in the future instrumental measurement of the different characteristics of cough might be used more routinely (Hammond et al., 2009).

GAG REFLEX

Either absent or weakened velar or pharyngeal wall contraction, unilaterally or bilaterally, in response to tactile stimulation of the posterior pharyngeal wall in patients with stroke was predictive of aspiration on a VFSS. Impaired gag reflex was one of the six indicators of increased risk of aspiration in patients with stroke (Daniels, Ballo, Mahoney, & Foundas, 2000). There is no one-to-one correspondence between an absent gag reflex and an inability to swallow (a false belief held by some nurses), but Mann and Hankey did find that palatal weakness or asymmetry was an independent predictor of dysphagia (Mann & Hankey, 2001).

VOCAL QUALITY/DYSPHONIA

In the Daniels study mentioned earlier (Daniels, Ballo, Mahoney, & Foundas, 2000), voice change after swallow was one of the six indicators studied. In another study there was no association between the presence of a wet voice and penetration or aspiration of material after a swallow. A wet voice may still be useful in identifying those with dysphagia who may have laryngeal dysfunction and therefore may be at risk of penetrating or aspirating any type of material, not just prandial material (Warms & Richards, 2000).

Another study explored the validity of clinician judgments of voice abnormalities as indicators of penetration, aspiration, or other swallowing abnormalities. These researchers concluded that a clear postswallow voice quality provides reasonable evidence that penetration, aspiration, and dysphagia are absent (specificity for penetration 75% and for aspiration 94%). However, observations of abnormal postswallow voice quality can be misleading and are not a valid indication that penetration, aspiration, or dysphagia exists (Waito, Bailey, Molfenter, Zoratto, & Steele, 2011). This is in contrast to findings in an earlier study with patients with stroke that the presence of dysphonia is a much stronger indicator of the presence of aspiration than the absence of dysphonia is for indicating the absence of aspiration. Particularly related to wet vocal quality (a more specific description than change in vocal quality), that study also found that the presence or absence of a wet vocal quality after swallowing appeared to be related to aspiration (McCullough et al., 2001).

HYOLARYNGEAL EXCURSION THROUGH LARYNGEAL PALPATION WITH FOUR-FINGER METHOD

In a study comparing judgments made on CSE to findings on VFSS, the only physiologic measure that was rated with some degree of reliability between CSE and VFSS was the hyolaryngeal elevation (a judgment of completeness). The measure was derived using the four-finger method, which involves placing the index finger under the chin on hyoid, the middle and ring fingers at top and bottom of the thyroid cartilage, and the little finger on the cricoid. Judgments regarding the extent, or completeness, of hyolaryngeal elevation were also best made on thin liquids (Rangarathnam & McCullough, 2016).

PITCH ELEVATION

A pilot study revealed that both maximum fundamental frequency (F_0) and perceptual evaluation of pitch elevation independently significantly predicted Penetration–Aspiration Scale scores for thin-liquid swallows. Vocal range (average pitch to falsetto) was not sensitive in predicting likelihood of oropharyngeal dysphagia. Instead, the study asked the speech–language pathologist rater to determine whether the patient had "normal maximum pitch elevation." These findings indicate that reduced pitch elevation can be indicative of reduced airway protection and swallowing impairment in some patients with dysphagia (Malandraki, Hind, Gangnon, Logemann, & Robbins, 2011).

The effortful pitch glide (EPG) was studied, and the biomechanics of the EPG and hyolaryngeal elevation for swallow were comparable. Therefore, asking the patient to produce an EPG during assessment might yield information about the movement of the hyolaryngeal complex for swallowing (Miloro, Pearson, & Langmore, 2014). However, another study showed that there was no significant relationship between laryngeal lift during a speech task and laryngeal lift during a swallow (Kennedy et al., 2018).

DYSARTHRIA

In the Daniels study (Daniels, Ballo, Mahoney, & Foundas, 2000), dysarthria was one of six features associated with increased risk of aspiration. In patients with stroke, any two of the six features predicted moderate to severe dysphagia and increased risk of aspiration. Dysarthria and reduced intelligibility were found to be indicators of aspiration (McCullough et al., 2001).

ORAL MOVEMENTS

In the McCullough et al., (2001) study, strength and range of motion of oral structures was not predictive of aspiration. However, Leder et al., (2013) found that the odds for liquid aspiration increased with decreased lingual ROM.

DELAYED ORAL TRANSIT AND ORAL CLEARANCE

Mann and Hankey have studied clinical indicators and demographic predictors of swallowing in patients with stroke. The clinical predictors of aspiration were found to be delayed oral transit and incomplete oral clearance (Mann & Hankey, 2001; Mann, Hankey, & Cameron, 1999).

MULTIPLE SWALLOWS

Residue in the pyriform sinuses and in the hypopharynx correlated with the number of swallows per bolus for thin liquids. This was not true for other consistencies but may be complicated by the fact that the patients had had a stroke, and thus sensation might have been impaired, reducing the patients' sensation that a second swallow was needed (Rangarathnam & McCullough, 2016). Number of swallows of pudding corresponded to amount of residue in the valleculae (Veis, Logemann, & Colangelo, 2000).

MANAGEMENT OF ORAL SECRETIONS

It is only logical to assume that if a patient is not able to manage oral secretions by swallowing completely and frequently enough, he or she would also have problems swallowing liquids and solids. Murray and colleagues, in a study with FEES, found that the accumulation of endoscopically visible oropharyngeal secretions located within the laryngeal vestibule was highly predictive of aspiration of food or liquid (Murray, Langmore, Ginsberg, & Dostie, 1996). The reduced ability to manage secretions can be observed. In acute-care settings, the nurse can also provide information about how frequently the patient is suctioned orally. In patients after stroke, reduced frequency of spontaneous swallowing of secretions was observed and found to correlate with severity of stroke and dysphagia (Crary, Carnaby, Sia, Khanna, & Waters, 2013; Crary, Sura, & Carnaby, 2013).

CERVICAL AUSCULTATION

Cervical auscultation is a general term that describes several techniques for listening to a patient's breath sounds. In research, a laryngeal microphone is used for cervical auscultation. In clinical settings, the flat diaphragm of a stethoscope is placed laterally below the thyroid cartilage on the side of the neck. Placement is adjusted until cervical breath sounds can be heard. Cervical breath sounds are generally hollow, or "tubular," as compared to breath sounds heard over the lungs. Some clinicians use cervical auscultation during CSE to listen to breath sounds but also to "hear" the swallow, although great caution must be taken in making summary statements on the basis of what is heard.

A normal swallow is thought to "sound" like this:

- Breath sounds are heard.

- Breathing stops (usually in the middle of an exhalation).

- A sound often described as a "clunk" or "swish" is heard.

- Breath sounds are heard again, similar to the way the breath sounded before the swallow.

The "clunk" and "swish" sounds heard through the stethoscope are considered the result of the pressure changes as the bolus passes through the pharynx and the upper esophageal sphincter (UES). A stethoscope does amplify sounds and may provide helpful information concerning the timing of the swallow and the breath sounds. Cervical auscultation (CA) is not, however, a reliable screening tool, and clinicians should not make judgments on the basis of what they hear.

Research does not indicate that the sounds heard on auscultation can reliably reveal whether aspiration has occurred solely on the basis of on cervical auscultation. In a study comparing cervical auscultation observation and results on VFSS, the individual reliability outcomes varied widely and thus agreement between judgments was poor. Raters' average percentage of sensitivity was 62% and that of specificity was 66%. However, when considering the decision made by the majority of each group, the group consensus, values improved to 90% specificity and 80% sensitivity. The authors therefore concluded that improving the poor raters would improve the overall accuracy of this technique in predicting abnormality in swallowing; in principle, CA should permit reliable classification (Leslie, Drinnan, Finn, Ford, & Wilson, 2004).

Another study found that comparison with radiologically defined aspiration/penetration for the group of experts (speech–language pathologists) yielded 70% specificity and 94% sensitivity. These researchers concluded that the swallowing sounds contain audible cues that should, in principle, permit reliable classification. If that were the case, then CA might be used as an early warning system for identifying patients with a high risk of aspiration/penetration; however, it is not appropriate as a stand-alone tool (Borr, Hielscher-Fastabend, & Lücking, 2007).

Note that each of these studies used the term *in principle*, which indicates some theoretical soundness to the use of this tool. Clinicians might gain some useful information from listening to swallows, but should not draw conclusions or make recommendations solely on these observations.

PULSE OXIMETRY AND OXYGEN SATURATION

It has been hypothesized that a drop in oxygen saturation indicates an aspiration event. In preliminary studies, Rogers, Msall, and Shucard (1993) and Zaidi et al. (1995) observed hypoxemic events during swallowing and hypothesized this might indicate aspiration. They thought that noninvasive monitors might yield important information about safety of swallowing at bedside. Sellars, Dunnet, and Carter (1998) performed pulse oximetry on six patients undergoing videofluoroscopic studies. The results indicated no clear-cut relationship between changes in arterial oxygenation and aspiration. The authors indicated that more research is needed on the relationship between respiratory status and dysphagia during oral feedings.

Studies by Colodny (2000) and Leder (2000) failed to support the use of oxygen saturation monitoring. Colodny (2000) concluded that desaturation seemed related to dysphagia but not to specific instances of aspiration. That is, events of aspiration were not responsible for any changes in the oxygen saturation levels; rather, individuals with dysphagia had compromised airway systems. Leder (2000) performed a fiberoptic endoscopic evaluation of swallowing while patients were monitored for arterial oxygen saturation as well as heart rate and blood pressure. He found no significant differences in SpO_2 levels based on aspiration status or oxygen requirements. Therefore, monitoring levels of oxygen is not a reliable way to determine whether a patient is aspirating.

Incidentally, the study also demonstrated that changes in heart rate and blood pressure were not reliable predictors of aspiration.

Ramsey and colleagues studied desaturation in patients with stroke, using a bedside assessment followed by chest radiograph to determine whether aspiration had occurred. Therefore, their definition of silent aspirators was that the patient had not demonstrated signs of airway compromise on the beside exam but were found to have aspirated material on the chest X-ray. Of the 85 patients with unsafe swallows, only 28 (32.9%) desaturated by >2% and 6 (7.1%) by >5%. Desaturation did not occur in any of the six silent aspirators (Ramsey, Smithard, & Kalra, 2006). In a study that simultaneously measured oxygen saturation during VFSS, Wang and colleagues found no significant correlation between desaturation measured by pulse oximetry and aspiration on VFSS. The positive predictive rate of pulse oximetry in detecting aspiration on VFSS was 39.1%, and the negative predictive rate was 59.4% (Wang, Chang, Chen, & Hsiao, 2005).

BLUE DYE TEST

This test is described in detail in Chapter 6. It involves suctioning the patient at the tracheostomy to determine whether there is evidence of aspirated material. Note: There is no evidence to support the assumption that watery eyes, sneezing or runny nose in any way indicate aspiration. It may indicate irritation of the trigeminal nerve. Runny nose or postnasal drip is experienced by some who have reflux.

Assessing Oral Health During CSE

Sometimes the only observations about oral health made during a CSE are whether the patient is edentulous and, if the patient has dentures, whether they were worn during the assessment. Studies suggest an association between poor oral hygiene and respiratory pathogens, and a decrease in the incidence of respiratory complications when patients are provided chemical or mechanical interventions for improved oral care (Pace & McCullough, 2010). The relationship of oral hygiene to overall health is well established. Langmore and colleagues analyzed risk factors for developing aspiration pneumonia in patients who were elderly in several settings: nursing homes, acutely ill, outpatients (Langmore et al., 1998; Langmore, Skarupski, Park, & Fries, 2002). In all settings, number of decayed teeth was associated with aspiration pneumonia. There was also a relationship between how often teeth were brushed and pneumonia, as well as being dependent on others for oral care. Other systematic reviews (Azarpazhooh & Leake, 2003; Scannapieco et al., 2003) have found a relationship between oral health and bacterial pneumonia.

Pneumonia is not the only disease associated with poor oral hygiene. Links have been established between periodontal inflammation and atherosclerosis and ischemic heart disease (Fowler et al., 2001), hypertension, and stroke. Exacerbation of COPD has also been demonstrated to be related to oral pathogens (Scannapieco et al., 1998).

Saliva plays an important role in eating, swallowing and digestion. It helps cleanse the oral cavity, form boluses, clear bacteria and lubricate the mucosa. Adequate saliva is also necessary to facilitate speech. Saliva also helps to protect the teeth by neutralizing acid, and it contributes to digestive actions (Pedersen, Bardow, Jensen, & Nauntofte, 2002). Xerostomia is known to have a negative impact on taste, eating, and swallowing, and can be caused by many medications. It is also a side effect of radiation therapy to the head and neck.

INFORMAL CHECKLISTS EXIST TO ASSESS ORAL HEALTH

The Kayser-Jones Brief Oral Health Status Examination (BOHSE) was specifically designed to evaluate the oral health of nursing home residents, with and without cognitive impairment, by varied nursing personnel (Kayser-Jones, Bird, Paul, Long, & Schell, 1995). It assesses oral tissue, saliva, and condition of natural teeth and artificial teeth. The speech–language pathologist does not need to perform a complete assessment of oral health but should at least comment on those areas.

Assessing Cranial Nerves

The CSE should include an examination of the five cranial nerves most involved in swallowing: V, VII, IX, X, and XII. The exam is performed to assess function related to eating and swallowing (see Table 2.3 for a quick reference guide to cranial nerve function).

If the speech–language pathologist wants to record the information on a specific form, Cranial Nerve Exam is provided in the Supplemental Materials (SLP Resources, Cranial Nerve Exam). In certain patients with complex neurological histories, the speech–language pathologist may want to assess other cranial nerves. A more complete table for cranial nerve assessment is included in the Supplemental Materials (see SLP Resources, Nerves and Muscles Involved in Swallowing).

Carnaby (2012) makes a strong case for including the assessment of cranial nerves to identify what remains intact, to direct the speech–language pathologist to muscles that can be used to support compensations and rehabilitative exercises. When an intact nerve is identified, the rehabilitation plan could use activities designed to maximize movement and strength on the intact side. If denervation is observed (e.g., atrophy on one side), then the plan would be to build strength on the opposite side to compensate.

Assessing Respiratory Function and Respiratory–Swallow Coordination

Assessing respiratory rate and the coordination between respiration and swallowing provides information about factors that could compromise the safety of swallowing. The normal respiratory

Table 2.3
Quick Reference Guide to Cranial Nerve Function for Swallowing

Cranial verve	Area of innervation	Effect on swallowing	Observation on task
V: Trigeminal	Anterior 2/3 of tongue Mandible	Loss of sensation Cannot use mandible for chewing	Bilateral impairment: cannot close mouth Unilateral: jaw deviates to weak side on opening
VII: Facial	Facial structures Lips and cheeks	Difficulty closing lips, controlling food in mouth Loss of taste	Unable to puff cheeks
IX: Glossopharyngeal	Posterior part of tongue and oropharynx	Loss of taste, sensation from posterior one-third Absent gag Delay in pharyngeal response	Changes in ability to taste bitter and sour
X: Vagus	Pharynx Larynx Upper esophagus	Impairment in closing or protecting airway Risk of aspiration Esophageal dismotility	Bilateral impairment: uvula doesn't lift on "ah" Unilateral: uvula deviates away from impaired side Gag reflex diminished or absent
XII: Hypoglossal	Tongue	Difficulty forming and manipulating bolus Difficulty propelling bolus	Tongue deviates to weak side Extrinsic muscles involved, will see on protrusion Intrinsic muscles involved, will see when lateralizing inside mouth Listen for imprecision in speech

Note. Adapted from Carnaby (2012); Humbert (2011); Shaw and Martino (2013).

rate for adults is 12–20 breaths per minute. Patients who are breathing more rapidly than that may tire easily during a meal because they are having to interrupt the respiration for swallowing. They may also alter their respiratory–swallow pattern. There are four patterns of coordination between breathing and swallowing: exhale–swallow–exhale (EX-EX), inhale–swallow–exhale (IN-EX), exhale-swallow-inhale (EX-IN), and inhale–swallow–inhale (IN-IN). The most common pattern, EX-EX, is reflected in Figure 2.1 (Martin-Harris, 2006; Martin-Harris, Brodsky, Price, Michel, & Walters, 2003).

A disruption of the normal breathing–swallowing pattern, such as inhaling after the swallow, could put patients at increased risk for aspiration. The pressure of inhalation has the potential to draw food and liquid residue toward the lungs. Abnormal patterns of swallowing have been observed in patients with COPD. In one study, they were observed to swallow more often during inhalation with masticated boluses. Pudding was followed by inhalation with increased frequency, and these participants swallowed at lower tidal volume (Gross, Atwood, Grayhack, & Shaiman, 2003).

Applying Critical Thinking With Use of Standardized Items on the CSE

Most SLPs do not use a standardized tool but instead use a tool they have developed themselves. There are standardized screening tools as described earlier in the chapter. The only clinical swallow exams standardized are the Mann Assessment of Swallowing Ability, standardized on stroke, and MASA-C, standardized on cancer (Mann, 2002).

One prospective study described the components included by SLPs when designing a standardized evidence-based dysphagia assessment protocol for acute-care patients. They then observed patterns of component use. The findings confirm that SLPs are highly variable in their use of certain components but also demonstrate consistent use of a core set. The authors recommend

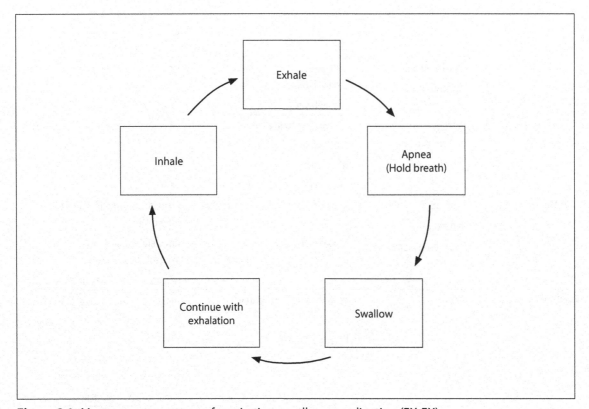

Figure 2.1 Most common pattern of respiration–swallow coordination (EX-EX).

that rather than promoting the standardization of strict item-based CSE protocols that constrain SLP practice, consideration be given to promoting the clinical reasoning process that supports the utility of the CSE for diagnosis, patient-centered management, and treatment planning (McAllister, Kruger, Doeltgen, & Tyler-Boltrek, 2016). McCullough et al. (2001) linked "global judgment" of the likelihood of aspiration to the presence of aspiration on VFSS.

Most experienced clinicians would agree that there should be core elements assessed during a CSE, though studies confirm there is variability in what is assessed (Bateman, Leslie, & Drinnan, 2007; Mathers-Schmidt & Kurlinski, 2003; Pettigrew & O'Toole, 2007; Vogels, Cartwright, & Cocks, 2015). They would also agree that applying clinical reasoning to customize the assessment to each particular patient is preferred over following a strict standardized protocol.

Engaging Patient and Family in the Exam

Patient and family education occurs every time the clinician interacts with the patient, whether during an evaluation or a treatment session. Explain what you are observing and your assessment of the patient's skills. A handout found in the Supplemental Materials may be useful: Education Materials, Patient/Family, Clinical or Bedside Swallowing Evaluation Information.

Clinical Swallow Evaluation Sample Forms

Given the information above, two examples of the Clinical Swallow Evaluation are shown below and provided in the Supplemental Materials (SLP Resources, CSE Form A, Form B, Summary). They are the components that many SLPs would agree form the core of a CSE as described in this chapter. In addition, presentation of liquid and food is included on the form, although for some patients the exam will be concluded before presenting PO if the patient is deemed too high risk for aspiration. The format of the sample forms can be altered for specific patient populations.

See Table 2.4 for an evaluation of which form to use. Each includes non-PO items described above, as well as a section for recording observations made during the presentation of liquid and food boluses.

The difference in the two forms is in the level of detail. Form A is more detailed, with information on individual items to be tested in each section, whereas Form B provides room for quick ratings and summary statements. Form A would likely be used as a clinician becomes familiar with all the steps needed for a CSE, and when this is mastered, Form B will be quicker and easier to use as the SLP has internalized the steps. Whether Form A or For B is used, there is a separate Summary Sheet for the diagnosis, recommendations, and a place to choose long- and short-term goals and treatment objectives for oral phase problems and compensatory strategies for use with PO. Pharyngeal phase goals and treatment objectives can be written in from hypotheses about possible pharyngeal deficits, but they cannot reliably be selected until an instrumental study has been completed.

At facilities using an electronic health record (EHR), the CSE can be used to help build and/or update the flow sheet in the EHR. In fact, all the short-term goals and treatment objectives could be built into the EHR for point-and-click selections.

The directions and tips provided below will be helpful when using either Form A or Form B. Citations to support the use of items are not repeated below as they have been provided earlier in this chapter. However, items that research suggests indicate increased risk of aspiration are listed with an asterisk. For example, in the Orientation section, the three questions (i.e., What is your name? Where are you right now? and What year is it?) each have an asterisk because failure to answer these questions indicates an increased risk of aspiration in at least one study.

Table 2.4
Form A and B of Clinical Swallow Evaluation

Best for...	Form A	Form B
Clinicians new to dysphagia	X	
Experienced clinicians		X
After training on detailed Form A		X
Greater detail	X	
Cranial nerve exam-	X	X
Note: more complete supplemental cranial nerve exam can be done with either form.		
Can be filled out more quickly		X
Can be used to build or revise EHR	X	X
Filled out in patient room	X	X
Information entered into EHR after completing in patient room	X	X
Paper form inserted into chart for MD review	Likely too detailed	X

Note. Summary Form to be used with either Form A or Form B.

Before Beginning the CSE

REVIEW OF CASE HISTORY INFORMATION

See Chapter 1 for a full discussion of the importance of gathering essential information from the patient's medical history.

REVIEW OF AUDITORY, VISUAL, AND MOTOR STATUS

This information may be obtained from the review of the history (see Chapter 1) or may be the first thing the SLP assesses when meeting the patient. Is the patient able to hear the SLP? Does the patient have hearing aids? If so, the SLP should be sure they are functioning and that the patient is wearing them. It is not unusual in inpatient settings that the family has taken home expensive hearing aids. Having an inexpensive amplification system available that the patient can borrow, although no substitute for the patient's own aids, can facilitate the evaluation. If the patient has glasses, be sure they are clean and that the patient is wearing them. A brief assessment of upper motor skills will help determine whether the patient will be able to self-feed. If the patient has been assessed by the occupational therapist, review the OT's findings.

POSITIONING THE PATIENT FOR THE EXAM

Before beginning the clinical exam, the patient should be positioned as upright as possible. If the patient is in a bed, a draw sheet (i.e., a sheet folded and placed under the torso of the patient) is likely in place that will facilitate positioning. With the patient lying flat, a staff member standing on one side of the patient holds the sheet and then draws the patient toward the head of the bed before elevating the bed into a sitting position. Extra pillows can be used to help stabilize the patient.

PERFORMING ORAL CARE

If the patient has not recently had oral hygiene performed, this would be a good time to do so.

Directions for Clinical Swallow Evaluation Form A

The Clinical Swallow Evaluation Form A is shown as Figure 2.2.

Clinical Swallow Evaluation Form A

Patient _____ Date _____

ALERTNESS/COOPERATION

Alert   ☐ Remained alert   ☐ Had to be aroused   ☐ Could not be kept awake   Other: _____

ORIENTATION*

What is your name?   Where are you now?   What year is it?   Answered all three   YES ☐   NO ☐

ORAL MOTOR EVALUATION   ☐ CNA

1. Structure   Note any abnormalities _____

Edentulous yes / no   Dentures yes / no   Wears dentures when eating yes / no   Dentures in during eval yes / no

Oral mucosa healthy   YES ☐   NO ☐

2. Awareness/Control of Secretions*

_____ Drooling   _____ Excess secretions in mouth   _____ Wet breath sounds

3. Assessing Jaw, Lip, and Tongue Function

Jaw Control CNA + / –	Lingual Function CNA
Labial Function CNA	protrusion + / –
	lick lips + / –
lip spread /i/ + / –	lateralization to buccal cavity R + / – L + / –
lip closure at rest	elevation of back (k ∧ k ∧ k ∧) + / –
symmetry + / –	repetitive elevation of back + / –
droop R L	final lingual shaping *(Say something nice to Susan on Sunday.)* + / –
Sentence *(Please put the paper by the back door.)* + / –	retraction + / –
lip round /u/ + / –	lateralization to corners R + / – L + / –
lip smacking + / –	elevation of tip (t ∧ t ∧ t ∧) + / –
lip closure on /p p p/ + / –	repetitive elevation of tip + / –
	Overall Lingual ROM* Adequate YES ☐ NO ☐

4. Velar Function   CNA

Prolonged /a/: symmetry during elevation   + / –

Resonance: _____ normal   _____ hypernasal   _____ hyponasal

5. Reflexes/Responses   CNA

Swallow response + / –   Gag reflex* + / –   Palatal reflex + / –

LARYNGEAL EXAMINATION   ☐ CNA

Tracheostomy Tube _____ yes / no

Cuffed   yes / no

Finger occluded   PM valve   Other _____

Figure 2.2 Clinical Swallow Evaluation Form A.   *(continues)*

Vocal Quality★   normal   hoarse   breathy   wet

Voluntary Cough★   strong   weak   absent

Throat Clearing   strong   weak   absent

Ability to Elevate Pitch★   adequate   YES ☐   NO ☐

Volume Control   Noticeable change in loudness   + / −   Ability to control loudness   + / −

QUICK CRANIAL NERVE CHART★

Cranial Nerve	Observation on Task	Observed to Be WNL or Impaired
V: Trigeminal	Bilateral impairment: cannot close mouth	
	Unilateral: jaw deviates to weak side on opening	
VII: Facial	Unable to puff cheeks	
IX: Glossopharyngeal	Changes in ability to taste bitter and sour	
X: Vagus	Bilateral impairment: uvula doesn't lift on "ah" sound	
	Unilateral: uvula deviates away from impaired side	
	Gag reflex diminished or absent	
XII: Hypoglossal	Tongue deviates to weak side	
	Extrinsic muscles involved, will see on protrusion	
	Intrinsic muscles involved, will see when lateralizing inside mouth	
	Listen for imprecision in speech	

RESPIRATORY STATUS★   ☐ **CNA**

BPM at rest _____   Patient swallows during inhalation / exhalation   BPM after assessment _____

COGNITION/COMMUNICATION   ☐ **CNA**

Follows One-Step Directions★   + / −   with cues   without cues

Open your mouth   Stick out your tongue   Smile   Follows all three   YES ☐   NO ☐

Follows Two-Step Directions   + / −   with cues   without cues

Expressive Language   gestures/points   uses single words   uses phrases

Intelligibility★   unintelligible   **Dysarthria★**   apraxia   confused speech

Short-Term Memory

Can patient retell techniques?   yes / no _____

HEARING ACUITY _____

Wears hearing aid(s)   yes / no   right _____ left _____

Hearing aid(s) in for eval   yes / no

Comments _____

Figure 2.2 *(continued)*

Alertness and Cooperation

Note whether the patient is alert, or had to be alerted or awakened. Does the patient remain alert throughout the evaluation? Is the patient cooperative, or does he or she refuse to participate in certain tasks?

Patient _____ Date _____

Swallowing

| + skill is adequate |
| - skill is inadequate |
| N/A not applicable for that texture |

OBSERVATION WITH TRIAL SWALLOWS

Texture				
Ability to Prepare Bolus				
labial closure				
lingual elevation				
lingual lateralization				
mastication				
Ability to Manipulate Bolus				
lingual function				
oral transit time				
Ability to Maintain Cohesive Bolus				
back-of-tongue control				
labial closure				
cheeks				
lingual lateralization				
Clears Oral Cavity in One Swallow				
No. of Swallows per Bolus				
Oropharyngeal Phase				
initiate response in _____ seconds				
Laryngeal Characteristics				
vocal quality/describe				
cough/throat clearing				
elevation of larynx				

Comments _____

Note. Citations to support the use of items have been explained in Chapter 2. Items that research suggests indicate increased risk of aspiration are listed on the CSE with an asterisk.

Clinical Swallow Evaluation Form A

Figure 2.2 (*continued*)

Orientation*

The patient's cognitive status will have implications for how well the patient can participate in therapy, remember precautions and compensatory strategies, and understand the results of the evaluation. In particular, an inability to answer these three questions indicated an increased risk of aspiration:

1. What is your name?

2. Where are you right now?

3. What year is it?

Oral Motor Evaluation

Examining a patient's oral motor skills in isolation does not necessarily reveal how the patient will be able to use these same structures for swallowing. Therefore, this oral motor examination is fairly brief but a good precursor to examining the use of the same structures when food is presented. Remember to perform hand hygiene and wear gloves when performing an oral motor evaluation. If the gloves used at the facility are latex, determine whether the patient has latex allergies, and use nonlatex gloves if necessary. Wear gloves that fit. It is difficult to palpate oral structures with gloves that are too big.

1. STRUCTURE/ORAL HEALTH

Carefully examine for any structural abnormalities of the lips, tongue, gums, and hard and soft palates.

Check the health of the oral mucosa. Look for signs of thrush or other lesions that might make eating painful. If the patient has teeth, observe for cavities or missing teeth. Poor oral hygiene indicates increased risk of aspiration pneumonia.

If the patient has no teeth (edentulous), note whether the patient has dentures and whether he usually eats with dentures. Many individuals who are edentulous can eat a variety of solid foods if they have been without teeth for a long period of time.

Note whether dentures are worn during the evaluation. If the patient wants to wear dentures, you may need to clean the dentures and help the patient put them in.

If the patient has had a stroke with hemiparesis, he or she will probably try to put the dentures in the side of the mouth that still has feeling, catching the denture on the side of the mouth in which there is no feeling. You may need to help the patient in getting the dentures in, starting on the weaker side.

Sometimes the patient does not want to put the dentures in for an evaluation. If he has not worn them for a while, they may not fit or they may even cause some gagging.

2. AWARENESS/CONTROL OF SECRETIONS*

Note whether the patient is unable to control secretions (e.g., drooling) or is retaining secretions in the mouth. Observe how often the patient spontaneously swallows saliva. Listen to the patient's quiet breathing before you begin your exam. Determine whether the patient has a gurgly, wet sound to breathing, possibly indicating that he or she is not swallowing secretions. Patients not managing their own secretions are at increased risk for aspiration.

3. ASSESSING JAW, LIPS, AND TONGUE FUNCTION

Circle the plus sign (+) if movements assessed appear within normal limits. Circle the minus sign (−) and note deficits. Circle CNA if you could not assess an area. Demonstrate any of the following lingual tasks if the patient does not understand your instructions.

Jaw control. Assess the patient's ability to open his jaw adequately and to maintain good jaw closure.

Labial function. Assess the patient's labial range of motion when asked to repeat /i/ and /u/. Note lip closure at rest, indicating whether there is symmetry or droop on either side. Have the patient repeat /p ∧ p ∧ p ∧ /. Note lip closure during this activity. Have the patient smack his or her lips. Observe for strength and symmetry.

Also note lip closure during repetition of sentences or in connected speech. Remember that the ability to use the articulators for speech does not have a direct correlation to the ability to use the same muscles for swallowing.

Lingual function: Protrusion, or retraction. Ask the patient to stick his or her tongue out as far as possible then retract it entirely into the mouth.

Lingual function: Lick lips. Ask the patient to lick his or her lips all the way around in a circular motion.

Lingual lateralization to buccal cavity. Ask the patient to put his or her tongue in the lower buccal cavity on either side.

Lingual back elevation. Have the patient produce /k/ with as much force as possible.

Lingual repetitive elevation of back. Ask the patient to repeat /k ∧ k ∧ k ∧ /, making each sound as sharp as possible.

Fine lingual shaping. Ask the patient to repeat a sentence such as "Say something nice to Susan on Sunday." Listen to how carefully the phrase is articulated. Remember that the ability to use the articulators for speech does not have a direct correlation to the ability to use the same structures for swallowing.

Lingual lateralization to corners. Ask the patient to touch the tip of his tongue to each corner of the lips.

Lingual elevation of tip. Ask the patient to place his or her tongue tip on the alveolar ridge with mouth open and jaw steady.

Lingual repetitive elevation of tip. Have the patient repeat /t ∧ t ∧ t ∧ / as sharply as possible.

*Overall lingual ROM.** Using the observations from these tasks, make a determination of lingual ROM. Reduced ROM indicates increased risk of aspiration.

4. VELAR FUNCTION

Using a tongue depressor to stabilize the tongue and a penlight to visualize the oral cavity, ask the patient to produce a prolonged /a/. Watch for symmetry on elevation of the velum. Remove the tongue depressor and listen to the patient's resonance in connected speech, or have the patient repeat "my pie" several times.

5. REFLEXES/RESPONSES

Swallow response. You have probably observed this already during the course of the evaluation. If not, and after providing oral hygiene, ask the patient to swallow saliva. If necessary, present a small ice chip or small amount of water on a spoon and ask the patient to swallow.

*Gag reflex.** The gag reflex is elicited by touching the back of the tongue or posterior pharyngeal wall with a tongue blade or laryngeal mirror. Watch for symmetrical contraction of the pharyngeal wall and soft palate. Any asymmetry may indicate a unilateral pharyngeal weakness (Logemann, 1999). If your patient is less than cooperative, you may want to forgo testing the gag reflex. The gag has not been shown to have a direct relationship to swallowing ability, but it is a measure of pharyngeal sensitivity; and impaired palatal movement may indicate increased risk of aspiration.

Palatal reflex. Test for the palatal reflex by touching a cold laryngeal mirror to the juncture of the hard and soft palates (DeJong, 1967). You should see the soft palate move up and back, but the pharyngeal walls should not move.

Laryngeal Function Examination

TRACHEOSTOMY TUBE

If the patient has a tracheostomy, identify the type of tracheostomy tube and whether it is cuffed. Also indicate whether you used finger occlusion or the patient had a Passy-Muir valve or other tracheostomy speaking valve on for the assessment.

VOCAL QUALITY*

Note the patient's vocal quality during conversation before any food is given. A breathy vocal quality may indicate decreased vocal fold closure. Wet quality may be related to poor management of secretions. Also note any change in vocal quality after PO intake. Ask the patient to say "ah."

VOLUNTARY COUGH*

Note whether the patient coughs spontaneously. If not, ask the patient to cough. Judge the strength of the cough. A weak or breathy cough may indicate poor vocal fold closure and may predict increased risk of aspiration.

THROAT CLEARING

Note whether the patient clears his throat spontaneously. If not, ask the patient to clear his throat. Judge the strength of the throat clearing. This may indicate the sensitivity of the larynx.

PITCH: ABILITY TO ELEVATE*

The patient's ability to elevate pitch may provide information about the ability to elevate the larynx. Have the patient follow this direction: "I want you to start saying the sound /ah/ at your normal voice or pitch and slowly glide your voice or pitch as high as you can." You are not assessing pitch range but rather whether the patient has normal maximal pitch elevation.

VOLUME CONTROL

Ask the patient to repeat a short phrase, then to repeat it again but loudly. You can also observe the patient's spontaneous ability to vary loudness. Observation of volume may give some information about vocal fold closure.

Cranial Nerves

There are two ways to gather information about cranial nerves. One is to complete the CSE Form A as shown in Figure 2.2, following all the steps for the oral motor exam and then filling in the information you have gained from that examination on the Quick Cranial Nerve Chart that appears on Form A after the Laryngeal Examination. The other is to skip Sections 3, 4, and 5 in the Oral Motor Evaluation and the Laryngeal Examination and use the Cranial Nerve Exam in the Supplemental Materials (SLP Resources, Cranial Nerve Exam).

Respiratory Status and Patterns*

Patients with respiratory disorders (e.g., chronic obstructive pulmonary disease, dyspnea) may have difficulty coordinating a swallow with their breathing and may fatigue very easily. They may exhibit better skills at the beginning of the meal and compromised skills as they fatigue.

DETERMINE RESTING BREATHS PER MINUTE*

Determining breaths per minute is easily done in most patients by watching the upper chest (or even resting your hand on the patient's upper chest) to count the breaths for 10 seconds and then multiplying by 6. Normal range for adults is 12–20 breaths per minute (bpm). Increased respiratory rate indicates increased risk of aspiration. Observe the respiratory rate again after the evaluation and note any changes.

APNEA AT WHAT PHASE OF RESPIRATORY CYCLE

Observe when in the inspiratory–expiratory phase the patient swallows. Most people with normal swallowing skills hold their breath for a swallow during the exhalation phase. Observe whether the patient is swallowing on exhalation or is stopping in the middle of an inhalation.

Cognition and Communication

Having completed the oral motor examination and/or the cranial nerve evaluation, you will have a good idea of the patient's ability to attend, comprehend, and follow directions. Therefore, it may not be necessary to administer all these items.

ONE-STEP DIRECTIONS*

Ask the patient to follow some basic one-step commands, such as "Close your eyes," "Point to the door," and "Pick up the spoon." Note whether the commands are followed accurately and whether cues are required. The items used by Leder et al. (2009) that showed increased risk of aspiration if unable to follow the directions were "Open your mouth," "Stick out your tongue," and "Smile."

TWO-STEP DIRECTIONS

Ask the patient to follow several two-step commands, such as "Open your mouth and touch your head" and "Point to the door and pick up the fork." Note whether the commands are followed accurately and whether cues are required.

EXPRESSIVE LANGUAGE

Provide a judgment about the patient's basic expressive skills.

INTELLIGIBILITY*

Indicate whether intelligibility is impaired by the presence of dysarthria, apraxia, or confused speech. The presence of dysarthria indicates increased risk of aspiration.

SHORT-TERM MEMORY

If the patient must use any techniques to ensure safe swallowing, indicate whether the patient is able to restate them and whether it seems he or she will be able to remember to use them.

HEARING ACUITY

Note whether the patient's hearing has been informally or formally assessed. Add any observation about hearing acuity that may interfere with dysphagia treatment. For example, does the patient fail to follow a direction because he or she cannot hear it accurately? Also note whether the patient wears hearing aids and is wearing them during the evaluation.

Observation With Trial Swallows

A CSE may or may not include presentation of liquids and foods. Much important information will have been gained when the non-PO sections of the CSE are completed. If it seems safe for the patient to try PO, then the speech–language pathologist proceeds with this section. For patients who are not deemed safe to try any PO, they may be made or kept NPO until an instrumental study can be performed or until a repeat CSE is indicated due to improved alertness or skills.

START WITH THIN OR THICK CONSISTENCY?

This decision is specific to each patient. Regardless of the consistency presented first, aggressive oral care should have been performed before beginning the exam. Then, should the patient aspirate some of the PO, there is less chance that oral bacteria will be aspirated as well. Some considerations for starting with thin or thick and whether or not to present other solids are outlined in Table 2.5.

TEST FOODS

Work with the dietary department at your facility to design a test tray or bag that includes samples of a variety of types and textures of foods and liquids. You may need to include a thickening agent if you do not have access to prethickened liquids. For example, a very complete tray might include the following:

¼ c. pureed fruit	1 c. Cheerios
¼ c. ground meat	1 c. 2% milk
¼ c. regular meat	1 c. juice
¼ c. cooked vegetables or fruit mixed with liquid	1 c. pudding

Table 2.5
Consistencies to Use During CSE

Considerations when starting with thin	Considerations when starting with thicker	Considerations for presenting other solids
Start with small sips of water if patient considered at high risk to aspirate	If very poor oral control, patient may have more success with thicker consistency	If information is needed about diet level, then trying different solids (e.g., ground meat, mixed consistencies) will provide important information
If no clinical signs with small sips, proceed to consecutive sips (e.g., 3 ounce water swallow) as silent aspirators on small amounts more likely to show signs on larger amounts	May not demonstrate any signs of aspiration with thicker, leading SLP to proceed to thins	If very poor oral control, may need to avoid things like mixed consistencies
There will be no (or little) oral residue after these swallows	Thicker materials may be harder to clear from the lungs if aspirated	
	Thicker materials may leave oral residue that could be aspirated later when thin liquid presented	

¼ c. food thickener that can be added to thin liquids to achieve desired consistency (or liquids prethickened to slightly, mildly, moderately)

1 soft cookie

WATER SWALLOWS

If the patient has already had a 3-ounce water swallow as part of a screening administered by nursing, the speech–language pathologist can decide whether or not to repeat this test. Repeating it can confirm the accuracy of the nurse-administered screen. See the section on screening in this chapter for more information on screening tests.

CSE Trial Swallows

If you have determined that it is safe to assess the patient's skills with food and liquid, proceed to this section. The grid provides room for you to note what was presented and any deficits in the patient's abilities. It is more important to note skill deficits and strengths than what happened with each bolus. If compensations were tried and seemed successful, note those.

ABILITY TO PREPARE BOLUS

Several specific skills are needed to prepare a bolus. The patient must be able to maintain adequate labial closure to prevent anterior loss of the bolus. In addition, adequate labial closure helps keep the bolus from falling into the anterior lateral sulcus (between gums and teeth). Lingual elevation is necessary to scoop the bolus, particularly liquid boluses, from the floor of the mouth so they are on the tongue. Lingual lateralization is necessary to move the bolus from midline to the chewing surface and from the chewing surface back to midline. Mastication skills are required for many textures to prepare an adequate bolus.

ABILITY TO MANIPULATE BOLUS

To manipulate the bolus from front to back, adequate lingual function is necessary. In addition, observe the patient's oral transit time. The average time to move a bolus from the front of the oral cavity to the back is 1 second or less.

ABILITY TO MAINTAIN A COHESIVE BOLUS
While the patient is preparing the bolus and manipulating the bolus, he or she must keep it on the tongue and avoid pocketing in the sulci. In addition, the patient must maintain the bolus to prevent either premature loss over the back of the tongue or anterior loss.

Observe any behaviors that might lead us to believe that the food is not remaining on the pharyngeal surface of the tongue but has prematurely fallen into the airway. Therefore, assess for back-of-tongue control and judge whether any of the material may be falling over the back of the tongue prematurely. This might be indicated by a cough before the swallow. You can only make a supposition about this. Labial closure is more easily assessed because you can observe for anterior loss. You can also observe for decreased tone in the cheeks, as the patient will demonstrate pocketing in the lateral sulci. Lingual lateralization skills allow the patient to return the bolus to the midline of the tongue.

ABILITY TO CLEAR THE BOLUS
After the swallow, check to see if the oral cavity is empty, to determine whether the patient is able to clear the oral cavity with one swallow. If not, note the number of swallows per bolus necessary for the patient to clear his oral cavity. Multiple swallows★ may indicate presence of pharyngeal residue.

Delayed or incomplete oral clearance★ is a predictor of risk for aspiration. A good way to monitor this is to place the forefinger of one hand immediately under the patient's chin, the middle finger under the chin near the base of the tongue on the hyoid, and the ring finger and small finger on the larynx to monitor laryngeal elevation, indicating a probable swallow. This digital palpation is somewhat supported in the literature as a way to judge laryngeal elevation. This method is better than using only a finger or two on the larynx. The fixed position of four fingers allows you to feel the larynx move past your fingers. Note that this method for assessing swallow and laryngeal elevation has never been validated.

ABILITY TO INITIATE PHARYNGEAL RESPONSE
When the head of the bolus passes over the back of the tongue, the swallowing response should occur within 1 second. Some patients exhibit a delay in the initiation of the response. When this occurs, the bolus falls to the valleculae and sometimes all the way to the pyriform sinuses before the response is initiated. A delayed response can be accurately judged only with an instrumental exam. During an instrumental, once the head of the bolus passes the base of the tongue at the point of the mandible, you can start counting the time before the swallow is initiated. At bedside, you can make a rough guess about swallow initiation by counting the time from when the patient stops moving his tongue until you feel laryngeal elevation.

LARYNGEAL CHARACTERISTICS
After the patient's swallow, assess vocal quality. A gurgly vocal quality can indicate possible penetration or aspiration.★ Also note any coughing or throat clearing and give an estimation of adequacy of elevation of the larynx This is very difficult to judge at bedside, but palpation can give a rough idea.

Directions for Clinical Swallow Evaluation Form B

The Clinical Swallow Evaluation Form B, shown as Figure 2.3, is more likely to be used by experienced clinicians who have performed many clinical swallow evaluations and have internalized the steps needed to draw conclusions about each area. Therefore, only section headers are included. Clinicians may wish to use Cranial Nerve Exam, or even Nerves and Muscles Involved in

Swallowing, found in the Supplemental Materials, if needed to complete the cranial nerve section on Form B.

Form B is a summary of all the tasks described on Form A. The clinician using this abbreviated version can refer to the directions for Form A if needed.

Drawing Conclusions and Making Recommendations

After your clinical assessment is complete, you'll have to draw conclusions and make recommendations. Your first decision is whether you have obtained enough information to make an informed

---

Clinical Swallow Evaluation Form B

As on Form A, items supported in the literature indicating an increased risk of aspiration appear with an asterisk. Additional information about some of those items is included on Form B (e.g., orientation questions to ask).

Patient _____ Date _____

AREA ASSESSED	WNL	ISSUES NOTED
Alertness/cooperation		
Orientation*		
Name, place, year		
ORAL MOTOR EVALUATION		
Structure/oral health		
Oral motor movements		
Control of secretions*		
Overall lingual ROM*		
Gag reflex*		
LARYNGEAL FUNCTION EXAM		
Vocal quality/change in quality*		
Strength of cough*		
Ability to elevate pitch*		
CRANIAL NERVE EXAM		
Trigeminal V		
Facial VI		
Glossopharyngeal IX		
Vagus X		
Hypoglossal XII		
RESPIRATORY STATUS/PATTERNS		
Breaths/minute baseline*		
Apnea location in respiratory cycle*		
COGNITION/COMMUNICATION		
One-step commands*		
Open mouth, stick out tongue, smile		
Dysarthria*		
Other communication		
Hearing		

Figure 2.3 Clinical Swallow Evaluation Form B.

Patient _____ Date _____

OBSERVATION WITH FOOD

	WNL	ISSUES NOTED:
ABILITY TO PREPARE BOLUS		
ABILITY TO MANIPULATE BOLUS		
ABILITY TO MAINTAIN COHESIVE BOLUS		
Multiple swallows*		
Delayed/incomplete clearance*		
ABILITY TO INITIATE PHARYNGEAL RESPONSE		
OTHER SIGNS OF PHARYNGEAL DYSPHAGIA/ASPIRATION		
Cough*		
Throat clear		

SLP Signature: _____ Date: _____ Time: _____

Figure 2.3 (continued)

decision about this patient's management. The following discussion pertains to patients expected to improve and regain swallowing function. There are different considerations for a patient at the end of life (see Chapter 7).

If You Do Not Have Enough Information After the CSE

IS AN INSTRUMENTAL ASSESSMENT OF SWALLOWING INDICATED?

An instrumental exam (MBS or FEES) is indicated if the patient showed clinical signs of aspiration or pharyngeal deficits. Perhaps it seemed that the sign was resolved with a compensatory technique at bedside. For example, did coughing stop with an increase in viscosity of the fluid? Did patient stop using multiple swallows exhibited on thin liquids when given a pureed texture? Even if you did eliminate the sign (e.g., chin-down eliminated coughing), you could not be sure there still was not some silent aspiration. And, of course, you would not know that the impaired physiology was causing the coughing. In a situation like that, an instrumental exam is indicated. An instrumental exam is also indicated if the patient is thought to be at high risk for aspiration even if no clinical signs were exhibited.

Instrumental assessments may not be readily available. In situations where an instrumental exam is not readily available, observations during the clinical exam may have to be used to manage the patient, but this should be on a short-term basis until the instrumental study can be obtained. For example, if the signs of pharyngeal dysphagia appeared to be eliminated with bolus and postural modifications, those compensatory strategies might be implemented and the patient placed on the modified diet for a short time until the instrumental exam can be scheduled. This may be preferable to making a patient NPO and placing an NG tube.

Ready access to instrumental exams. In acute-care and inpatient rehabilitation situations with ready access to VFSS and often the FEES, there is no compelling reason to make diet recommendations based on the CSE. Patients who are acutely ill are often more fragile and need to be managed conservatively. If the patient demonstrates signs of pharyngeal dysphagia, and especially signs of aspiration, it is advisable to keep the patient NPO and schedule the instrumental exam expeditiously. Mobile VFSS and FEES units have made instrumental exams more accessible to patients in skilled nursing facilities.

WHAT RISKS FOR PHARYNGEAL DYSPHAGIA SHOULD YOU CONSIDER WHEN DECIDING WHETHER TO REFER FOR AN INSTRUMENTAL EXAM?

- Coughing or throat clearing during CSE
- Multiple swallows
- Wet vocal quality or breath sounds
- Other change in vocal quality
- Reduced laryngeal elevation on trial swallows
- Not managing own secretions
- History of pneumonia
- Significant fatigability
- Recent extubation
- Presence of tracheostomy

There may be times when the patient is not ready for an instrumental study:

- If the patient is not alert enough to eat anyway
- If all problems appear to be in the oral phase and you do not suspect aspiration or pharyngeal problems
- If the patient refuses to eat
- If the patient will not open mouth for food or liquid (Some patients may need work to get ready for an instrumental study—if they are orally defensive, in the advanced stages of dementia, or very apraxic.)

WHAT IS THE SOURCE OF THE PATIENT'S NUTRITION WHILE AWAITING AN INSTRUMENTAL STUDY?

If the patient is ready for an instrumental study but needs to be NPO until then, what will the source of nutrition be? If it will be a short wait (e.g., study to be scheduled the next day) the physician may just leave the patient NPO with instructions on how medications are to be given. If the patient is not ready for an instrumental study, then there is likely a need for short-term alternative nutrition. It is up to the physician to make that determination, but the speech–language pathologist should provide the physician with information about prognosis for when the patient might be ready to participate in an instrumental study.

IS THERE A NEED TO CONSULT WITH OTHER PHYSICIANS OR HEALTH-CARE PROFESSIONALS?

Perhaps there are questions that need to be answered by another health-care professional based on your observations and findings. The consultation might be needed before you can draw accurate conclusions. In contrast, these consultations could take place independent of implementing your recommendations. Examples of referrals and consultations that might be needed include the following:

- Gastroenterologist if the patient presents symptoms that seem more esophageal in nature
- Neurologist if the change in swallowing seems related to a change in overall cognitive or neurological status
- Otolaryngologist if more information is needed about laryngeal structures
- Dietitian if the patient is not taking in adequate calories, or if questions arise concerning best ways to modify diet

- Physical or occupational therapy if deficits in mobility, trunk or head control, or fine motor
- Audiologist if patient had obvious difficulty hearing

Be sure to discuss any findings with the patient's primary care physician before making a referral.

If You Have Enough Information to Determine Management

If you think the clinical swallow evaluation has yielded all necessary information, then the first considerations are:

Whether patient is a candidate to begin rehabilitative techniques

Whether the patient can take any PO safely

Whether patient can maintain nutrition and hydration via PO alone (see Figure 2.4).

IS THE PATIENT READY FOR REHABILITATIVE TECHNIQUES?

Whether the patient is ready or not to eat by mouth, you may be able to begin therapy for obvious oral phase deficits and for suspected pharyngeal phase deficits. If the patient is going to have an instrumental study, it can be helpful to teach the patient techniques that might be tried during the study. For example, if it is suspected that the patient has reduced laryngeal elevation, teach the Mendelsohn, and this could then be tried during the instrumental study.

IS IT SAFE FOR THE PATIENT TO EAT BY MOUTH?

If the answer is yes, determine the type of diet the patient can tolerate as well as any compensatory techniques that will help the patient eat safely. Consider the following compensatory techniques when recommending a diet.

ARE BOLUS MODIFICATIONS NEEDED?

Bolus modifications can include many different ways to adapt a bolus such as the following:

Texture changes

Temperature changes

Viscosity changes

Sensory changes (e.g., sour, carbonation)

Size of bolus

How bolus is presented (e.g., small sips, place bolus on strong side)

DOES THE PATIENT NEED POSTURAL STRATEGIES TO CHANGE FLOW OF BOLUS?

- Feeding position for the patient: Upright at 90° is standard
- Head turn, tilt

WILL THE PATIENT NEED TO USE TECHNIQUES TO INCREASE CONTROL?

- Hold bolus and prepare to swallow
- Presentation of the food or liquid can also be used to increase control

In addition to making determinations about diet, other questions will need to be addressed. These are reflected in Figure 2.4 and discussed below.

CAN THE PATIENT MAINTAIN ADEQUATE NUTRITION AND HYDRATION WHEN EATING BY MOUTH?

Some patients may be able to eat safely by mouth but may fatigue easily or may be on such a restrictive diet (e.g., pureed with no sticky foods, no eggs, pudding-thick liquids) that they cannot get

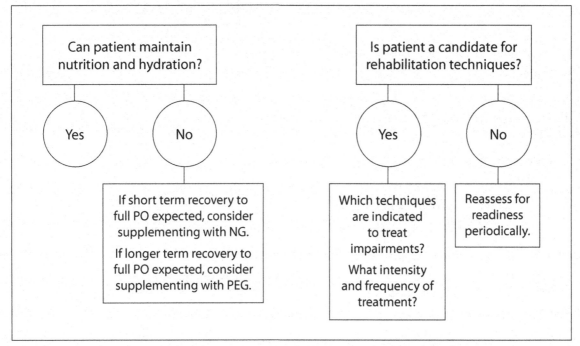

Figure 2.4 The patient can safely take some PO after CSE: other considerations.

adequate nutrition or hydration by mouth. Consult with the dietitian and physician to help make this determination. It certainly is not appropriate to recommend that a patient eat by mouth and to select a diet, yet not mention the concern that the patient may not be able to eat enough by mouth. Very shortly, you may find that the patient is dehydrated and in the early stages of malnutrition.

If you have concerns about the patient not being able to eat or drink enough, request a 3-day calorie count. Then the dietitian can determine whether the patient is getting adequate intake. Some patients may just need oral supplements to reach adequate nutritional levels.

CAN A PATIENT RECEIVE SOME PO FEEDINGS AND BE TUBE FED?
The most important consideration is to maintain the patient's health. The physician and the dietitian will determine the dietary specifics, such as type of tube feeding, type of tube, and rate of tube feeding.

As the patient gains strength and seems ready to eat more, you may want to speak to the dietitian about turning off the tube feeding an hour before meals or running it only at night. Even if the patient is never able to take enough food or liquid by mouth to maintain nutrition, he may still be able to have periodic oral feedings. Oral feedings are pleasurable and often enhance the quality of a patient's life.

If Medicare is the payment source, keep the payment guidelines in mind. Medicare will pay for tube feeding if ordered by the physician to maintain adequate nutrition and hydration. Medicare will also pay for swallowing therapy if the patient meets certain guidelines (e.g., there is a reasonable expectation that the patient will improve, the patient's safety is an issue if treatment is not initiated, the patient is alert enough to participate). It's *not* true that Medicare will stop paying for tube feeding when swallowing therapy is initiated.

WHEN SHOULD A PATIENT BE NPO?
There are no hard-and-fast rules about who should and should not be NPO. The general guidelines are that if you cannot find any consistency the patient can eat without aspiration, then the patient should be NPO until an instrumental study can be done. The SLP also has to determine

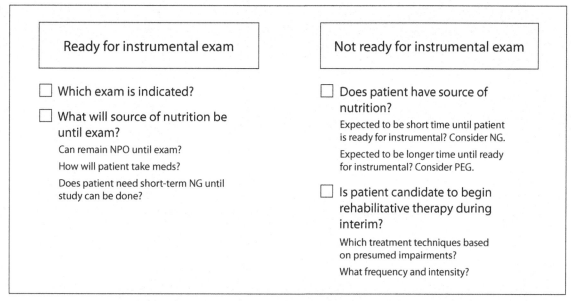

Figure 2.5 The SLP has obtained enough information during CSE to make patient NPO.

whether the patient is even ready for an instrumental exam (Figure 2.5). This guideline is different for patients in palliative and hospice care (see Chapter 7).

Keep in mind the situation in which the patient will normally be fed. Perhaps during a modified barium swallow it's determined that the patient can safely take pudding-thick liquids with chin down and head rotation to the right, swallowing twice to clear the residue. If these techniques are for a patient who cannot self-feed and will be fed most meals by staff who may not follow your recommendations, the patient might be safer NPO with enteral feeding (except for feeding therapeutically when you are present).

HOW TO WORD THE RECOMMENDATION THAT A PATIENT BE NPO

It is ultimately up to the physician to make a patient NPO, considering the patient's wishes. Therefore, rather than making a recommendation for NPO, you may need to give your findings and offer options such as the following:

"Clinical evaluation of the patient reveals significantly impaired oral skills. The patient is not able to masticate and form a bolus with any materials. Of more concern is the fact that aspiration is strongly suspected. The patient showed the following clinical signs of aspiration:

- Coughed with thin liquids despite a variety of compensatory techniques
- Showed intermittent throat clearing with foods of mixed textures
- Showed occasional throat clearing with pureed textures

Consider making the patient NPO until an instrumental exam can be completed to rule out the possibility of aspiration. However, if the patient is to continue eating, a diet of pureed texture and pudding-thick liquids may reduce, but not entirely eliminate, the risk for aspiration."

On the other hand, you may want to leave it even more open-ended like this:

"Patient has significantly impaired oral skills, and the pharyngeal phase is also suspected to be impaired. Patient has many clinical signs of aspiration. An instrumental exam is needed to confirm or rule out aspiration. Safer textures for the patient appear to be pudding-thick liquids and purees, although aspiration of these materials cannot be entirely ruled out."

If you are making a recommendation of NPO, have a prognosis in mind. If you think the patient is likely to regain enough skills to be able to take the majority of nutrition and hydration by mouth within weeks, consider recommending placement of an NG tube:

> "This patient shows clinical signs of aspiration of all materials. These signs could not be eliminated with a variety of compensatory techniques. This needs to be confirmed via an instrumental exam, but it appears that the patient is not safe for any PO at this time. Because the prognosis is good for a return to safe intake of some PO within _____ weeks, consideration might be given to placement of an NG tube while intensive indirect therapy (therapy without presentation of foods) proceeds."

If the patient is not expected to improve, or the improvement will take longer, then a PEG tube or PEJ tube is probably indicated:

> "This patient shows clinical signs of aspiration on all consistencies that could not be eliminated with postural or diet texture changes. The aspiration can be confirmed or ruled out via an instrumental exam. The instrumental exam will also allow us to identify the impairments in physiology causing these signs. Patient's decreased cognitive skills preclude using other compensatory techniques. Therefore, pending the results of an instrumental exam, it is recommended that the patient be NPO and consideration be given to an alternative form of nutrition and hydration. Since this dysphagia is not likely to resolve quickly, a PEG tube is suggested if the instrumental study confirms the findings."

CAN ANY RECOMMENDATIONS FOR REHABILITATIVE TREATMENT BE MADE?

If the patient has oral deficits, then recommendations for specific rehabilitative techniques for those oral deficits can be made (see Chapter 4). Although impaired physiology of the pharyngeal phase cannot be determined without the instrumental exam, the SLP still might be able to make some recommendations for pharyngeal rehabilitative techniques.

This might be done to prepare a patient for the instrumental exam, in case any of the techniques (that are both rehabilitative and compensatory) would be tried during the instrumental exam. For example, if it is suspected that the patient has reduced closure of the larynx, the patient might be taught the super-supraglottic swallow so that it can be tried during the instrumental exam.

The SLP might also recommend that a patient begin treatment with rehabilitative techniques that would be likely to be beneficial regardless of which specific physiological deficits are found on the instrumental exam. For example, the effortful swallow and lingual strengthening exercises would be beneficial for many patients. The recommended techniques could be adjusted after the instrumental study is completed.

BESIDES DIET, WHAT OTHER THINGS MIGHT BE RECOMMENDED FOR A PATIENT?

Who can safely feed the patient. Does the patient need a trained nursing assistant to feed him or her or to provide standby assistance? If family members are going to help with feeding, what training is required?

Family training. Which family members are involved in the patient's care, and when are they available for training? What kind of training will be most appropriate for each family member? Not all adults learn in the same manner, so consider appropriate methods and materials. The following need to be included in the family training: general information about dysphagia, and this patient's prognosis, diet restrictions, specific techniques for feeding, and so on.

Where the patient should eat. If the patient is in a facility, can the patient eat in the dining room with other patients, or is the patient too distractible? The social aspect of eating is important and should be balanced with the need to safely feed the patient.

Contextual factors. Consider which personal and environmental factors might be barriers to or facilitators of the patient's successful participation in dysphagia therapy.

How to give medications. If the patient is on thickened liquids, he or she will need to take medications with other than a thin liquid like water. However, thickened fluids, prepared using commercial powder thickeners, can significantly delay dissolution of drugs mixed into them. Yogurt is the most appropriate of the products tested in one study because it is easy for patients with oral dysphagia to manipulate without severely limiting drug dissolution. However, variability in composition and textural attributes between brands needs to be considered (Manrique-Torres et al., 2014).

Many times patients can swallow a pill whole in a spoon of yogurt, pudding, or applesauce. However, just using a thickening agent with medications can change how the medication is absorbed and metabolized. Provision of "spoon-thick" or "extremely thick liquids" is particularly likely to contribute to dehydration and poor bioavailability of solid-dose medication. Clinicians are encouraged to prescribe the minimal level of thickness needed for swallowing safety. Consultation with pharmacy is suggested before recommending crushing or using thickened fluids with medications (Cichero, 2013).

How to position patients with NG tubes and PEG. Patients with feeding tubes should be kept elevated at least 30°, even when sleeping, to reduce the chance of reflux. Just turning off the tube feeding before laying the patient flat (e.g., for bathing, for changing linens) does not accomplish this, because there is still tube feeding in the stomach.

How and when to perform oral care. Facilities may have a policy about what "standard" oral care is (e.g., perform oral care BID and PRN). You may want to change this timing. You may want to have the oral care performed before meals to clear bacteria before the patient eats, for example. Patients, family members, and some nursing staff may not understand how to brush teeth and clean the oral cavity. Some are under the impression that "teeth" brushing is not necessary if the patient is edentulous. However, proper teeth brushing should include brushing not only the teeth but also other surfaces in the mouth (roof of mouth, tongue, gums). A toothbrush should be used, not a Toothette, along with a dentifrice to provide proper cleaning. A patient/family handout, Oral Care, is provided in the Supplemental Materials (Education Materials, Patient/Family).

The status of the tracheostomy cuff during feeding. If the patient has a tracheostomy tube, is there a recommendation that the cuff be inflated or deflated during PO? See Chapter 6, Critical Care, for more information.

Directions for Clinical Swallow Evaluation Summary Sheet

After completing the evaluation (either Form A or Form B), and going through the decision-making as described above, the Summary Sheet should be completed (Figure 2.6).

This form serves as an overview of the findings and includes a place for recommendations as well as for selecting long- and short-term goals. Only short-term goals for the oral phases are listed, as goals for the pharyngeal phase cannot be reliably selected from the clinical exam alone.

This front page can serve as a summary of the findings. It is a one-page sheet that might be placed in the front of the medical chart, as the level of detail on the CSE evaluation form may be more than the physician wants to read. Also, this summary sheet can be used to build or revise the EHR.

Clinical Swallow Evaluation Summary Sheet

Patient _____ Date _____

Admit Date _____ Physician _____

Admit Diagnosis _____

Medical History _____

Pertinent Medications _____

Current Method of Nutrition: ☐ PO _____ diet   ☐ NPO   NG/PEG/TPN

History/Duration of Swallowing Problems _____

Swallowing Function Prior to Onset/Recent Change _____

_____

_____

Previous Evaluation/Treatment _____

Dysphagia Diagnosis _____

Positive Expectation to Begin Service _____

_____

_____

Need for Skilled Service _____

_____

_____

Long-Term/Functional Goals (Circle goals to be addressed.)

These goals are set for a _____ time period.

1. Patient will safely consume _____ diet with _____ liquids without complications such as aspiration pneumonia.

2. Patient will maintain adequate nutrition and hydration through oral diet.

3. Patient will be able to complete a meal in fewer than _____ minutes.

4. Patient will maintain nutrition/hydration via alternative means.

5. Patient's quality of life will be enhanced through eating and drinking small amounts of food and liquid.

6. Patient will be able to eat meals with family and friends in controlled environment.

7. Patient will be able to eat meals in public places.

Figure 2.6 Clinical Swallow Evaluation Summary Sheet.

The top part of the summary sheet contains the history you should obtain from the patient's chart (see Chapter 1 for more detailed information). The bottom of the form is completed at the conclusion of the evaluation.

Short-Term Goals—Oral Phases

Patient _____ Date _____

Short-Term Goal 1—Anterior Loss/lip closure (AL//lc)
- Patient will improve lip closure to reduce anterior loss and keep food or liquid in the mouth while eating.
- Patient will improve lip closure for more efficient removal of bolus from utensil.

Short-Term Goal 2—Anterior Loss/jaw closure (AL//jc)
- Patient will improve jaw closure to reduce anterior loss and keep food or liquid in the mouth while eating.
- Patient will improve jaw closure to improve ability to masticate a bolus and increase efficiency of swallowing.

Short-Term Goal 3—Bolus Formation and Propulsion/tongue movement (BFP//tm)
- Patient will increase tongue movement to improve the ability to put food or liquid into a cohesive bolus and reduce the risk of food residue falling into the airway.
- Patient will increase tongue movement to improve the ability to move a bolus to the back of the mouth in a coordinated fashion and reduce the risk of its falling into the airway.
- Patient will increase tongue movement to improve the ability to move a bolus to the back of the mouth in a coordinated fashion for more efficient swallowing.

Short Term Goal 4—Bolus Formation and Propulsion/Motor planning, agnosia (BFP//mp,a)
- Patient will increase oral coordination/improve motor planning to improve the ability to form a bolus for a more efficient swallow.
- Patient will increase oral coordination/improve motor planning to improve the ability to move a bolus to the back of the mouth in a coordinated fashion for a more efficient swallow.
- Patient will increase oral coordination/improve motor planning to improve the ability to move a bolus to the back of the mouth in a coordinated fashion and reduce the risk of its falling into the airway.

Short-Term Goal 5—Bolus Formation/tone in cheeks (BFP//tc)
- The tone in patient's cheek(s) will increase to improve the ability to put food or liquid into a cohesive bolus and increase the efficiency of the swallow.

Short-Term Goal 6 Oral Range of Motion (OPROM/LC)
- Patient will complete oral range of motion exercises to reduce impact of fibrosis on safety of swallow.
- Patient will complete oral range of motion exercises to reduce impact of fibrosis on efficiency of swallow.

Figure 2.6 *(continued)* *(continues)*

Identifying Information

- Admit date—When was the patient admitted to your facility or first seen as OP?
- Physician—Who ordered the dysphagia consult?
- Admit diagnosis—What caused the patient to be admitted/referred to the facility?
- Medical history—Include information pertinent to the assessment you are about to perform, including the diagnosis related to the swallowing problem.

Patient _____ Date _____

RECOMMENDATIONS

____ **NPO**	____ **DIET**
____ Consider alternative feeding	____ Diet Level: _____
____ Short term NG	____ Liquids: _____
____ Long term PEG	____ Meds: _____
____ NPO until instrumental exam	____ Other info re: diet: _____
	____ **SUPPLEMENTAL NUTRITION**
____ **REEVALUATION OF SWALLOWING:**	____ Oral supplements
____ When patient more alert	____ Short term NG
____ Other: _____	____ Longer term PEG
____ **REHABILITATIVE TREATMENT BY SLP**	____ **THERAPEUTIC PO WITH SLP**
	____ **REHABILITATIVE TX BY SLP**
____ **INSTRUMENTAL EXAM**	**COMPENSATORY STRATEGIES WITH PO**
____ Ready for FEES/VFSS	____ Postural: _____
____ To be scheduled when patient is more alert/_____	____ Bolus control: _____
____ **OTHER EXAMS**	____ **SUPERVISION WITH PO**
____ Speech-language-cognition	____ Direct 1:1 supervision
____ OT	____ Assist as needed
____ PT	
____ Clinical nutrition	
____ ENT	
____ Other: _____	

Figure 2.6 (continued)

- Pertinent medications—Note whether the patient is currently on, or has been on in the past, any medications that might reduce the level of alertness, cause confusion, or cause dry mouth.
- Current method of nutrition—Check whether the patient is receiving a PO diet, and indicate the diet. If the patient is NPO, check that box and indicate that the patient is receiving nutrition via NG, PEG/PEJ, or total parenteral nutrition (TPN).
- History or duration of swallowing problems—If the patient is in an acute-care facility, and it is a new onset of dysphagia, simply state "since admit." If the patient is in another type of facility, note the date and related cause of the swallowing disorder, for example, "Patient has been unable to swallow (food/liquid) w/o choking since CVA on 2/12/17."

Swallowing Function Before Onset/Recent Change
Describe how the patient was able to eat before this most recent change.

Previous Evaluation and Treatment
Describe any treatment the patient has previously received for dysphagia.

Dysphagia Diagnosis

List your diagnosis and the swallowing phases affected. For example, you might write, "Moderate oral dysphagia with anterior loss and pocketing. Suspected pharyngeal dysphagia with clinical signs of aspiration including coughing and wet vocal quality."

Positive Expectation to Begin Service

Describe why you think this patient is a good candidate for intervention. Is the patient alert, motivated to eat, cooperative?

Need for Skilled Service

Document why this patient needs your level of intervention to improve swallowing skills. List what could happen to the patient without your intervention.

Long-Term and Functional Goals

Circle all goals appropriate for the patient. More than one goal may be appropriate. For example, Goals 1 and 3 might be addressed at the same time. Also indicate the period of time for which the goals are being set.

Short-Term Goals and Treatment Objectives

Circle the appropriate oral phase short-term goal(s) and then write in the abbreviation codes for the treatment objectives you have chosen or write out the objectives if abbreviations are not allowed. (See Chapter 5 for more information on goals. A complete list of goals and treatment objectives is included in the Supplemental Materials.) Indicate the period of time for which these goals apply. Pharyngeal-phase goals are not included on this bedside form because they cannot accurately be determined without an instrumental exam.

You may write some pharyngeal goals if you want to begin to work on them while you await the instrumental exam. For instance, if the patient presents with a very breathy vocal quality and weak cough, you might choose to begin work on laryngeal closure activities or teach the super-supraglottic swallow so that the patient will be able to perform the technique if needed during the instrumental exam.

Recommendations

The recommendations are formatted to first make the decision about PO versus NPO status. Other categories of recommendations include whether an instrumental exam is needed, other exams, strategies to use with PO, and so on.

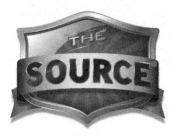

Chapter 3

Instrumental Assessment of Swallowing

A bedside, or clinical, evaluation of swallowing has significant limitations. Regardless of how astute your observation skills are at bedside, you can only hypothesize about possible pharyngeal problems. If there is reason to suspect a pharyngeal problem, you should complete an instrumental assessment of swallowing on the patient or refer him or her for such an assessment.

Of course, there are limitations to instrumental exams as well, as these exams are not performed in a natural setting. It is certainly not a realistic situation for the patient to be swallowing barium in a dark room sitting between a hard table and a large camera. Nor is it realistic to swallow with an endoscope in the nose or throat. Neither situation is able to capture the effects of fatigue, although the FEES certainly comes closest because there is no time limitation on the study. Neither really captures what swallowing is like in different positions, although again the FEES comes closest.

Indications and Preparations for Instrumental Exam

Any time you suspect that the patient presents with a pharyngeal disorder, you should refer for an instrumental exam. Current Medicare regulations state that medical workup and professional assessments must document history, current eating status, and clinical observations. This information is used to determine necessity for further medical testing, such as videofluoroscopy or endoscopy. Medicare regulations do not require an instrumental exam, but some Medicare administrative contractors (MACs) may require an instrumental examination to reimburse for treatment of dysphagia. In addition, some facilities require an instrumental exam before they proceed with a recommendation for the placement of a PEG tube.

The overriding consideration in recommending an instrumental exam is that you suspect a pharyngeal dysphagia. (See Chapter 2 for information on indicators of pharyngeal problems.) The following indications for an instrumental exam are listed on the ASHA Practice Portal:

- Concerns regarding the safety and efficiency of swallow function

- How dysphagia might be contributing to nutritional and pulmonary compromise

- Assess swallowing physiology to guide management and treatment

- Inconsistent signs and symptoms in the findings of the CSE

- The need to assist in differential medical diagnosis related to the presence of disordered swallowing

- Patient has a medical condition or diagnosis associated with a high risk of dysphagia

- Previously identified dysphagia with a suspected change in swallow function that may also change recommendations (this might be an improvement or decline in function; ASHA, 2000; Practice Portal: Adult Dysphagia, 2017).

Determining Whether the Patient Will Be Able to Participate

Before you refer a patient for an instrumental exam, carefully assess whether the patient will be able to participate fully. Physicians are sometimes reluctant to order repeated studies, so if your patient is being fed by an alternative means and is not very alert or did not participate well on the clinical swallow evaluation, it may not be the best time to refer for an instrumental exam. It may be more beneficial for the patient to remain NPO with the alternative feeding source until he or she is more alert and fully able to participate in the study.

An exception to this might be a patient for whom you do not expect to see improvement in the swallow but for whom the payer or facility is requiring an instrumental exam to document your prognosis. In this case, referral for the exam may be appropriate while the patient is still less than optimally alert.

Preparing the Patient for the Exam

If you have a patient for whom a specific compensatory technique may be helpful, you may want to defer the study until you can teach the patient that technique (if the patient is not in any danger of aspiration from PO feeding in the meantime). It is much better that the patient begins to learn any helpful techniques before arriving for the instrumental exam than trying to learn a very difficult maneuver in a few minutes. For example:

1. Your patient presents with a very breathy vocal quality and a wet voice, so you suspect decreased laryngeal closure. You begin working on laryngeal adduction exercises and teaching the patient the supraglottic and super-supraglottic swallow because the examiner might want to try these during the instrumental exam.

2. Your patient shows reduced laryngeal elevation on palpation with a wet vocal quality and delayed cough, so you suspect some aspiration after the swallow coming from residue in the pyriform sinuses. You begin to teach the patient the Mendelsohn maneuver.

EXPLAINING INSTRUMENTAL STUDIES TO THE PATIENT

Fact sheets in the Supplemental Materials may be helpful when providing the patient with information before she comes in for the study. (See Education Materials, Patient/Family: Fiberoptic Endoscopic Evaluation of Swallowing [FEES] Information; Modified Barium Swallow/VFSS Information; Phases of Swallow; Modified Barium Swallow/VFSS FAQs; and Endoscopic Evaluation of Swallowing FAQs.) Answer all the patient's questions about the procedure.

Essential Information Needed for the Exam

Before you perform the VFSS or FEES, obtain a complete history (see Chapter 1 for information on history taking). It is also important to determine the diagnostic question. For example, does the referring SLP want to know if the patient can upgrade the diet to allow for safe swallowing of thin liquids? Does the physician want to know the safest diet for the patient? Knowing the referring question will help you determine the information you need to obtain in the history and help you focus your instrumental examination. If you are the referring speech–language pathologist, be sure to elaborate the questions you need to have answered. The Outpatient Instrumental Exam Referral Form in the Supplemental Materials (SLP Resources) will help you gather the following information. You can complete this form during a phone call with the referring site, or you can send to the site to complete and return to you.

MEDICAL HISTORY

Pertinent information about the patient's medical history may include any diagnoses that could be the etiology for dysphagia, weight loss (which may signal dysphagia), and recent hospitalization.

CODE STATUS

It is not likely that a patient will experience cardiac arrest during the exam, but it is critical that you know what to do should this occur. This information is provided in an advance directive.

RESPIRATORY STATUS AND TRACHEOSTOMY

Does the patient have any respiratory deficits (e.g., COPD)? Is the patient on oxygen, and if so, which delivery method and percentage or flow rate? If the patient has a tracheostomy, note which type of tracheostomy tube the patient has and whether it has a cuff. It is also important to know whether the cuff can be deflated and whether the patient is routinely fed with the cuff up or down. If the patient is fed with the cuff down, find out whether the patient has a tracheostomy speaking valve.

MEDICATIONS

Some medications can alter the patient's level of alertness during the study or otherwise impact swallowing

PRESENT/HISTORY OF PNEUMONIA/ASPIRATION

Decreased lung sounds or any recent hospitalizations for pneumonia may indicate aspiration.

PRESENT COMPLAINT

The patient's or referring clinician's description of the problem in the oral phase and suspicions about pharyngeal problems provide diagnostic clues. In addition, although the esophageal phase cannot be assessed at bedside, valuable information can be gained about the possible interaction with the esophageal phase through observation and patient report.

ESOPHAGEAL SYMPTOMS

The patient may complain of a fullness or feeling like there is a lump in her throat. This is a more common symptom of GERD than heartburn. The patient may burp a lot or state that food "comes back up." The patient may cough when lying down or complain of feeling like she is smothering at night. If the patient is reporting any of these symptoms, you may want to complete an esophageal screening at the same time the MBS study is completed.

ONSET OF DYSPHAGIA

Note information about the onset of dysphagia as sudden versus gradual and any other related medical problems that occurred around the same time as the onset.

PREVIOUS INSTRUMENTAL EXAM OR CLINICAL EVALUATION RESULTS

Note the results of any previous instrumental exams or bedside evaluations of swallowing. Specify the dates, locations, and results.

CURRENT DIET AND INTAKE

Note which kinds of foods and liquids the patient is eating and which special techniques or positions the patient has to use. If the patient is receiving alternative feeding, note whether this feeding is occurring continuously or via bolus feeding.

COMPENSATORY STRATEGIES

Does the patient require the use of compensatory strategies to eat and drink safely? If so, which ones, and how reliably does the patient use them?

INDEPENDENT SITTING BALANCE AND TRANSFERS

Information about the patient's ability to sit and maintain balance and difficulty of transfer is crucial to determine appropriate seating for the study. Note whether specialized seating is needed. Also note whether the patient is wearing any restraints and the reason for the restraints.

The Role of the SLP in Instrumental Assessments

At present, two procedures are widely used by speech–language pathologists (SLPs) to assess the pharyngeal phase of the swallow: the videofluoroscopic swallowing study (VFSS) (or modified barium swallow, MBS) and the fiberoptic endoscopic evaluation of swallowing (FEES). Most of this chapter focuses on the VFSS and the FEES. (Note: A derivation of the FEES, the FEESST, includes sensory testing.) High-resolution manometry, described below as used in research, is moving into the clinical realm, though at this time typically only in large university, multidisciplinary clinics.

The ASHA Preferred Practice Patterns state that videofluoroscopy, endoscopy, ultrasound, manometry, and electromyography are within the scope of practice for SLPs (ASHA, 2004). The scope of practice also supports use of endoscopy, videofluoroscopy, and other instrumentation to assess aspects of voice, resonance, velopharyngeal function, and swallowing (*Scope of Practice SLP*, 2016). Several policy documents exist to provide information and guidance concerning instrumental assessments:

- Knowledge and skills needed by speech–language pathologists performing videofluoroscopic swallowing studies (Knowledge and Skills VFSS, 2004)

- The role of the speech–language pathologist in the performance and interpretation of endoscopic evaluation of swallowing: technical report *[Technical Report](Role of SLP in FEES, 2005)*

- Knowledge and skills for speech–language pathologists performing endoscopic assessment of swallowing functions *[Knowledge and Skills](Knowledge and Skills Endoscopy, 2002)*

- Guidelines for speech–language pathologists performing videofluoroscopic swallowing studies *[Guidelines]. (Guidelines SLP VFSS, 2004)*

The ASHA Practice Portal is also a good site to visit for up-to-date information about management of dysphagia (Practice Portal: Adult Dysphagia, 2017).

Becoming Proficient at Instrumental Studies

It is not the purpose of this chapter to teach you how to perform and interpret these procedures. Becoming proficient at performing, interpreting, and documenting an instrumental study requires extensive reading, study, hands-on practice, and mentoring. ASHA recommends multiple steps to achieve competence in administering and interpreting VFSS studies:

1. Observe and participate in the VFSS with an experienced clinician. The number of supervised studies required is at the discretion of the mentor or supervisor, based on the trainee's competence.
2. Once conducting the VFSS, meet with an experienced clinician on a regular basis to review the accuracy of observations and therapeutic management. Meetings should include review and discussion of written reports.
3. Attend continuing education courses that focus on interpretation of the VFSS.
4. Review current literature about the VFSS.
5. Participate in study groups with other SLPs who perform the VFSS (*Guidelines SLP VFSS*, 2004).

Although a guideline document does not exist for performing FEES, similar steps are recommended. But in addition to "conducting" the endoscopic study, the speech–language pathologist must master the technical skill of passing the endoscope.

This chapter, then, provides information about each procedure, along with forms that may be useful when performing these procedures.

VFSS or FEES: Is There a Gold Standard?

SLPs routinely perform the FEES and the VFSS to assess the pharyngeal phase of the swallow. The VFSS has been called the "gold standard" for assessing dysphagia. A gold standard test is considered the best available tool to compare measures. The term does not imply that the VFSS is perfect (Claassen, 2005).

Although the VFSS has long been considered the gold standard for pharyngeal assessment, in a recent historical review of FEES, Langmore (2017) asserted that perhaps the FEES should be considered the gold standard. She cites four studies that used simultaneous FEES and VFSS and found that FEES consistently yielded a worse score in terms of increasing severity of the finding of interest: PAS scores and ratings of residue. Langmore (2017) states, "The gold standard should represent the truth as close as we can ascertain. FEES is more sensitive to bolus findings, and in the case of detecting the presence of a bolus, it is clearly superior" (p. 28).

Some facilities utilize both procedures. For example, many acute-care and inpatient rehabilitation hospitals provide both services to inpatients. Mobile VFSS and FEES studies are becoming increasingly prevalent, making both tests more accessible to residents of skilled nursing facilities.

Videofluoroscopic Swallowing Study/ Modified Barium Swallow

The videofluoroscopic swallowing study, or modified barium swallow, is the most frequently used procedure to assess the pharyngeal phase of the swallow. Logemann (1993) was the leader in the development of this procedure and in training SLPs in its use, resulting in widespread acceptance of the VFSS.

Roles During the VFSS

The primary role of the speech–language pathologist during the study is to "run the show." However, because each fluoroscopy suite is designed differently, staff roles may differ. In some situations the speech–language pathologist must present the materials to the patient and manage the study (e.g., determine what to present next, interact with patient and radiologist, watch video capture of the swallow). Playing all those roles may mean that the speech–language pathologist misses crucial information about the swallow because he or she cannot see the monitor at all times. Some swallows may be missed as the speech–language pathologist steps back from presenting materials to the patient, or the patient may swallow before the speech–language pathologist is in front of the monitor. Also, if the speech–language pathologist is presenting the materials to the patient, the SLP may be exposed to more radiation, especially if feeding the patient. Carefully consider the setup in the fluoroscopy suite to allow for the speech–language pathologist to visualize the monitor at all times while still interacting with the patient as needed. Ideally, someone other than the speech–language pathologist running the study should be the one to present materials to the patient.

Collaborate with the staff of the radiology department to delineate roles and responsibilities. Establishing a close working relationship with the radiology technologist results in a more efficiently run study. The radiology technologist becomes familiar with how the speech–language pathologist would like the materials to be presented and can keep an eye on the patient for changes in position, for example, while the speech–language pathologist watches the monitor. In this way, the radiology technologist can convey information to the speech–language pathologist, such as, "Patient is holding his mouth shut" or "Patient is becoming fatigued." Who mixes and sets up the tray of materials is something else that can be worked out in this collaboration. A good relationship between the two departments means that the speech–language pathologist should be willing to jump in and help as needed on other tasks, like transferring the patient from stretcher to chair or locating portable oxygen-tank holders.

RADIOLOGIST PRESENT DURING STUDY

Current ASHA policy does not require that a radiologist or other physician be present in the examination room during the completion of a VFSS by a competent SLP. The American College of Radiology (2017) indicates that the study should be done with a physician. Some local coverage determinations (LCDs) cite the professional guidelines. Typically, the VFSS is performed with the speech–language pathologist and the radiologist present.

This allows for the speech–language pathologist to focus on swallowing physiology and functioning and the radiologist to make medical diagnoses relative to anatomy. In some cases, the study may be done with the SLP and radiology technologist, with the radiologist available for consultation as needed. Such consultation is a good idea so that the report generated by the radiologist and the report from the speech–language pathologist contain consistent findings. When a radiologist is not present during the VFSS, the SLP assesses and comments on only swallowing physiology and function. The speech–language pathologist should check state and regulatory issues and any third-party-payer requirements regarding the presence of a physician in the study (*Guidelines SLP VFSS*, 2004).

Materials Used in the Study

The materials needed to perform the study include the following:

- Barium sulfate powder mixed into a liquid form
- Thickener (to be mixed with the barium to derive slightly, mildly, moderately, and extremely thick consistencies; a smoother liquid will be obtained if the dry thickener and dry barium powder are mixed together before adding the water)
- Barium paste (e.g., Esophatrast)
- Cookie spread with barium
- Empty capsules that can be filled with barium powder. If the patient complains about the inability to swallow pills, use these to see why the patient is having trouble. (Note: when presenting a barium-filled capsule, have the patient drink water instead of liquid barium so that the movement of the capsule is not obscured by the liquid barium.)

Bracco produces Varibar, the only premixed barium sulfate designed specifically for use in VFSS. Varibar is available in five consistencies: thin, nectar, thin honey, honey, and pudding (Bracco Varibar, 2017). Barium paste or liquid can also be mixed with or applied to specific foods (e.g., particulate matter like rice) if the patient presents with a very specific complaint about difficulty with certain foods. However, research using the MBSImP standardized procedures and scoring reveals that a cookie-swallowing task was the most likely to yield the overall impairment score for oral clearance, and that large-volume, thin-liquid swallowing tasks had the highest probabilities of yielding the overall impairment scores for oral containment and airway protection (Hazelwood, Armeson, Hill, Bonilha, & Martin-Harris, 2017). That is to say, the point of the VFSS is to identify impaired physiology, not test every imaginable texture the patient will eat. Gaining information about physiology allows the speech–language pathologist to predict how the patient will perform in situations outside fluoroscopy and with a variety of foods.

Views Obtained

The MBS allows for visualization of all phases of the swallow, from the oral phase through the esophageal phase. This dynamic view is captured on a recording device for later review (frame by frame if necessary).

Typically, two views are obtained: lateral and anterior-posterior (A-P). The study begins in the lateral view with thin liquids given in small amounts (e.g., 3 cc, 5 cc, 10 cc) and progresses to uncontrolled amounts if the patient is swallowing safely. Liquids are tried from both a cup and a straw (the initial small boluses are often presented on a spoon). The sequence of thick liquids (e.g., nectar, honey, pudding) should be premixed and ready to use in case the patient aspirates thin liquids and you want to try texture changes. The patient is also given paste bolus (although this material is stickier than many "real" foods, with the possible exception of peanut butter), so a pudding-thick liquid may give a more accurate representation of what the patient will be able to do with pureed foods. The Varibar pudding is more similar in consistency to pudding-like foods. Patients who are able to masticate are given a cookie with contrast material.

The lateral view allows for visualization of the oral phase as the patient manipulates the bolus. You can see problems such as anterior loss, material falling to the floor of the mouth or anterior or lateral sulci, residue on the hard palate, and premature spill of the bolus over the back of the tongue. Be sure the radiologist opens the frame of the fluoroscopy view so that you can see the oral cavity and the pharynx in the same view. The camera should not have to move to "follow the bolus" if the picture is framed appropriately. The lateral view also allows you to assess the oropharyngeal phase, where you can observe problems such as increased stage transition duration (delay in initiation of the pharyngeal swallow); penetration into the upper laryngeal vestibule; aspiration before, during, or after the swallow; residue in valleculae and/or pyriforms; and so on. It is crucial to determine which anatomical or physiological impairment is causing the problem(s). Clinicians new to interpreting videofluoroscopic studies often see the sign (e.g., residue) and then deduct the impaired physiology. For example, they might notice residue in the valleculae and recall that this can be caused by reduced tongue base and/or pharyngeal wall movement and perhaps limited elevation. As speech–language pathologists gain more experience, their trained eye sees the impaired movement first. They would note, for example, that the pharyngeal walls are not moving well, and as a result, there is residue in the valleculae.

The A-P view provides a way to visualize symmetry of residue in the valleculae and pyriforms, shows whether the bolus moves symmetrically through the hypopharynx, and provides a view of the movement of the vocal folds toward midline. It is very difficult to visualize aspiration in this view because the trachea is immediately in front of the esophagus.

PHARYNGOESOPHAGEAL ASSESSMENT

The lateral view also allows for screening of the esophageal phase of the swallow. Because many esophageal problems have symptoms manifested in the pharyngeal region, it is important to screen this phase. It is the physician's responsibility to diagnose problems in the esophageal phase, but the speech–language pathologist must understand symptoms and signs that point to esophageal disorders (Table 3.1).

The speech–language pathologist must also be familiar with the function of the upper third of the esophagus and be able to discuss with the radiologist any relationship between problems in the esophageal phase and the pharyngeal phase (*Guidelines SLP VFSS*, 2004). Oropharyngeal swallowing function can be altered in patients with esophageal motility disorders and other esophageal dysphagia. Slow esophageal clearance has implications for eating and drinking and, when revealed on a VFSS, warrants referral for further medical evaluation, such as to a gastroenterologist (Martin-Harris et al., 2000). Patients with complaint of globus, or a sensation of a lump in the throat, may represent up to 10% of patients referred to an otolaryngologist (Dworkin et al., 2015). It is

Table 3.1
Esophageal Symptoms

- Feels like food is "sticking" during swallowing anywhere from mid-chest to the neck
- Difficult to swallow solids
- Report of coughing up food or pills after the swallow
- Use of liquids to "wash down" foods to complete a meal
- Report of pain with swallowing (e.g., base of throat, chest, substernal)
- Complaints of heartburn
- Sensation of lump in throat after eating
- Related symptoms of potential laryngopharyngeal reflux, esophageal reflux (e.g., nighttime halitosis, voice change, chronic respiratory, sinus problems)
- Regurgitation
- Report of unexplained weight loss, altered hunger, and appetite changes

Note. Adapted from *Guidelines SLP VFSS* (2004).

not uncommon for the ENT to refer the patient to the speech–language pathologist for a VFSS study. It is interesting to note that the retrospective review by Dworkin et al. (2015) found that the VFSS and barium swallow for patients with globus sensation are most often negative and fail to add significant diagnostic information for the physician.

Because of the relationship between esophageal and pharyngeal function, it should be a routine part of a VFSS to screen the upper third of the esophagus with the patient in the upright position. If, before the exam, the patient is complaining of any symptoms pointing to an esophageal disorder, the speech–language pathologist might consider getting an order for a barium swallow or upper GI to be completed immediately after the VFSS. There are reimbursement restrictions (coding edits) that prevent the radiologist from billing a VFSS and barium swallow on the same date. At present, there is no similar restriction on VFSS and UGI performed on the same date.

Compensatory Strategies During the VFSS

The purpose of the VFSS is to analyze the physiology of the oropharyngeal swallow. In patients who present with relatively intact function, the study is straightforward. However, for patients with impaired structure or physiology that results in deficits in timing and/or bolus clearance, the most important part of the MBS is further analyzing these deficits and exploring ways to reduce the impact of the deficits. Therefore, as soon as the patient begins to exhibit timing or bolus clearance difficulty, you must try compensatory techniques (e.g., posture changes, changes in texture, techniques such as supraglottic swallow). The charts in the Supplemental Materials (SLP Resources, MBS/VFSS Interpretation) will help you interpret findings and choose compensatory techniques to attempt during the study, based on the sign you see as well as the impaired physiology causing the sign. The charts also list other rehabilitative techniques you might try in therapy, but these are not appropriate as compensations during the study because immediate effects are not expected.

Radiology Equipment and Recording

There are many different brands of fluoroscopy equipment and methods of recording VFS studies. There may be limitations based on the electronic health record system in use, age of fluoroscopy equipment, and storage capacity. Many SLP departments invest in equipment specifically for recording these studies. Work closely with the engineer in the radiology department when selecting any equipment that will need to interface with the fluoroscopy unit and the storage system.

ACCURATELY CAPTURING THE IMAGES

Accurately capturing the images requires close coordination between the speech–language pathologist conducting the study and the radiology staff operating the fluoro equipment. The patient must first be positioned so that the view needed is captured. The boundaries are front of the patient's face showing the lips, top of the oral cavity, cervical vertebrae C-2 through C-5, pharyngoesophageal segment, and upper third of esophagus.

The X-ray should be turned on when the patient has the bolus in the mouth (if the patient is able to hold the bolus until instructed to swallow) or when the bolus is presented if the patient is told to take a natural sip. The X-ray should be turned off after the patient has swallowed, but turned on again if there is residue that needs to be observed (to see whether it is going to spill into the airway) or if the patient is initiating a clearing swallow.

Cued swallows. Although cueing the patient to hold the bolus until ready to swallow makes it easier to time the fluoro on or off, studies with healthy adults have found that cued swallows change several aspects of the swallow. Verbal cue affected bolus position at onset of timing measures, thereby influencing duration. The bolus was positioned farther back in the oral cavity at onset of oral transit for cued as compared with noncued swallows. Durations of the cued swallows were significantly shorter than for noncued swallows for all timing measures (Daniels, Schroeder, DeGeorge, Corey, & Rosenbek, 2007). Another study confirmed the same findings in young adults. Swallow-onset patterns and timing differ between cued and noncued conditions. In particular, bolus advancement to more distal locations in the pharynx at the time of swallow onset is seen more frequently in noncued conditions (Nagy et al., 2013).

Frames rate, fluoroscopy rate and pulse rate. The SLP should be familiar with several different terms related to how video images are captured and recorded. Frame rate typically applies to the number of images recorded per second and usually includes choices of 2, 4 7.5, 15 and 30. Fluoroscopy rate is the number of images produced by the fluoroscope each second. Fluoroscopy equipment can produce continuous or pulsed images. Pulsed means there is no radiation exposure in between pulses. Pulse rates typically include 2, 4, 7.5, 15 and 30 pulses/second. When a pulse rate of 30 pulses per second is used to generate 30 images per second, and these images are recorded at a frame rate of 30 frames per second, the visual results are the same as they would have been when continuous fluoroscopy was captured at a frame rate of 30 frames per second.

Reducing pulse rate reduces the amount of radiation exposure. However, several studies have demonstrated that VFSS should be conducted at the highest available pulse rate in order to capture essential elements. There are differences in both judgment of swallowing impairment and treatment recommendations when pulse rates are reduced from 30 to 15 pps to minimize radiation exposure. (Bonilha, Blair, et al., 2013)Measures of timing events are rated differently if seen at a slower frame rate. (Mulheren, 2017)The lowest recording rate should also be 30 fps.

Hospital recording systems (e.g., PACS) may be set to record at a lower frames/second to save space. The speech-language pathologist should talk to the appropriate person at their facility (e.g. Radiology Engineer, Radiology IT) to determine the rate being used. The goal is 30 unique frames per second. Some recording equipment may indicate that it is capturing 30 frames per second, but each frame is not unique. If the video is reviewed in frame-by-frame, what is seen is a unique image, followed by another frame with that same image, then a unique image followed by another frame of that same image. In other words, only every other image is unique. The equipment is essentially "pasting" a copy of the previous image. The SLP may think he is seeing everything that is happening with the swallow when instead they are actually only seeing a half of what is happening.

The SLP should also be aware that some systems use a "video loop". A video loop stores a set number of frames in a working memory on the fluoroscopy equipment. Near the end of the loop, the operator needs to use a save function to transfer the contents of the loop to the recording archive. If the save function is not used, the video loop maintains the set number of frames in working memory but drops the earliest frames in the loop as it captures new frames on the opposite end. For a more comprehensive discussion of these issues, visit: http://steeleswallowinglab.ca/srrl/best-practice/videofluoroscopy-frame-rate/

Correcting Common Mistakes in Reviewing and Interpreting the Study

Regardless of the amount of experience or expertise in conducting and interpreting VFSS, the speech–language pathologist should make time to review the study, taking advantage of features like slow motion and frame by frame, before drawing conclusions and making final recommendations.

As mentioned earlier, the intent of this chapter is not to have the reader achieve competence in interpreting studies. However, several facts are shared here to address common mistakes made by those new to interpreting VFSS studies.

PENETRATION IS NORMAL

Normal subjects of all ages demonstrated penetration, and significantly more penetration occurred on liquid boluses. The frequency of penetration of thin liquids increased after the age of 50, and thick viscosities were penetrated only by older subjects (Daggett, Logemann, Rademaker, & Pauloski, 2006). Another study confirmed that penetration is present in 11.4% of normal adults and is more common with a liquid bolus (Allen, White, Leonard, & Belafsky, 2010).

THE EPIGLOTTIS DOES NOT MOVE ON ITS OWN, NOR CAN IT BE "PARALYZED"

The epiglottis is a cartilage. It is brought to the horizontal position during swallowing by three actions: the elevation of the larynx, tongue-base retraction, and pharygeal squeeze. The full inversion to cover the airway is also helped by the pressure of the bolus (Ekberg & Sigurjónsson, 1982). Therefore, when problems are noted in the movement of the epiglottis, analyze the movement of the larynx and the pressure the tongue base and pharyngeal walls put on the bolus (Kendall, Leonard, & McKenzie, 2004; Paik et al., 2008).

BOLUS MOVING OVER THE BACK OF THE TONGUE "BEFORE" SWALLOW DOES NOT NECESSARILY MEAN "DELAY"

Using FEES as the tool, Dua and colleagues studied natural eating and drinking in young healthy subjects as they ate an entire meal. Spillage of part of the bolus was even more pronounced than in cued or noncued swallowing of single boluses. In fact, for 60% of liquid swallows and 76% of solid food swallows, the bolus entered the pharynx before initiation of the swallow (Dua, Ren, Bardan, Xie, & Shaker, 1997).

BACK-OF-TONGUE CONTROL ISSUE AND TIMING ARE DIFFERENT PROBLEMS

One of the more difficult determinations to make when first starting to interpret VFSS is the reason for part of a bolus (usually liquid) moving over the back of the tongue before the patient seems ready to swallow. Logemann (1993) stressed watching the head of the cohesive bolus. If most of the bolus is still in the oral cavity and some seems to slip over the back of the tongue, then it is probably a back-of-tongue control issue. If the bolus is pushed over the back of the tongue in a cohesive fashion and rests briefly in the valleculae, or even falls to the pyriform sinuses, then that is likely a timing issue and not related to tongue control. Differentiating these is important because two different interventions are indicated.

TRUE "DELAY" (INCREASED STAGE TRANSITION DURATION) DIFFERS FROM "MISTIMING"

If it appears the patient has purposely propelled the entire cohesive bolus over the back of the tongue but the pharyngeal response does not start when the head of the bolus passes the ramus of the mandible, is it characterized as a "delay" (increased stage transition duration, or delay in pharyngeal response), or is it mistiming? The delay seems to be a motor response problem. That is, the sensory input to swallow (the bolus in the pharynx) does not initiate the motor response of closure and lifting of the larynx. Mistiming is harder to characterize. It appears as if all the elements are moving as they should, that the movements have been initiated, but the airway closure is not timed correctly and part of the bolus enters the airway. Perhaps the best way to summarize the difference is as follows:

- Delayed initiation of the pharyngeal response (with the bolus too low in the hypopharynx before closure starts)
- Mistiming of the pharyngeal response (such that closure does not occur at the correct time during bolus movement, but the bolus does not dwell long enough in the pharynx to be considered a delay)

A CERTAIN AMOUNT OF RESIDUE IS "NORMAL"

This is another problem difficult to define. Residue is a measure of efficiency of the swallow. An efficient swallow clears all, or nearly all, of the bolus with the first swallow. Some residue is normal, but residue may put the patient at risk for later aspiration of the remaining residue. Using scintigraphy, Logemann et al. (2005) determined that experienced clinicians were accurate in describing the percentage of residue in the mouth and pharynx. The absolute volume of residue cannot be approximated from videofluorography. The authors argued that clinical observations of percentage residue are particularly accurate when used to compare the patient's own performance across times or bolus types. There are attempts to develop a more standardized way to measure the amount of residue that incorporates both the ratio of residue relative to the available pharyngeal space and the residue proportionate to the size of the individual.

It is reassuring that clinicians can estimate the percentage of residue, but that does not answer the question of how much is too much. This is dependent on several factors: viscosity, where in the pharynx the residue is, patient's physical characteristics, patient's sensation, and effectiveness of multiple clearing swallows.

Viscosity. Thicker materials are more likely to leave residue. However, a large amount of thin residue may be more likely to spill after the swallow.

Location of residue. Residue is seen in the valleculae and pyriform sinuses and on pharyngeal walls. Postswallow residue in one or both pharyngeal spaces was significantly associated with impaired swallowing safety on the subsequent clearing swallow for the same bolus. However, when analyzed separately by residue location, only vallecular residue was significantly associated with impaired swallowing safety on the next clearing swallow (Molfenter & Steele, 2013).

Patient's physical characteristics. The size and shape of each patient's valleculae and pyriform sinuses differ (Pearson, Molfenter, Smith, & Steele, 2013). Some patients appear to have pyriform sinuses large enough to hold several milliliters of material; others have pyriform sinuses so tiny that no residue can be retained. The angle of the epiglottis on patients varies as well, changing the size and shape of the valleculae.

Clearing swallows. A patient with good sensation may realize there is residue after the swallow and spontaneously swallow again. The clearing swallows may or may not safely clear the residue. This should be observed during the VFSS.

How residue will affect recommendations. The final consideration regarding residue is how it will affect your recommendations for diet. For example, if the patient has a lot of residue with solids, even though he or she can safely clear with multiple swallows, and perhaps even a liquid wash, the patient is very aware of the residue. Such a patient might become fatigued with multiple swallows, and might be more comfortable with a diet that results in less residue.

Inter- and Intrarater Reliability

Several studies have examined inter- and intrarater reliability in scoring elements of the VFSS. These findings consistently support the finding that reliability is generally not good (McCullough et al., 2001; Pauloski, Rademaker, Kern, Shaker, & Logemann, 2009; Sia, Carvajal, Carnaby-Mann, & Crary, 2012; Stoeckli, Huisman, Seifert, & Martin-Harris, 2003). A systematic review of those studies found that to achieve reliable measurements in videofluoroscopy of swallowing, it is recommended that raters use well-defined guidelines for the levels of ordinal visuoperceptual variables (Baijens, Barikroo, & Pilz, 2013).

Standardizing Administration and Scoring of the VFSS

Given the evidence that SLPs are generally not reliable in making judgments and scoring components of the VFSS, developing standards for the administration and scoring of the exam is essential to accurate management of dysphagia. The most significant advance toward standardization is the development of the Modified Barium Swallow Impairment Profile (MBSImP). The MBSImP standardizes both the procedure (which materials to present, the amount, and the order in which they are presented) and the scoring of the exam. Seventeen oral, pharyngeal, and esophageal components are carefully defined and a scoring metric is provided for each to objectively profile physiologic impairment of swallowing function (Martin-Harris et al., 2008). To reliably use the instrument, the speech–language pathologist must undergo extensive training in interrater reliability. The training is available online, and when clinicians pass the test (achieve acceptable level of reliability), they are a "registered user" for 5 years in the tool. Even experienced clinicians have found the training to be extremely valuable—and challenging! When all clinicians at a facility are registered users, there is increased confidence in the accuracy of interpretation as well as consistency across clinicians (Standardizing the MBS Study, 2017).

Studies have demonstrated that using the MBSImP protocol minimizes radiation exposure to an average of less than 3 minutes (Bonilha, Humphries, et al., 2013), and the swallowing tasks on the standardized protocol have high probability for capturing impairment (Hazelwood et al., 2017). Using such a standardized protocol eliminates the need to present many different food consistencies to the patient.

A recent study confirmed that SLPs can reliably learn and incorporate objective VFSS measures within a reasonable period. Level of experience has limited influence on the learning curve, so that both novice and experienced SLPs improved their accuracy (Nordin, Miles, & Allen, 2017).

Radiation Safety

Speech–language pathologists who work in facilities where VFSS are performed will typically complete multiple studies in a day or a week, depending on the size of the facility. The speech–language pathologist should be familiar with radiation safety. The most important safety factors are related to time, distance, and shielding.

TIME

Keep the study as short as possible. It would be unusual for a VFSS study to exceed 3 minutes of fluoro time (Bonilha, Humphries, et al., 2013). The radiologist should turn off the fluoro between swallows but turn the fluoro back to on to capture clearing swallows.

DISTANCE

The speech–language pathologist should stand as far from the patient and X-ray tube as practical. Having the radiology technologist present the materials to the patient allows the speech–language pathologist to remain farther back. The amount of radiation exposure received is inversely related to the distance from the source.

SHIELDING

The speech–language pathologist should wear protective lead apparel during the study. This includes lead apron (or skirt and vest), thyroid shield, and eye shield. The staff member presenting materials to the patient should ideally wear lead gloves and get hands out of the X-ray field before fluoro is turned on.

The speech–language pathologist should wear a film badge (dosimetry badge) on the outside of the lead apron at the neck area. A second badge to be worn under the apron may be required by some facilities and when the staff member is pregnant. Consult the facility's radiation safety officer for more information on precautions for pregnant staff members. More information is also found in the ASHA Guidelines document (*Guidelines SLP VFSS*, 2004; Kelchner, 2004).

Documenting Your Findings in a Report

Different institutions will have different formats for reporting findings of the VFSS. A sample format for reporting findings (SLP Resources, MBS/VFSS Report Form) is provided in the Supplemental Materials along with two sample reports (SLP Resources, MBS/VFSS Report Samples).

Efficacy of the VFSS

Many studies in the literature show that the VFSS allows the SLP to identify specific problems in the anatomy and physiology of the swallow and to try appropriate treatment or compensatory techniques. For example, it was demonstrated that tucking the chin provides better airway protection (Welch, Logemann, Rademaker, & Kahrilas, 1993). The chin-tuck strategy results in a posterior shift of anterior pharyngeal structures and a narrowing of the laryngeal entrance and the distance from the epiglottis to both the pharyngeal wall and the laryngeal entrance, widening the angle of the epiglottis to the anterior tracheal wall. Logemann et al. (1992) demonstrated that postural techniques are effective in eliminating aspiration of liquids, as they were successful in eliminating aspiration on at least one volume of liquid in 81% of patients studied after head and neck surgery.

Several studies indicate that the VFSS is more accurate than the bedside or clinical exam in identifying whether aspiration is occurring as well as identifying the cause of the aspiration (Martin-Harris, McMahon, & Haynes, 1998). Some studies attempt to demonstrate that the use of the VFSS changes the number of patients who ultimately get aspiration pneumonia (Daniels et al., 1998; Nilsson, Ekberg, Olsson, & Hindfelt, 1998; Odderson, Keaton, & McKenna, 1995). The problem with these studies is that the patients got treatment between the assessment and the follow-up to determine whether they acquired pneumonia, which makes it difficult to determine the role of the VFSS in the prevention of pneumonia.

The VFSS can prevent unneeded or trial-and-error therapy for patients who are able to eat safely, as such trial-and-error therapy can be more costly in the long run. In an interesting study of patients with head and neck cancer, Logemann et al. (1992) found that patients who had initially been assessed with videofluoroscopy (vs. bedside assessment alone) had better swallow times and more efficient swallows. The authors conclude that this occurred "because the patients' swallowing therapy was more accurately directed at the nature of the physiologic impairment" (p. 184).

Martin-Harris et al. (1998) found that swallowing therapy was warranted in only 37% of 608 patients seen for videofluoroscopic evaluations. Strategies that improved the safety of the swallow and/or efficiency of the swallow were identified on 48% of the exams, and diet modifications were determined on 45% of the patients, with most of the diets being upgraded (Martin-Harris et al., 1998).

Fiberoptic Endoscopic Evaluation of Swallowing

The FEES is a procedure initially developed by Susan Langmore (Schatz, Langmore, & Olson, 1991); it requires a flexible endoscope, which is passed transnasally into the pharynx. Therefore, the clinician must develop skill in not only interpreting the exam, as for the VFSS, but also passing the scope. Throughout most of the study, the tip of the scope hangs just above the epiglottis so that the hypopharynx and larynx can be seen. The scope is left in this position most of the time, but after each swallow, it is moved lower into the laryngeal vestibule to display the vocal folds and the subglottic region and reveal whether any material has been aspirated. The FEES examination has two basic parts: examining structure and function of the pharynx and larynx, and assessing swallowing function.

Part 1: Structure and Function

The first part of the procedure is completed with the tip of the scope resting in the nasopharynx, so closure of the velopharyngeal port can be observed. With the tip in the hypopharynx, movement of the back and base of tongue can be seen. With the tip of the scope over the top of the epiglottis, an excellent view of the larynx, including the vocal folds, can be obtained. The speech–language pathologist may observe abnormalities in structure or function of the vocal folds but should be careful to describe only what is seen, not to make a medical diagnosis. Table 3.2 provides suggestions on how to word observations.

EVALUATING ACCUMULATED ORAL SECRETIONS

During the first part of the exam, the patient's ability to manage secretions can be observed. Murray and colleagues developed the rating scale found in Table 3.3 to predict which patients are at risk for aspiration based on the location of secretions (Murray, Langmore, Ginsberg, & Dostie, 1996).

The Murray et al. (1996) study involved 49 patients. The authors concluded that using the FEES to visualize excess secretions and the place of secretions could predict aspiration. They found that 100% of patients rated as 2 or 3 aspirated foods or liquids, and 53% of patients rated as 1 aspirated foods or liquids. However, 21% of patients rated as 0 also aspirated. Therefore, visualization of secretions alone cannot be used to determine whether the patient will aspirate. Certainly patients rated as 2 or 3 would be considered at high risk to aspirate foods or liquids, but those rated 1 or 2 also have to be considered at risk. As a result, the FEES should not be stopped after this part of the exam (unless the patient is aspirating secretions and does not appear able to follow compensatory techniques) because you would have no information about how the patient might do with different textures. The Murray scale was later validated and found to have good and very good intra- and interrater reliability, respectively (Pluschinski et al., 2016).

Donzelli and colleagues developed a 5-point scale to measure accumulated secretions (Donzelli, Wesling, Brady, & Craney, 2003). When studying 100 consecutive patients, they found that their 5-point secretion-severity scale correlated highly to aspiration and to diet recommendation outcomes. Patients who received tube feedings were more likely to demonstrate a higher secretion level than patients who received oral feedings. In another study, these researchers looked at what accumulated secretions tell us. Donzelli and colleagues confirmed that reduced swallowing frequency leads to increased accumulation of secretions.

Table 3.2
Describing Vocal Fold Lesions

If you see what you think is/are	Try describing it like this
Vocal fold nodules	Bilateral swelling, fullness, or lesions on anterior third of true vocal folds
	Lesions appear to be soft and pliable
	Glottal closure was compromised
Polyps	Pedunculated or sessile-based lesion noted on _____ (describe R/L and location anterior/posterior)
	Lesion(s) resembling a blister
	Lesion(s) appear to be filled with blood
Cysts	A spherical lesion is noted on R/L mid-membranous vocal fold
Paralysis or paresis	Absent or reduced adduction or abduction of R/L vocal fold
	L/R vocal fold appears fixed in midline, paramedian, or lateral position
	Movement is absent or sluggish
	Complete, incomplete, touch closure of glottis
	Glottal gap noted (small, large)
Hemorrhage	The R/L vocal fold demonstrates a yellow or red appearance
	Patient reports that sudden-onset voice loss is suggestive of recent or resolving hemorrhage
Granuloma	Unilateral/bilateral lesion(s) on vocal process
	Describe size of lesion(s)
	Mention any complaints of shortness of air
Papilloma	Clusters of small cauliflower-like growths observed on vocal folds, ventricular folds, airway

Note. Adapted from Branski, Verdolini, Sandulache, Rosen, and Hebda (2006); Reder and Franco (2015); Rosen and Murry (2000).

Table 3.3
Murray Secretion Scale for FEES

Score	Description	Percentage of patients who aspirated food or liquid
0	No excess secretions	21%
1	Secretions in valleculae, pyriforms, lateral channels	53%
2	Transitional rating (changed from 1 to 3 during the observation)	100%
3	Secretions in laryngeal vestibule, not cleared	100%

Note. Adapted from Murray, Langmore, Ginsberg, and Dostie (1996).

Part 2: Swallowing Assessment

During the second part of the exam, the patient's swallowing is assessed using a variety of textures and sizes of food and liquid boluses. The scope is usually at the level above the back of the tongue for the swallowing portion.

During this part of the exam, some problems that may be observed include premature spilling of the bolus over the back of the tongue, penetration of the material into the upper laryngeal vestibule, residue in the valleculae or pyriforms, delay in the initiation of a swallow, and poor timing of the airway closure or increased stage transition duration.

WHITEOUT

During the FEES, at the moment of swallow when the larynx closes, the tip of the scope is obliterated for approximately a half second. This is called *whiteout*. One might think this period of whiteout would mean the examiner is missing critical information. However, more than 90% of all events of aspiration occur before or after the swallow (or whiteout) (Colodny, 2002; Smith, Logemann, Colangelo, Rademaker, & Pauloski, 1999). In addition, if the patient expels material after the swallow, the expelled bolus is evidence of aspiration. And if the bolus entered the airway from the anterior commissure, there will likely be a coating of residue on the subglottic shelf. In fact, this small amount of material would probably not be visualized on fluoroscopy at all, as confirmed from viewing simultaneous studies (Pisegna & Langmore, 2016). After the swallow, when the patient opens the larynx to breathe, the area can again be visualized. Because only a small percentage of aspiration occurs during the swallow, this is not a significant problem.

BLUE DYE

Some clinicians choose to add blue or green food coloring to test materials used during the FEES. Is the dye necessary to make reliable judgments about the patient's swallowing? One study compared the ratings of studies done with and without food coloring and concluded that FEES maintains both high intra- and interrater reliability in detecting the critical features of pharyngeal dysphagia and aspiration using either blue-dyed or non-dyed (Leder, Acton, Lisitano, & Murray, 2005). Contradictory findings using a within-participant design demonstrated a difference in the detection of airway invasion between green and white milk boluses, suggesting that assessment of aspiration may be enhanced by the use of dye (Marvin, Gustafson, & Thibeault, 2016).

However, concerns have been raised regarding the use of blue dye to assist in the detection and/or monitoring of pulmonary aspiration in patients being fed via enteral feeding tubes; therefore, the same concerns were raised about the small amount of dye used during endoscopic exams (Lucarelli, Shirk, Julian, & Crouser, 2004). The safety concerns were that, in patients with gut permeability, the blue dye was "leaking" from the gut to other organs and there was a risk that the blue dye bottles or vials were becoming contaminated with bacteria (File, Tan, Thomson, Stephens, & Thompson, 1995; Knoll, 1993).

Given these concerns, and the difficulty in obtaining single-use sterile vials of blue food coloring, it seems advisable to avoid the use of food coloring. Instead, use foods that naturally reflect the light from the scope and are distinct from the color of the mucosa—milk, vanilla pudding, sugar cookie, and so forth (Swigert, 2002, 2003).

COMPENSATORY STRATEGIES

As with the VFSS, an important aspect of the FEES is to try compensatory strategies when problems are observed. The patient's response to these compensatory strategies yields important information to help you make recommendations and develop a treatment plan. Similarly, a chart is provided in the Supplemental Materials (SLP Resources, FEES Interpretation) specific to use with FEES to help interpret what you see and to determine which compensatory strategies to try during FEES. The effect of some of those strategies (e.g., head rotation, change in bolus consistency) may be easier to observe on FEES than others (e.g., supraglottic swallow).

SENSORY TESTING

Aviv et al. described the Fiberoptic Endoscopic Evaluation of Swallowing with Sensory Testing (FEESST) as a technique to determine laryngopharyngeal sensory discrimination thresholds by endoscopically delivering a pulse of air to the anterior wall of the pyriform sinus or to the aryepiglottic folds (innervated by superior laryngeal nerve) (Aviv et al., 1998; Aviv et al., 2000). Karnell and Langmore (1998) performed sensory testing by touching the tip of the scope lightly to the pharyngeal mucosa, the base of the tongue, or the tip of the epiglottis.

NEGLIGIBLE RISKS

The risks of an endoscopic swallowing procedure are negligible. In large cohorts of patients, less than 1% are reported to have minor, self-limiting nosebleeds (Aviv et al., 2000).

In addition, endoscopic procedures may be difficult to use with patients who are agitated, aggressive, or hostile, as well as with patients with movement disorders or septal deviations.

RESIDUE SCALES

As previously described, there are rating scales to measure the amount of accumulated secretions. There are also rating scales to measure and describe the amount of residue after the swallow. One example is the Yale Pharyngeal Residue Rating Scale, which uses a 5-point scale (*none, trace, mild, moderate,* and *severe*) and provides visual images of each for valleculae and pyriform sinuses (Neubauer, Rademaker, & Leder, 2015).

TOPICAL ANESTHETIC AND NASAL DECONGESTANTS

There have been several studies investigating the effect of topical anesthetic on swallowing skills and on patient comfort and tolerance of the exam. Those studies had equivocal results. In a large, randomized double-blind study with patients, no significant differences in patient comfort levels were observed when a topical anesthetic, vasoconstrictor, or placebo was administered to the nasal mucosa before endoscopy. In addition, no significant differences in patient comfort levels were found when nothing was administered to the nasal mucosa before endoscopy (Leder, Ross, Briskin, & Sasaki, 1997). Another study showed higher penetration-aspiration scores in healthy subjects with the anesthetized swallows (Lester et al., 2013).

The most recent study by Fife et al. (2015), with 25 consecutively referred patients, found, the use of 0.5 ml of 4% lidocaine applied topically to the nares before FEES did not significantly impair swallowing in patients with dysphagia but did increase the odds of a higher PAS score by 33%. Topical nasal anesthesia significantly reduced perceived pain and discomfort during all aspects of FEES and improved overall patient tolerance when administered before examination (Fife et al., 2015). In another study, the dose of lidocaine was reduced to 0.2 ml. Results showed no significant difference in the anesthetized versus nonanesthetized conditions for PAS or residue scores. Patients did rate the exams done with lidocaine significantly more comfortable, especially on insertion of the scope (O'Dea et al., 2015).

Vasoconstrictors cause constriction of the small blood vessels, resulting in the tissue in that area shrinking. In the case of nasal decongestant, the tissues in the nasal passages shrink, which may make it easier to pass the scope.

If topical lidocaine or nasal decongestants are to be used, the speech–language pathologist will need to determine the facility's policy about who can "administer" medications and how they must be stored and secured. They must also know what the state licensure board says about SLPs administering medications. The anesthetic should be applied only to the nasal passage, preferably in jelly form and with a cotton-tipped applicator. It should not be sprayed into the nose, as some of the anesthetic can reach the back of the pharynx and interfere with the swallow. Before administering the medication(s), the speech–language pathologist should check the patient's medical record for drug allergies, should question the patient about drug allergies, and should query the patient's physician if necessary about the safety of administering the drugs. There should be provisions for medical treatment in the case of adverse patient reaction to the test or medication.

Interpretation of the FEES Exam

One of the best ways to develop skill in interpreting the exam is to accompany an experienced speech–language pathologist and discuss structure and function during the exam. That way, skilled endoscopists can explain what they see, why they are presenting certain materials, and why they are attempting certain compensatory strategies.

Another source that has been very helpful to clinicians in mastering the interpretation of endoscopic swallow exams is *Training and Interpretation of FEES in Adults* by Edie Hapner. This set of three DVDs and a CD contains didactic lectures and actual FEES exams to aid in the diagnosis of swallowing problems as seen through endoscopy. The package includes a FEES documentation template, completed FEES documentation forms for exams featured on the DVDs, a scope-passing and FEES competency checklist, and resources in addition to the three training DVDs (Hapner, 2010).

Documenting Your Findings in a Report

The FEES Examination Protocol, in the Supplemental Materials, reflects the examination as originally described by Karnell and Langmore and provides guidance for the speech–language pathologist in how to administer the exam. When the protocol is followed precisely as described by them, the procedure is called FEES.

Observations of the structures and functions of the larynx and pharynx and of swallowing can be recorded on the FEES Report Form found in the Supplemental Materials (SLP Resources). There is also a sample report included in the Supplemental Materials (SLP Resources, FEES Report Sample).

FEES Equipment

CLEANING THE EQUIPMENT

The speech–language pathologist should work closely with specialists in infection control and staff safety at the facility when determining what the guidelines will be for cleaning, disinfecting, and storing the endoscopy equipment. There are specific requirements for the room in which the scope will be cleaned, as well as how it will be stored. Cleaning and high-level disinfection are required. A consideration is whether the speech–language pathology staff will complete the cleaning and disinfecting, or whether it will be done by the central sterilization department at the facility. Some facilities choose to use endosheaths, but the scope still needs to be cleaned and sterilized. It was this author's experience that use of the endosheath had two distinct disadvantages: It sometimes made it hard to visualize the swallow because the endosheath clouded the view, and the sheath was tricky to remove at the end of the study. More than once the scope was damaged during removal of the sheath.

RETURN ON INVESTMENT FOR FEES EQUIPMENT

If a facility is interested in purchasing FEES equipment, the speech–language pathologist can play a key role by gathering information on return on investment. If the facility already provides VFSS, the cost of the two studies can be compared. For example, staff costs should be lower with the FEES, as typically there is a speech–language pathologist's time and a nursing assistant's time (to present the foods to the patient), whereas for a VFSS the staff involved are a speech–language pathologist, radiology technologist, radiologist, transporter, and nurse if the patient's condition requires the nurse to accompany the patient off the floor or unit.

For facilities considering implementing FEES as part of their dysphagia management program, Leder and Murray (2008) provide an overview of FEES.

Efficacy of the FEES

Leder, Sasaki, and Burrell (1998) and Leder (1998) contributed two articles to the research base supporting the effectiveness of the FEES in the evaluation and management of patients with dysphagia. Leder et al. (1998) performed the FEES on 400 consecutive patients referred because of their dysphagia. On the first 56 patients, both the FEES and the MBS were performed, and 96% agreement was reached on identifying patients with silent aspiration. Leder (1998) detailed the advantages of using the FEES multiple times during a patient's admission to help make decisions about changes in the management of the patient. Specifically, 47% of the subjects received the FEES 3–5 times within 6–22 days. Leder (1998) stated, "Timely serial FEES (Leder, Sasaki, & Burrell, 1998) allowed 22 of 32 (69%) subjects to resume an oral diet as early and safely as possible" (Leder, 1998).

Cranial Nerve Exam, Penetration–Aspiration Scale, and Contextual Factors: VFSS and FEES

Cranial Nerve Evaluation During VFSS or FEES

Whether performing the VFSS or the FEES, the speech–language pathologist can assess function of cranial nerves during the exam. Understanding which cranial nerve is responsible for movements in the oropharynx and larynx allows the clinician to make judgments about cranial nerves. The Cranial Nerve Assessment During Instrumental Exam, found in the Supplemental Materials (SLP Resources), can be used during an instrumental exam to gather this information.

Rating Scales

A number of rating scales can be used with VFSS or FEES, and some have been designed specifically for one of the exams (Brady, 2007). Residue scales, typically used with FEES, have already been described. Objective rating scales can provide detailed information about different aspects of the physiology of the swallow and can be particularly useful when comparing physiology changes in patients who receive repeat studies.

PENETRATION–ASPIRATION SCALE (PAS)

The Penetration–Aspiration Scale can be used with either exam (Rosenbek, Robbins, Roecker, Coyle, & Wood, 1996). The PAS is an 8-point penetration–aspiration scale designed to describe penetration and aspiration during videofluoroscopic studies. The scores describe the depth to which material enters the airway and indicate whether the material was expelled and swallowed with the rest of the bolus.

The PAS scale has been used in numerous research studies when scoring the VFSS and in research on normal swallowing in young and elderly (Allen et al., 2010; Bingjie, Tong, Xinting, Jianmin, & Guijun, 2010; Cvejic et al., 2011; Daggett et al., 2006; Gillespie et al., 2005).

The PAS has also been used in scoring the FEES. Two studies examined reliability and sensitivity. Using 79 swallows and four judges, Colodny reported that interrater reliability was equally good when visualized endoscopically as had been reported for fluoroscopy studies (Colodny, 2002). A subsequent study found excellent interrater reliability among clinicians assigning a PAS score whether the clinicians were new or experienced in FEES (Butler, Markley, Sanders, & Stuart, 2015).

It is probably more common for the speech–language pathologist to review the recording of a VFSS than it is to review the recording of a FEES. This may be in part because of the length of each study. The VFSS may be a few minutes long, and even watching it in its entirety and using slow motion might only take 10 minutes. In contrast, the FEES may be 10–15 minutes of recording to review, and searching and reversing to find the points of interest can take quite some time. However, one study revealed better reliability in scoring the PAS with FEES when frame-by-frame review of recording was used compared to real time (Hey et al., 2015).

Contextual Factors

As during the clinical evaluation, during an instrumental study, the speech–language pathologist should be evaluating factors that will have an influence on the success of the intervention strategies being recommended. In the recommendations section of the report, the clinician should comment on things like fatigue, motivation, alertness, distractibility, level of cueing needed, and any cultural or language differences.

Comparison of the VFSS and the FEES

These two procedures yield similar but not identical information. Each is a valuable tool for assessing the pharyngeal phase.

Several studies provide comparative information about the FEES and the MBS. Briani et al. (1998) examined 23 patients with motor neuron disease using three instrumental procedures: videofluoroscopy, videopharyngolaryngoscopy, and pharyngoesophageal manometry. They concluded: "Videofluoroscopy was the most sensitive technique in identifying oropharyngeal alterations of swallowing." They also stated, "Videofluoroscopy was also capable of detecting preclinical abnormalities in patients without dysphagia who later developed dysphagia" (Briani et al., 1998, p. 211).

Périé et al. (1998) evaluated the ability of videoendoscopic swallowing studies to assess pharyngeal propulsion and aspiration episodes when compared with videofluoroscopy and manometry. They examined 34 patients with each of the procedures and found total agreement between videoendoscopy and videofluoroscopy in 76.4% of the patients for pharyngeal propulsion and 82.3% for aspiration (Périé et al., 1998).

Langmore et al. (1991) tested 21 subjects with both the FEES and the MBS within a 48-hour period. The FEES was found to be reliable for detecting some of the major pharyngeal symptoms. They found that 75% of subjects who had penetration on the FEES also had penetration on the MBS. Eighty-eight percent of subjects who aspirated on the FEES also aspirated on the MBS (Schatz et al., 1991).

Kelly et al. compared clinician ratings of PAS from recorded swallows visualized endoscopically and fluoroscopically taken from simultaneous studies. They found the PAS score was significantly different when scored from a FEES versus a fluoroscopy exam. The PAS scores from the FEES tended to be worse. That is, FEES was detecting more events of penetration than the MBS study—and more events of aspiration (Kelly, Drinnan, & Leslie, 2007). Four studies were done using simultaneous fluoroscopy and endoscopy, and the same bolus and same swallow were compared. Multiple raters were used to judge presence or absence of the bolus findings (Rao, Brady, Chaudhuri, Donzelli, & Wesling, 2003), or asked to rate severity of residue (Kelly, Leslie, Beale, Payten, & Drinnan, 2006; Pisegna & Langmore, 2016) or to score penetration or aspiration on the PAS (Kelly et al., 2007). These studies found that agreement for presence or absence of findings was very high but that FEES consistently yielded a worse score in terms of increasing severity of penetration or aspiration and residue.

Considerations in Recommending VFSS or FEES

Whether you recommend the VFSS or FEES is specific to each patient. If the facility offers each, or if there are mobile services for either, the decision can be made solely according to which exam will give you the best information about the patient's specific problem. Table 3.4 lists some considerations for each.

Table 3.4
Comparing VFSS and FEES

Considerations in selecting VFSS or FEES	VFSS	FEES
Visualize structures of pharynx and larynx	X	X
Visualize closure of velopharyngeal port	X	X
Visualize vocal fold movement at rest and in breath-hold tasks		X
Assess secretions in hypopharynx		X
Two-dimensional image	X	
Three-dimensional image		X
Black-and-white image	X	
Full-color image		X
Assess oral phase with specific movements of the tongue	X	
Assess pharyngeal phase	X	X
Assess pharyngeal or laryngeal sensitivity		X
Assess coordination of breathing and swallowing		X
Use "real" food to assess		X
Does not use contrast material (patient may refuse contrast)		X
Assess effects of fatigue (i.e., exam is not time limited)		X
Assess swallowing in position in which patient eats (e.g., semireclined) if needed		X
Assessment more closely mimics mealtime function		X
Mobile unit to assess patient at SNF	X	X
Can be performed by SLP without physician (only other staff needed is someone to feed patient)		X
Can be performed at bedside		X
Exposes patient to radiation	X	
Agitated or combative patient may pull at scope		X
Can predict safety of swallowing by visualizing secretions		X
Can observe swallow with ice chip		X
Observe residue in lateral channels, valleculae, and pyriforms	X	X
Observe tongue-base retraction to posterior pharyngeal wall during the swallow	X	
Observe forward movement of posterior pharyngeal wall during the swallow	X	
Observe anterior and superior movement of the hyoid	X	
Observe laryngeal elevation	X	
Observe opening of the cricopharyngeus	X	
Observe closure at entrance to airway between arytenoids and epiglottis during the swallow	X	
Observe tipping of the epiglottis during the swallow	X	
Assess movement of bolus in upper third of esophagus	X	
Patient complaints indicate esophageal involvement	X	
Visualize movement of the bolus during the swallow	X	
Judge effectiveness of Mendelsohn maneuver	X	
Observe movement of pharyngeal walls on phonation		X
Observe airway closure by true vocal folds, false vocal folds, arytenoid movement		X
Visualize reflux into the hypopharynx	X	X

Note. Some items adapted from Kidder, Langmore, and Martin (1994).

Sample Cases for Selecting Appropriate Exam

Case Examples: Choosing the Appropriate Exam is provided in the Supplemental Materials (SLP Resources) elaborating reasons one might choose VFSS or FEES, or in some cases only the clinical exam.

Other Instrumental Procedures

Four other instrumental techniques are often used by physicians to assess other aspects of swallowing (e.g., those related to the esophageal phase). Although some SLPs in multidisciplinary medical settings have begun to use high-resolution pharyngeal manometry (HRM), this and other procedures are not in widespread use as diagnostic tools in most clinical settings. Following is a brief description of each technique.

ELECTROMYOGRAPHY (EMG)

This technique uses surface electrodes (sEMG), or hooked wire electrodes, to provide information about the contraction of a muscle or muscle group. The surface electrodes are usually placed under the patient's chin to measure activity of the floor of mouth muscles, which contribute to anterior and superior movement of the hyolaryngeal complex. The sEMG technique has been used in research to gather information about hyoid movement during certain therapeutic maneuvers (Crary, Carnaby, & Groher, 2006, 2007; Wheeler-Hegland, Rosenbek, & Sapienza, 2008). Hooked wire electrodes have been used to study laryngeal muscles and pharyngeal constrictors (Burnett, Mann, Stoklosa, & Ludlow, 2005; Palmer, McCulloch, Jaffe, & Neel, 2005). At present, such procedures are not easily applied outside the laboratory for diagnosis of swallowing disorders (although surface electromyographic stimulation, sEMG, is used as a biofeedback technique in treatment, as described in Chapter 4).

HIGH-RESOLUTION PHARYNGEAL MANOMETRY (HRM)

Manometry and impedance-pH manometry are more commonly used to measure pressure in the upper and lower esophageal sphincters (Kahrilas & Sifrim, 2008). HRM is also used to assess pressures in the pharynx (Hoffman et al., 2012; McCulloch, Hoffman, & Ciucci, 2010). A flexible tube containing sensors is passed transnasally into the pharynx, where the sensors measure pressure at specific points (e.g., base of tongue, cricopharyngeus). This procedure is often done in conjunction with a videofluoroscopic study so that the material passing through the pharynx can be viewed at the same time the manometric readings are taken. HRM for assessing pharyngeal function is currently used in some large, multidisciplinary medical settings (Knigge, Thibeault, & McCulloch, 2014). For more information, the review article by Cock and Omari (2017) provides detailed information.

SCINTIGRAPHY

This test, completed by nuclear medicine, allows for the measurement of the amount of material aspirated. It is the only test that accurately measures amount of aspiration. It can also determine when aspiration is occurring. For instance, if aspiration of reflux material is suspected, the patient is scanned at intervals over a time period and the amount of aspirated material is measured at each interval. Scintigraphy is also considered more of a research tool than a clinical procedure.

ULTRASOUND

This procedure uses high-frequency sounds to produce dynamic images of soft tissues and is considered completely noninvasive. It is completed by holding a transducer under the chin. This procedure is useful in studying the oral and oral preparatory phases of swallowing, but it does not allow for observation of aspiration or thorough analysis of the pharyngeal phase.

Instrumental Exam Reports

Refer to the reports in the Supplemental Materials to help you collect, organize, and report information. (See SLP Resources, MBS/VFSS Report Form and MBS/VFSS Report Samples, FEES Report Form and FEES Report Sample.)

Medicare Guidelines for Components of Evaluation Report

A report on an evaluation, based on Medicare guidelines, should include the following information.

HISTORY

The history section should include some information about the patient's prior level of function. Medicare in particular will not pay for therapy designed to take patients above their prior level of function.

The history should also include information about the results of any previous treatment or evaluations. If a patient showed little progress with previous therapy, a claims reviewer will probably not see the need for further intervention. However, if you can determine why the patient made limited progress, your chances of continuing therapy are improved. For example, you might find that the patient's level of alertness changed as a result of a medication change or that a previous therapist neglected to try an appropriate technique.

NEED FOR SERVICE

The report should clearly indicate why this particular evaluation is needed.

EFFECTS OF ANY STRATEGIES ATTEMPTED

The report should describe any compensatory techniques, rehabilitative strategies, or diet changes tried during the exam and the patient's responses.

POSITIVE EXPECTATION

The report should indicate expectation that the patient will be able to change swallowing behaviors. Include information about skills the patient exhibited on the swallow study, the patient's level of cooperation, and the patient's alertness. If the patient showed extremely poor performance during the study, was not alert, or had many complicating diagnoses, it would be difficult to justify intensive therapeutic intervention that requires a lot of the patient's cooperation.

DESCRIPTIVE INFORMATION

Reports should provide information about each phase of the swallow assessed. For the VFSS, this will include oral, oropharyngeal, pharyngoesophageal, and esophageal. For the FEES, only the oropharyngeal and pharyngoesophageal phases are assessed. An objective rating scale may be used to provide more information.

SPECIFIC RECOMMENDATIONS

The report should include recommendations about the following:

- Diet
- Food presentation
- Food placement
- Positioning
- Status
- Presentation of medications
- Nutrition
- Charting and monitoring

- Compensatory techniques to use during meals
- Facilitation and treatment techniques
- Prognosis
- Reevaluation

DIAGNOSIS
The report also must identify a specific diagnosis and the phase(s) of swallow affected.

NEED FOR REEVALUATION
The report must indicate whether the patient needs to come back for a repeat exam before any changes can be made in the recommendations. For example, if the patient was aspirating, it will almost certainly be necessary for the patient to have another study before the recommendations can be altered.

It is apparent that a silent aspirator will need a repeat exam before trying any food. Some SLPs think that a patient who coughs with aspiration on a study can be upgraded at bedside because a cough can be used to judge whether aspiration is occurring. Unfortunately, the patient's larynx may become desensitized so that he or she no longer coughs with aspiration. In addition, patients are often inconsistent with coughing on aspiration.

Strategies for Collaboration Between Referring SLP and Study SLP

If an SLP sends a patient to another facility for an instrumental study and does not receive reports or verbal indications concerning the results of the evaluation, the referring SLP should make an effort to establish contact with the person performing the study. The following strategies may facilitate better collaboration:

- Telephoning the facility and requesting its records
- Sending a signed medical release form requesting the records
- Indicating that a complete written report is expected by a certain date

If schedule permits, the referring SLP may also want to attend the study. It is impossible to plan effective treatment for the patient without the complete results of the study.

Documenting If Not Following Recommendations From the Report

After the referring or treating SLP has received a report from the instrumental exam and is implementing intervention, it is important to document any changes that occur in the patient's status and whether they are positive or negative. For example, within a week of a patient's instrumental exam, the patient may experience a neurological event, such as a CVA or TIA. This change in medical status may render the recommendations of the previous instrumental exam invalid. This should be clearly indicated in documentation, including the rationale for changing the treatment plan originally recommended, based on the instrumental exam.

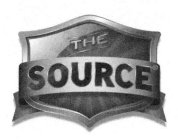

Chapter 4

Dysphagia Treatment: Theoretical Basis, Planning, and Implementing

What Needs to Be Considered When Treating Dysphagia?

The clinical and instrumental evaluations provide the speech–language pathologist with a picture of the patient's physiologic impairments that are responsible for the signs and symptoms of dysphagia, as well as the impact these deficits have on the patient's activities and participation. After the evaluations have been completed, the speech–language pathologist, in collaboration with the patient and family, establishes a treatment plan. The decisions about the treatment will be influenced by client-specific factors such as etiology of the dysphagia; comorbidities, overall health, and cognitive status of the patient; setting in which patient is seen; and family support. Collaboration with the patient is essential, as the speech–language pathologist should keep the focus on function as decisions are made about the patient's course of treatment (Figure 4.1).

The first decision will be whether the patient is a candidate for treatment of the impaired physiology causing the functional deficits. Whether or not the patient is a candidate for rehabilitative treatment, the next important decision is to determine whether the patient will be able to eat, and if so, what kind of diet (bolus modifications) and with which compensatory strategies (e.g., postural, increasing control of bolus). If the patient is not a candidate for rehabilitation, then the decision making is complete at that point. If the patient is a candidate for rehabilitative treatment, the decision also needs to be made as to which rehabilitative treatment techniques will be used and in what combination with the compensatory strategies.

Specific compensatory and rehabilitative techniques must be selected to address the physiologic and functional impairments. If rehabilitative techniques will be used, then the speech–language pathologist must also apply knowledge of underlying principles of neuroplasticity and motor learning in order to establish an appropriate treatment regimen. Consider first the focus on function and the importance of collaborating with the patient and family in planning treatment. Then focus will shift to each of these decision points and the things that can influence the decision.

Keeping the Focus on Function

As diagnosticians, speech–language pathologists focus on the impaired physiology and consider how, or whether, it can be "fixed." In fact, a later section in this chapter highlights the importance of addressing impairments at that level. However, the speech–language pathologist must first and foremost consider the person with dysphagia and how impairments are affecting the individual's ability to function. Each treatment decision should be made in collaboration with the patient, to the extent that the patient has the ability to participate, and with the patient's family. These collaborations will help the clinician stay focused on what is important to the patient.

Without this important collaboration, the speech–language pathologist may think that the selected goals were appropriate and feel at the end of treatment that this case is a "win." For example, perhaps for a patient who is NPO, after treatment the patient is able to eat a pureed diet with small

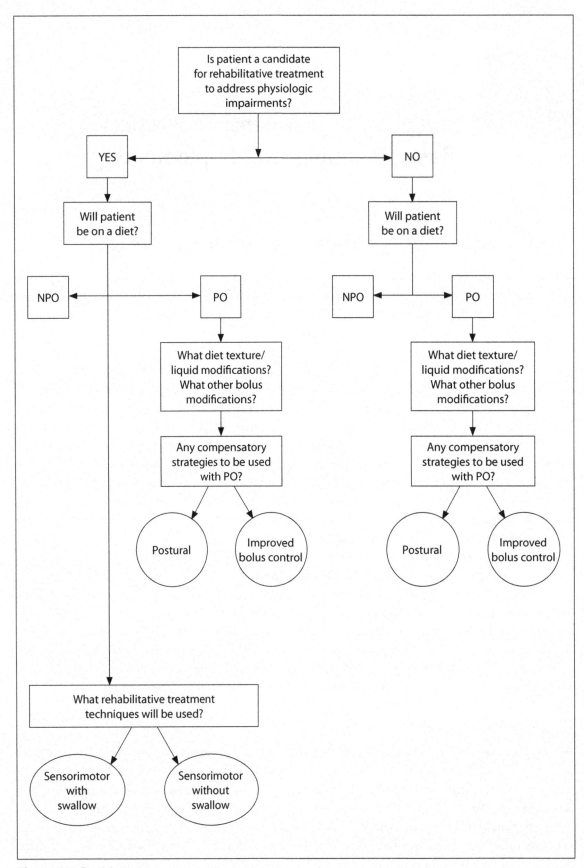

Figure 4.1 Decision tree.

sips of thickened liquid while using three different compensatory techniques. Eating this way takes 50 minutes to complete a meal, and the patient is still losing weight. From the patient's perspective, would this be a "win"? From the patient's perspective, function is still significantly impaired.

The ICF Model

The International Classification of Functioning, Disability, and Health (ICF) model helps the clinician focus on the client as a whole. The model is constructed around two main components, health conditions and contextual factors (Figure 4.2). Health conditions include body structure and function, activities, and participation. Contextual factors include environmental and personal factors. Traditionally, speech–language pathologists have focused on assessing and treating the deficit at the level of body structure and function (e.g., improve laryngeal closure, reduce stage transition duration). Applying the ICF model results in a more holistic, person-centered approach to care. It is all about the client. When clinicians keep that in mind, everything else falls into place. The ICF is a framework for classifying the consequences of disease, which then focuses on function. That is, how is the disease affecting the client?

In 2001, the World Health Organization (WHO) approved the ICF model (see WHO, 2016). The ICF is structured around two comprehensive components:

- Health conditions

  - Body functions and structure (functioning at the level of the body; in an earlier model called *impairment*). These describe the anatomy, physiology, and psychology of the human body.

  - Activities (functioning at the level of the individual) and the activity limitations an individual experiences.

  - Participation in all areas of life (functioning of a person in society) and the restrictions he or she experiences.

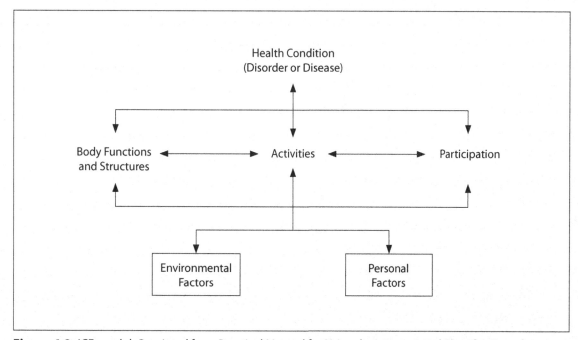

Figure 4.2 ICF model. *Reprinted from Practical Manual for Using the International Classification of Functioning Disability,* WHO, page 7. Copyright 2013.

- Contextual factors
  - Environmental factors that affect these experiences and whether these factors act as barriers or facilitators. These factors are not within the person's control, and they can include family, work, government agencies, laws, and cultural beliefs.
  - Personal factors influence how an individual experiences the disability and include age, race, gender, food preferences, habits, lifestyle, social background, and coping styles. Personal factors are represented in the framework because they may have an influence on how a person functions. Personal factors can have a positive or negative impact on a person's function (Üstün, 2001).

To help users further understand these factors, WHO has developed definitions explaining how these terms are used in the context of health (Figure 4.3).

The ICF model does not ignore the health condition and focus only on its impact, but it does relate the health condition to functioning and disability. Functioning and disability are considered part of a complex interaction between the health condition of the individual and the contextual factors of the environment and personal factors. The model was designed to be relevant across cultures as well as age groups and genders, making it useful across heterogeneous populations (International Classification of Functioning, Disability and Health, 2015).

Example of applying the ICF in dysphagia. An example of how two patients with the same impairment look very different according to the ICF model will help illustrate the importance of considering the whole person (Table 4.1). The patients have had a similar stroke, and their swallow impairment is almost identical. However, considering the contextual factors, both environmental and personal, makes it clear that the two patients will need to be managed differently and may indeed have very different goals.

Is the Patient a Candidate for Rehabilitative Treatment?

Part of the evaluation process is determining prognosis, which should be further delineated as the question "Prognosis for what?" For example, what is the prognosis that the patient will eat enough

---

In the context of health:

Functioning is an umbrella term for body functions, body structures, activities and participation. It denotes the positive aspects of the interaction between an individual (with a health condition) and that individual's contextual factors (environmental and personal factors).

Disability is an umbrella term for impairments, activity limitations and participation restrictions. It denotes the negative aspects of the interaction between an individual (with a health condition) and that individual's contextual factors (environmental and personal factors).

Body functions—The physiological functions of body systems (including psychological functions).

Body structures—Anatomical parts of the body such as organs, limbs and their components.

Impairments—Problems in body function and structure such as significant deviation or loss.

Activity—The execution of a task or action by an individual.

Participation—Involvement in a life situation.

Activity limitations—Difficulties an individual may have in executing activities.

Participation restrictions—Problems an individual may experience in involvement in life situations.

Environmental factors—The physical, social and attitudinal environment in which people live and conduct their lives. These are either barriers to or facilitators of the person's functioning.

Figure 4.3 WHO definitions for the ICF. Reprinted from *Practical Manual for Using the International Classification of Functioning Disability*, WHO, page 8. Copyright 2013.

Table 4.1
Using the ICF Model

ICF component		Patient A	Patient B
Health condition (disorder or disease) Each patient suffered a similar type of stroke	Body structures and functions	Moderate pharyngeal dysphagia with reduced laryngeal elevation resulting in residue in pyriform sinuses with thicker foods clears with second spontaneous swallow	Moderate pharyngeal dysphagia with reduced laryngeal elevation resulting in residue in pyriform sinuses with thicker foods and aspiration after swallow; cued swallow clears residue
	Activity	Able to safely eat runny, pureed foods and thin liquids in small amounts with multiple swallows	Able to safely eat runny, pureed foods and thin liquids in small amounts with multiple swallows requiring cues
	Participation	Will go to dining room for meals	Does not like to go to dining room because the aide has to be with him to cue
Contextual factors	Environmental factors	Patient's daughter present at each meal	No family close by to visit
	Personal factors	76 years old; otherwise good health; able to remember to use multiple swallows; outgoing personality; very motivated to improve	93 years old; hard of hearing; mild-moderate dementia and cannot follow complex directions; does not enjoy interacting with fellow residents

of the modified diet to maintain nutritional status? Or, what is the prognosis that the patient's medical condition will improve enough to be able to participate fully in therapy or to experience some spontaneous recovery? Determining the prognosis for rehabilitative treatment requires predicting whether the patient after treatment will exhibit a lasting change in physiology. Not all patients are candidates for active treatment of their disorder. Although the decision whether to try rehabilitative therapy versus compensations must be specific to each patient, certain factors would likely make a patient *not* a good candidate for rehabilitation:

- Patient has significant cognitive impairments that would prevent understanding and following directions for swallowing exercise.

- Etiology for the dysphagia is attributed to a progressive disorder such as advanced dementia or ALS. (See the information in Chapter 9, Reimbursement: Coding and Documenting Dysphagia Services, on Medicare guidelines for maintenance therapy for patients not expected to improve.)

- Patient refuses to participate in therapy.

When in doubt as to whether the patient can benefit from rehabilitative techniques, a short period of trial therapy with carefully designed, measurable goals can help make that determination in some cases.

Will the Patient Take PO or Be NPO?

The determination about oral intake is often decided after an instrumental evaluation, although there are situations in which it is clear from the clinical exam that it either will or will not be safe for a patient to take an oral diet. The results of either type of exam must be considered along with the patient's personal and environmental factors when making this recommendation. It is ultimately the patients' decision, if they are capable of deciding, whether they will comply with any medical recommendations. If they are not capable, their surrogate decides in their place.

The speech–language pathologist considers multiple factors in formulating a recommendation about safe intake of PO. In a discussion with the patient and family about the recommendation, the speech–language pathologist should highlight the factors that influenced the recommendation (Table 4.2). For more information on how management of dysphagia changes in palliative and hospice care, see Chapter 7.

IS TUBE FEEDING RECOMMENDED?

If the recommendation is made that the patient be NPO, then the patient will need an alternative form of nutrition and hydration. If the prognosis for return to safe PO intake is good, then a short-term solution (NG tube) is usually recommended. If the prognosis is poor for patient returning to full or partial PO, or if it is predicted that it will take some time for the patient to reach that goal, then the more permanent PEG is recommended.

CAN PATIENT MAINTAIN NUTRITIONAL STATUS?

At times it will be recommended that a patient take PO but there is a concern that the patient will not be able to eat and drink enough to maintain nutrition and hydration. In those cases, the speech–language pathologist should discuss this concern with the physician and dietitian. Sometimes the dietitian can recommend oral supplements to augment the recommended diet. Other times the patient may need tube feeding to supplement oral intake. Discuss this with the physician to help determine whether a short-term option (NG tube) or long-term option (PEG) is more appropriate.

DISCUSSING NPO RECOMMENDATION WITH PHYSICIAN

If a conversation with the physician is not possible at the time the recommendation is being made, then the speech–language pathologist should avoid using wording prescribing to the physician what type of tube should be used. However, it is incumbent on the speech–language pathologist to provide enough information about the patient's dysphagia for the physician to make the determination (Table 4.3).

WILL A WATER OR ICE CHIP PROTOCOL BE RECOMMENDED FOR THE PATIENT?

It is sometimes thought that dysphagia increases the risk of dehydration because patients are restricted from thin liquids. Therefore, it is surmised that patients cannot get enough fluids when taking only thickened liquids. Some programs try to counteract this fact by providing free water to their patients with dysphagia. The Frazier Rehabilitation Hospital in Louisville, Kentucky, pioneered this technique in 1984, called the Frazier Free Water Protocol (FFWP; Panther, 2005). The protocol, as implemented at Frazier, is included in the Supplemental Materials (SLP Resources, Frazier Free Water Protocol Guidelines).

Garon, Engle, and Ormiston (1997) tested the hypothesis that patients become dehydrated on thickened liquids in a randomized controlled trial that examined two groups of stroke patients who had previously been identified as aspirating thin liquids. Control group subjects were given only thickened liquids and, over the course of the study, had a mean intake of 1210 cc per day of thickened liquids. The study group subjects were allowed thickened liquids with additional thin water intake. They averaged a combined fluid intake of 1318 cc per day. No patient developed pneumonia, dehydration, or complications during the course of the study or during a 30-day follow-up period. The patients, as expected, reported dissatisfaction with thick liquids and high satisfaction with access to water. The authors expressed surprise that the study subjects did not drink less thickened liquid and more thin liquid (Garon, Engle, & Ormiston, 1997).

In follow-up satisfaction surveys, most of the study patients reported drinking water generally for oral dryness and to quench thirst (Garon, Engle, & Ormiston, 1997). The authors recommended that water and ice chips be given only in instances of patient refusal to drink thickened liquids or when hydration issues cause medical concerns. They urged staff making decisions

Table 4.2
Factors to Consider When Recommending PO or NPO

Factor	Things to consider
Results of instrumental exam	How severe is the pharyngeal dysphagia?
	Was the aspirated material partially or fully expelled (Pen-Asp scores)
	How much pharyngeal residue was present and with which consistencies?
	What is the risk the residue will be aspirated?
	Were there any consistencies the patient swallowed safely?
	Did the patient aspirate?
	How much of any consistency was aspirated?
	Did the patient aspirate silently or have a productive cough?
If recommending PO, impact of diet restrictions on nutrition	Is the diet that can be eaten safely so restrictive that the patient will not be able to maintain nutrition?
	If the liquids need to be thickened, will the patient drink enough to maintain hydration?
Patient's medical condition	Is the patient acutely or critically ill?
	Is the patient stable and recovering?
	Is the patient in palliative or hospice care?
	Is patient mobile or bed bound?
Risk factors for developing aspiration pneumonia	Dependent for feeding
	Multiple medical diagnoses
	Current smoker
	Tube fed
	Dependent for oral care
	Number of decayed teeth or poor oral health
	Number of meds
	Admitted from nursing home
	Takes sedative medication
	Has feeding tube or on mechanically altered diet
Patient's cognitive status	If the patient can eat safely only with specific compensations (e.g., small sips), will the patient be able to remember to use these?
	Will patient be compliant with recommended diet and restrictions?
	Does the patient have fluctuating alertness?
	Is patient able to comprehend the disorder and why the recommendations are necessary?
Patient setting	Is the patient in a facility, and if so, what structure is in place to ensure that recommendations for safe intake are followed?
	If the diet is modified, can the kitchen consistently produce trays that match the recommendation?
	Can the patient eat in a social setting with others?
Patient's support system	If the patient is not able to independently remember and follow necessary compensations, are there staff or family members present for each meal who can help?
	How much cueing will be necessary?
	Can an oral hygiene plan be implemented for the patient?
	Does the patient self-feed or require assistance?

Table 4.3
Wording in Recommendations About NG or PEG

Do not make recommendations that prescribe to the physician	Instead provide the physician with enough information to make the determination	Should it be short term or long term?
This patient needs an NG tube to supplement oral feeding.	Results of the evaluation reveal patient appears safe to eat a _____ diet with _____ liquids with these compensations: _____. However, due to patient's [lethargy, fatigue, severity of impairment, need for multiple compensatory strategies], it is suspected he will not be able to eat enough to maintain nutrition.	Because it is likely the patient will [experience spontaneous recovery, gain strength quickly] consider NG tube for short term supplementation.
This patient needs a PEG tube to supplement oral feeding.		Because it is likely the patient will take some time (e.g., weeks, months) to [regain strength, see results from exercise to improve impaired physiology] consider longer term form of supplementation such as PEG.
This patient should be NPO and needs NG.	Results of the evaluation reveal patient is not able to consume any consistencies safely, with [aspiration, silent aspiration, significant risk for aspiration of residue] due to [describe impaired physiology]	Prognosis for [return of some function, responding to treatment of the impairments] is good, consider short term form of alternative nutrition such as NG.
This patient should be NPO and needs PEG.		Prognosis for [return of some function, responding to treatment of the impairments] is poor or will take some time (e.g., weeks, months), consider more permanent form of alternative nutrition, such as PEG.*

*See Chapter 7 for information on use of PEG at end of life.

regarding water intake to follow a set protocol and examine outcomes. They also concluded that a larger-scale study was needed to assess the safety of such a protocol, as at the time of publication, in 1997, there was insufficient literature supporting widespread use of this approach, particularly with very ill, nonambulatory patients.

Other studies have since been completed, and the results of a few are summarized here. Carlaw et al. (2012) modified the FFWP to specify in more detail how the patient could take water and the oral hygiene regimen; they called this the GF Strong Water Protocol. In their trial with 15 patients in an inpatient rehabilitation setting, study participants remained free of adverse events, including pneumonia, over the course of an initial 14-day trial and continuing until discharge from the facility (range = 13–108 days).

Karagiannis and Karagiannis (2014) completed two studies. In their earlier study, six of 42 patients randomly assigned to a free water protocol developed pneumonia or respiratory symptoms, compared to none of the patients assigned to the thickened-liquid-only control group. In that study, most participants had multiple medical diagnoses including disease other than CVA, and patients with degenerative neurologic dysfunction and patients who were immobile were included. In a 2014 study by Karagiannis and Karagiannis, only patients who were ambulatory and had relatively good cognitive status were recruited. In this relatively small study ($N = 16$), patients with acute stroke (within 3 weeks) served as their own control, and the authors found that aspiration pneumonia did not develop when the free water protocol was used. That is, access to water did not result in any instances of pneumonia, dehydration, or other complications during the short study period. Patients indicated improved quality of life on three measures: quality of drinks, hydration, and oral mouth care.

Murray and colleagues conducted a similar study with a small number of patients ($N = 14$) poststroke in a rehabilitation setting (Murray, Doeltgen, Miller, & Scholten, 2016). These authors excluded patients who were poststroke who also had a condition that put them at increased risk of respiratory complications, such as a chronically suppressed immune system or chronic obstructive pulmonary disease (COPD). There was no difference in the total amount of beverages consumed between the water protocol group and the thickened-liquids-only group. Participants in the water protocol group drank water, but their total amount did not differ because it was offset by drinking less thickened liquids. This is similar to the Garon et al. (1997) findings, whose patients' hydration improved over time compared with participants in the thickened-liquids-only group, but differences between groups were not significant.

A systematic review of the literature concerning free water protocols was conducted by Gillman, Winkler, and Taylor (2016), who found

> low-quality evidence indicating that carefully selected adult rehabilitation inpatients, who do not have degenerative neurological conditions and who are relatively mobile with reasonably intact cognition (or access to supervision to compensate for a cognitive deficit), should be given the choice to implement the Free Water Protocol, and that this may increase their fluid intake levels. Swallow-related quality of life may also improve. This body of evidence highlights the importance of managing other risk factors for acquiring lung complications such as aggressive oral hygiene. It is recommended that clinicians carefully consider the limitations discussed above before implementing this protocol with patients and ensure that the guidelines . . . are closely adhered to. (p. 14)

The principles used in the studies reviewed included the following:

- Access allowed to water before and 30 minutes after meals
- Oral hygiene before drinking water
- Thickened fluids with meals
- Ice chips are considered thin liquid
- Meds not given with water
- Compensatory techniques used when indicated
- Supervision may be required for patients with impulsivity
- Family educated
- Well-trained staff

Gillman et al. (2016) also pointed out that "further research is also required to identify an appropriate oral hygiene program and to determine if this protocol can be implemented within other settings such as the acute, outpatient and residential care settings" (p. 14).

Coyle (2011) challenged the results of studies supporting the use of a free water protocol, indicating that because of the design of the studies, it is difficult to determine the impact of the aggressive oral hygiene program on the outcomes of patients in the water protocols.

In the same journal issue where Panther (2005) described the Frazier Free Water Protocol, Brady-Wagner (2005) discussed legal and ethical considerations for facilities considering instituting such a protocol. She indicates that facilities should consider the following:

- Professionals should employ a full informed consent process.
- Facilities should utilize the highest level of evidence-based care.
- Facilities should involve all appropriate clinical disciplines when considering the legal implications to instituting such a program (Wagner, 2005).

These recommendations are still appropriate, although there is more research to consider now than when the article was written in 2005. If speech–language pathologists want to let a single patient in their facility follow a free water protocol, they should consider all risk factors involved (e.g., patient's overall health, ambulation status, oral hygiene, training and compliance of staff).

If the Patient Is to Take PO, What Are the Diet Recommendations?

Dysphagia diets should address the texture of foods, including their cohesiveness, and the thickness or flow properties of liquids. There is a great variation among facilities concerning how they name and describe different dysphagia diets. There is also typically a great deal of inconsistency in how a particular food is prepared from day to day. For example, a pureed vegetable may be quite thick on one day and runny another, depending on the kitchen staff who prepare the food. Previous editions of this manual have included diet levels and foods on each level. Those diet levels have been eliminated in this edition for many reasons. For example, there are various ways to prepare food, and something described as "cohesive" on a diet level may be cohesive when prepared in one kitchen but not another. This lack of standardization could lead to confusion when trying to implement diet levels. Clinicians are instead encouraged to consult the International Dysphagia Diet Standardisation Initiative (IDDSI) guidelines to see how those descriptions compare to the diet levels used at their facilities (Cichero et al., 2017; Initiative, 2017; Lam, Stanschus, Zaman, & Cichero, 2016). See below for more information on the IDDSI.

TEXTURES OF FOODS

Patients with pharyngeal problems who are at risk of aspiration sometimes have more difficulty with thinned, runny purees because the disordered mechanism cannot respond in time with sufficient control to protect the airway. For such individuals, foods like macaroni and cheese or baked potato maintain a cohesive texture and do not easily break up in the mouth. They can typically be swallowed as a single bolus and are probably tolerated better than runny purees. These kinds of foods may trigger a weak swallow response better than runny, pureed foods do.

As the patient progresses, food items that require more manipulation are added, and the consistency of the liquids is thinned. Generally, avoid foods that fall or break apart in the mouth (e.g., dried muffins; pound cake; plain rice; coconut; foods with multiple consistencies, such as fruit cocktail or soup with pieces). This precaution helps prevent small pieces of food from entering the airway.

Keep in mind that a pureed diet is usually not very palatable or visually appealing. A creative clinical nutrition specialist can be a big help in changing the way foods look. Molds are available to shape pureed fruits and vegetables. For example, a mold can be used to change a bowl of pureed peas into what appears to be a pile of little round peas. Pureed meats can be molded in a loaf pan and then sliced. In addition, a slurry (made by mixing milk and a food thickener) can be poured over bread and cake products. The bread retains its shape but takes on a pureed texture.

THICKNESS AND FLOW PROPERTIES OF LIQUIDS

Thickness of liquids is a complex issue that involves not only viscosity but also how the liquid flows. The goal should be to keep the patient on thin liquids if possible. Thin liquids are more palatable, and therefore the patient may drink more fluids and stay hydrated. However, for many patients with dysphagia a change in consistency of liquids may be needed to ensure safety.

If a patient has extremely poor tongue control, particularly of the back of the tongue, liquids will roll over the back of the tongue before the patient has control of the bolus and is ready to begin a swallow. Thin liquids may be aspirated more easily. Thicker liquids reduce the risk of penetration and aspiration. Although it cannot be assumed to apply to all patient populations, one study found that patients with Parkinson's who aspirated honey-thick liquids developed pneumonia more often than those that aspirated nectar, prompting one to consider that thicker may not always be the better recommendation. In addition, because they are thicker, these materials result in more pharyngeal residue, which may place the patient at risk for later aspiration (Robbins, Gensler, et al., 2008).

One of the most difficult challenges when working with patients is getting them to take enough thickened liquids to meet their fluid needs. The dietitian can help you incorporate high-fluid-content foods into the patient's diet, such as pureed fruits, custard, gelatins, and frozen juice. Work closely with the dietitian regarding the patient's nutritional needs and calorie counts. Liquids are not just beverages but also soups and broth. Also, things that liquefy in the mouth before being swallowed are considered a liquid, such as ice cream and gelatin.

Numerous studies have confirmed that inter- and intrarater reliability in mixing thickened liquids is not good. What an individual SLP considers "nectar thick" or mildly thick one day is different from what that same SLP considers as such another day (Garcia, Chambers, Matta, & Clark, 2005; Glassburn & Deem, 1998; Steele, Van Lieshout, & Goff, 2003). Commercially available prethickened liquids are used in some facilities, which then increases consistency of viscosity from day to day. However, these are more expensive than buying thickener and mixing, and so even facilities that purchase some prethickened liquids also mix to thicken others. For example, they might stock prethickened liquids on nursing floors but mix in the kitchen for meals.

STARCH VERSUS GUM THICKENERS

Starch-based powder thickeners are usually made of modified cornstarch or maltodextrin, which is also derived from corn. These thickeners can be mixed with most beverages to reach a desired consistency. Clear liquids will appear cloudy, and beverages will have a slightly grainy texture. For best results, and to avoid over- or underthickening, measure the amounts of liquid and starch per the manufacturer's directions.

Gum-based thickeners usually contain xanthan and/or cellulose gums. Gum thickeners work well in all types of hot and cold beverages. Clear beverages remain clear and do not become cloudy. Gum thickeners require accurate measuring and vigorous mixing to get them into solution. They will require about 5 minutes to reach consistency but then will remain at that same consistency. Gum powders or gels can be used to thicken pureed foods; however, they do not "stiffen" as well as starch thickeners do. Because they result in a softer puree, they do not work as well for molded foods or when a food is intended to hold its shape (Purchasing Guide for Thickeners, 2012).

Foods other than commercial thickeners can also be used to change the consistency of liquids, but they may change the food flavor or texture. These foods include instant or mashed potatoes, unflavored gelatin, and baby rice cereal.

International Dysphagia Diet Standardisation Initiative

In 2015, the IDDSI published a framework to standardize the way diet levels and thickness of liquids were described (Figure 4.4). The framework uses thin liquid and four levels of thickness to describe the flow properties of drinks, from thin to extremely thick. The framework for food texture includes regular and four levels of modification, from soft and bite-sized to liquid. The drink and food frameworks, in the form of triangles, overlap, so that moderately thick drinks align with liquid foods and extremely thick drinks with pureed foods because of the similarity of their flow behavior.

IDDSI Method for Testing Texture

The IDDSI has developed methods to standardize how to determine the texture of a particular food. Their measurement of foods captures mechanical properties (e.g., hardness, cohesiveness,

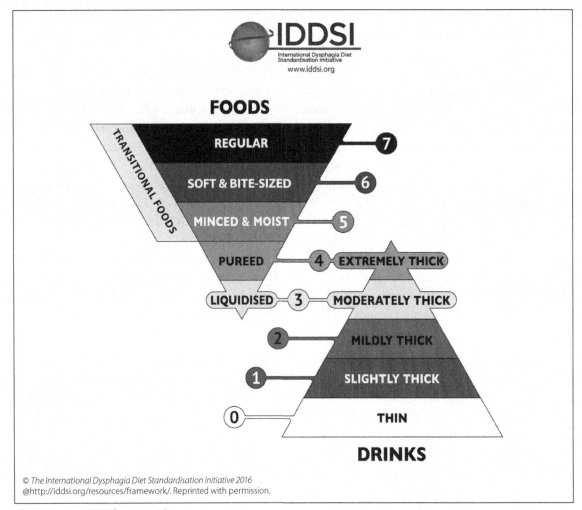

Figure 4.4 IDDSI framework.

adhesiveness) and particle size as well as geometrical or shape attributes, particularly relevant with respect to choking risks. The IDDSI recommends a combination of tests for pureed, soft, firm, and solid foods, including fork drip, spoon tilt, fork or spoon pressure, chopstick, and finger tests. Directions and videos are available on the IDDSI website regarding how to perform the test (Food Testing Methods, 2018).

IDDSI Method for Testing Thickness of Liquids

The IDDSI does not include a measure of viscosity; it states that viscosity is only one of the parameters that measure liquid thickness and flow. Instead, the IDDSI devised a gravity flow test that can be performed easily with the use of a 10-cc syringe. When using the IDDSI classifications, it is important that the barrel length of the syringe measures 61.5 mm from the 0–10-cc markers on the syringe. Using this method, a facility or individual SLP can ensure uniformity when preparing and classifying thickened drinks. Directions and videos are available on the IDDSI website regarding how to perform the test (Drink Testing Methods, 2018).

Implementing the IDDSI Framework

The IDDSI website (https://www.iddsi.org) has information on how one might implement the framework at his or her facility.

Types of Treatment Techniques and Strategies

When developing a treatment plan, it is imperative to think of the types of strategies that can be used in addition to any needed diet and bolus modifications (which are certainly compensatory) (Figure 4.5). These additional techniques are compensatory (which include postural changes and techniques to help patients gain more control over the bolus) and rehabilitative. Some strategies are both rehabilitative and compensatory. For example, the super-supraglottic swallow can be used during meals to increase purposeful closure of the airway to keep food from entering the laryngeal vestibule. This same technique, when practiced repetitively, may actually restore function so that the laryngeal vestibule closes more effectively even when the technique is no longer used. In most cases, the treatment plan will utilize a combination of these strategies, and the combinations may change over time.

Compensatory Strategies

Compensatory strategies are those designed to compensate for lost or impaired function. They are designed not to improve the impaired anatomy or physiology but to help patients have a more functional, effective, safe, or efficient swallow. Bolus modifications are a type of compensatory strategy that overlaps with diet texture and liquid flow, as described above. Two other types of compensation are postural and techniques designed to give the patient more control of the bolus. Bolus modifications and techniques to gain control of the bolus are related. Compensatory strategies are effective only when in use and when immediate response to compensation can be observed. In fact, many of the techniques we consider rehabilitative have been shown to have only short-term effects, and thus they are more accurately described as compensatory.

DIET AND BOLUS MODIFICATIONS

In addition to recommending appropriate textures of foods and thickness of liquids, dysphagia treatment must address any other bolus modifications needed, including how boluses are presented, such as liquids only per spoon. Things like temperature, touch, and taste are used to lead to changes in motor output. If the change in motor output is only temporary (e.g., improvement on one swallow), then the technique can appropriately be considered compensatory. There is not much data on sensory stimulation to indicate anything but a transient effect (Sapienza, Wheeler-Hegland,

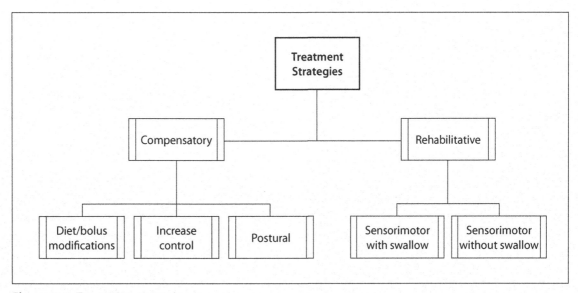

Figure 4.5 Treatment strategies.

Stewart, & Nocera, 2008). Most sensory strategies involve changes in bolus presentation (e.g., taste, temperature).

CONTROL COMPENSATORY STRATEGIES

An example of a compensatory strategy to help patients gain control of the bolus might be applying external pressure to the impaired side of the lips if the patient is losing liquids from the front of the mouth. Another example might be to have a patient with unilateral lingual weakness place the bolus of food into the oral cavity on the stronger side. This will help keep the bolus on the chewing surface, where the patient has more control. Presentation of a bolus is also considered a compensatory strategy, designed to help the patient gain control. For example, some patients may handle a bolus of thin liquid more efficiently or safely when delivered from a cup instead of a straw.

POSTURAL COMPENSATORY STRATEGIES

An example of a postural compensatory strategy is to have a patient with unilateral pharyngeal weakness turn the head toward the weak side when swallowing a bolus. This directs the bolus through the strong side of the pharynx and may result in less residue. In general, postural changes are designed to redirect bolus flow in the oral and/or pharyngeal phases.

None of these compensatory strategies will have any impact on the actual function of the lips, tongue, or pharynx. They might, however, help individuals eat and drink more efficiently, thus compensating for the impairment.

PRESCRIBING COMPENSATIONS TO BE USED DURING MEALS

When selecting strategies for the patient to use during meals, consider the impact that the use of the strategies will have on the individual. Is the strategy hard to remember? Will the person remember to use it with every swallow? Does the strategy require physical effort (e.g., effortful swallow, super-supraglottic swallow) that might fatigue the person? If it requires too much effort and work, will the patient not finish the meal, compromising nutritional status? Will the patient be able to consistently use the strategy throughout the meal, or will he or she need cues? If cues are needed, who will consistently provide them?

PHYSICAL THERAPY EXAMPLE OF COMPENSATIONS

A physical therapy example might help solidify the concept of compensation. If a person injured her knee and could not bear weight on that leg, the physical therapist might have the person use crutches while the knee is healing. The crutches would certainly allow the individual to get around, but the use of the crutches in no way will actively help improve function of the knee.

A physical therapy example of a postural change might be a person suffering a back injury who complains of pain while sitting. The physical therapist might suggest that the person sit with a pillow behind the lower back and both feet planted on the floor. This posture might provide relief from the pain. Does it actually help with healing the injury? It likely does not, but one might argue that sitting with a better posture might facilitate a better balance between the flexors and extensors in the back and aid in healing.

Rehabilitative Techniques

Rehabilitative techniques are designed to, and in some cases have been demonstrated to, effectively change the physiology of the swallow, not just when the strategy is in use but also to make the swallow more efficient and safe after therapy has ended. The effortful swallow, for example, has been shown to result in clinical improvement in the swallow (Huckabee, Butler, Barclay, & Jit, 2005). The effortful swallow is also a good example of a rehabilitative strategy that improves more than one aspect of physiology. It has been shown to improve linguapalatal pressure, tongue base to pharyngeal wall pressure, hyolaryngeal excursion, and submental muscle activity (Hind,

Nicosia, Roecker, Carnes, & Robbins, 2001; Huckabee et al., 2005; Lazarus, Logemann, Song, Rademaker, & Kahrilas, 2002). The strategies should target underlying physiologic impairment identified during assessment. Strategies thought to be rehabilitative in nature should have evidence to support the claims of a change in physiology. However, many strategies have some evidence of change with healthy individuals but not with patients. Other strategies have evidence related to one population but not another. For example, one can read studies that were performed with individuals recovering from stroke but did not include patients with other neurological disorders (Hagg & Aniko, 2008; McCullough et al., 2012). Still others do not have evidence to support their use, but clinicians use them because they are based on principles of neuroplasticity or motor learning and address physiological impairment.

Unlike compensatory strategies (e.g., bolus modification, postural and increasing control), which can sometimes be applied or used without the patient's active participation, rehabilitative techniques require that the person be able to understand, follow directions, and perform sometimes very complex actions. For example, the super-supraglottic swallow requires that the individual do the following: take a breath, let a little out, hold the breath tightly in the throat, swallow hard, breathe out, cough, swallow again. There are certainly many adults for whom following such a multistep command might be far too challenging.

PHYSICAL THERAPY EXAMPLES OF REHABILITATIVE TECHNIQUES

These are often described as modalities: hot packs, strengthening exercises, ultrasound, iontophoresis, moist heat, and so on. In contrast to the rehabilitative techniques for swallowing, some of these physical therapy techniques are passive and do not require active participation by the individual.

SWALLOWING REHABILITATIVE STRATEGIES USED AS COMPENSATIONS.

Rehabilitative strategies are typically used during a treatment session and not during meals, although some can also be used as compensations. For example, the Mendelsohn maneuver can be used on each swallow of pureed food to sustain hyolaryngeal elevation, thus reducing pyriform sinus residue and allowing for a safe swallow. In this way, it is a compensation. In addition to this application as a compensation, studies have also shown that in some populations, use of the Mendelsohn maneuver as a rehabilitative strategy results in actual long-term improvement in hyolaryngeal excursion and an improved, functional swallow (McCullough et al., 2012; McCullough & Kim, 2013).

Theoretical Basis for Rehabilitative Techniques and Exercises

Planning and implementing dysphagia therapy is not like following a recipe in a cookbook. The clinician must understand the basis for rehabilitative exercise, including thorough knowledge of the following:

- Physiology of swallowing
  - Normal swallow
  - Abnormal swallow
- Evidence for techniques
- Related principles
  - Neural plasticity
  - Motor control and motor learning

Although this book supplies many charts to help clinicians organize and structure decision making during treatment planning to keep a focus on physiology, skilled dysphagia clinicians also use tools like the Chapter 4 Appendix, together with knowledge of evidence for each technique and an understanding of muscle function and related principles. When evidence has demonstrated that a treatment technique *does* work, that evidence should help the clinician determine whether the technique will be beneficial to a particular client. However, the clinician should also use the knowledge of related principles to understand why a particular exercise was attempted for that impaired physiology in the first place. When there is lack of evidence, the clinician uses information about these related principles to determine whether a treatment strategy *should* work. The treatment technique should make sense when the clinician applies knowledge of physiology, evidence, and related principles. Consider these important questions that will require such information to answer:

- Given the etiology of dysphagia, can the impaired physiology in this patient actually be changed?
- Could a certain exercise do more harm than good?
- How frequently should the exercise be practiced?
- How many repetitions of the exercise are needed to obtain a benefit?
- Should the practice sessions be spaced out or massed together?

Principles of Neural Plasticity

Neural plasticity describes the brain's ability to change, to alter neuronal systems in response to changes in input (Burke & Barnes, 2006; Huttenlocher, 2009; Kleim & Jones, 2008). Neural plastic changes indicate that a change has taken place in synaptic function in a specific neural substrate. These changes occur as a result of input. Some input achieves neural plastic changes resulting in improved behavioral response (e.g., training, cues, experience), whereas other input (e.g., aging, disease, injury) may result in neural plastic changes resulting in impaired behavioral response. Some input is designed not to change a neural pathway but to use a different neural pathway to compensate for loss. Compensatory strategies such as postural changes are an example of utilizing a different neural pathway (Robbins, Butler, et al., 2008).

When utilizing specific rehabilitation strategies for improved swallowing, the clinician intends to achieve not only a change in strength, speed, and coordination of specific muscle movements or sensorimotor responses, resulting in a behavioral change, but also a change in the underlying neural pathways that guide that movement. Martin (2009) points out that there is mounting evidence that "(1) swallowing neural substrates can undergo plastic changes as a function of experience, and (2) these swallowing neuroplastic changes may be associated with modulated swallowing behavior" (p. 219).

Ten principles of neural plasticity have been described and related to rehabilitation strategies used in swallowing. These principles as they pertain to swallowing are being studied in some translational research, but there is not definitive information (Kleim & Jones, 2008; Robbins, Butler, et al., 2008). However, the clinician should consider these principles in decision making regarding dysphagia management. Much of what is known about these principles comes from the study of change in skeletal muscle in large-muscle groups. A simple example of each principle is provided in Table 4.4. For an in-depth review of swallowing literature related to the principles, readers are referred to the Robbins, Butler, et al. (2008) article.

A brief highlight of these principles, summarized from the referenced articles, follows.

USE IT OR LOSE IT

If a certain brain function is not used, then the behavioral response can degrade. If a person is kept NPO, using the swallowing mechanism only for swallowing saliva, does this disuse of the mechanism result in reduced cortical representation for swallowing?

Table 4.4
Examples of Principles of Neural Plasticity

Principle	Example in physical activity	Consideration in swallowing
Use it or lose it	Individual was excellent golfer in high school but has not played in 20 years. Putting ability would not be as good now as it was.	What is the implication for a patient made NPO?
Use it and improve it	Individual plays golf daily and applies what golf coach has taught each time to improve swing.	Providing cues and instructions for improved swallowing is important during treatment, not just swallowing repetitively.
Specificity (experience specific)	Practicing a golf swing would likely not result in a change in the neural substrates for a swing of a tennis racket.	The exercise should be closely related to the movement needed for swallowing.
Repetition matters	If a person wants to improve strength in biceps, he or she would perform multiple bicep curls, not just one.	Swallowing exercises must be practiced enough.
Intensity matters	The bicep curls would involve a weight heavy enough the person would have to work hard to lift, not performing curls with a very light weight.	Swallowing exercises should perhaps be performed not a specific number of times but until fatigue.
Time matters	Weight training at the gym would involve a lengthy session (e.g., 25, not 5, minutes) and would occur consistently (e.g., several times/week rather than once a month).	How many times a day should the client practice? How many days per week?
Salience matters	If the person desires to do more hiking, and needs stronger leg muscles to do so, practicing squats and leg presses at the gym would make the exercise more salient.	If the client understands that a certain exercise may improve function and help return to eating, then the exercise might be more salient.
Age matters	Learning a sport as a youth is easier than picking it up at an older age, although you *can* teach an old dog new tricks.	Is prognosis for improvement in swallowing better for a younger client?
Transference	Training improved backhand swing in tennis might also improve backhand in racquetball.	Will improved lingual motion for swallowing liquids transfer to improved lingual motion with solids?
Interference	Skills learned for downhill skiing could interfere with learning skills for snowboarding, which requires different movements and positions.	Could a swallowing exercise interfere with the neural pathway necessary for another swallow movement?

Note. Adapted from Martin (2009) and Robbins et al. (2008).

USE IT AND IMPROVE IT

Function can be improved through use. This is especially true if the activity involves practice designed to improve the performance of the activity. That is, repetitive swallowing alone might not result in a change, but that the practice should involve working to change some aspect of the swallow, such as increased strength or coordination.

SPECIFICITY

Plasticity is related to the specific skill being practiced. Practicing one skill will not necessarily result in a change to a different area of the brain. Specificity indicates that the movement being trained should be close to the movement needed during the functional target task. For example, training lingual strength on an isotonic endurance task did not increase endurance on an isometric endurance task (Clark, 2012).

REPETITION MATTERS

To change neural substrates, practice must be extensive and continue for a period of time. What is not known is how many repetitions of an exercise should be performed or how long an isometric position (e.g., tongue press) should be sustained.

INTENSITY MATTERS

To achieve neural change, practice must occur frequently and the activity must force the body beyond the typical level of activity in order to achieve neuromuscular adaptation. When the term *intensity* is used relative to weight training for skeletal muscles (e.g., bicep curls), intensity can be adjusted by increasing the weight and/or number of repetitions. When using an instrument such as the Iowa Performance Instrument (IOPI), the intensity can be increased, but with most swallowing exercises that do not use instrumentation, the "weight" or resistance cannot be increased. Therefore, intensity is addressed by increasing the number of repetitions. Related to specific swallowing rehabilitation strategies, although we do not know how many repetitions are enough, Burkhead (2009) suggests that patients work to the point of fatigue rather than perform a specific number of repetitions or sets. When the term *intensity* is used related to sensory treatment, the meaning does not refer to resistance or number of repetitions but to the intensity of the sensory stimulus being applied.

TIME MATTERS

Long periods of training and continuous training (rather than intermittent) may result in maximal neural change (Fisher & Sullivan, 2001). The clinician must apply this concept at the right time during the course of treatment. For example, in the early days after a stroke, the individual may not be able to participate in long treatment sessions. At that point in the continuum, compensatory strategies could be used until the individual can fully participate in therapy and benefit most from the use of rehabilitation strategies. Conversely, the concept of time being important might also indicate that the rehabilitation strategies should be initiated earlier in the recovery phase.

SALIENCE MATTERS

The movement being practiced has to be functional, important to the individual, and related to the behavior being trained (Morgen et al., 2004; Remple, Bruneau, VandenBerg, Goertzen, & Kleim, 2001). If the clinician intends to change swallowing, then the exercises taught must be related to swallowing.

AGE MATTERS

The younger brain is more adaptive and plastic, so that training behaviors in a young adult is more likely to result in neural plasticity than training in an individual who is elderly. Neural plasticity does occur across the life span, although the response decreases with age (Kramer, Erickson, & Colcombe, 2006; Sawaki, Yaseen, Kopylev, & Cohen, 2003).

TRANSFERENCE

Plasticity in response to training one behavior can enhance acquisition of similar behaviors. Training tongue lateralization to clear the sulci might enhance acquisition of tongue lateralization to place food on the chewing surface.

INTERFERENCE

Plasticity within a given neural structure can impede that structure from other, more beneficial plasticity. A person might learn a maladaptive compensation, which then might impede them using the same neural circuitry to learn an appropriate behavior.

Neuromuscular Treatments and Motor Learning

Rehabilitative therapy techniques for swallowing largely involve attempts to teach a muscle or group of muscles to produce highly skilled movements, and hope that the change in a behavior (how a muscle works) also results in a change in neural circuitry. Much of the work on neuromuscular treatments is derived from the work of physical therapists, who work on large muscles in the limbs. Muscle fiber types in these large muscles often differ from the muscle fiber types found in the small muscles of the lips, tongue, cheek, and soft palate, and therefore the same types of treatments cannot be applied to the oral musculature, hoping to achieve the same results. Another difference in limb muscles and muscles of the oral mechanism is that in the limb system, it is fairly easy to identify a single muscle group (e.g., bicep) and work just on that muscle. In the oral mechanism and pharynx, many muscle groups overlap in structure and function. In addition, there is less lateralization in function of the brain for oropharyngeal function compared to limb function (Burkhead, 2009; Martin, 2009).

There is a difference between *motor performance* and *motor learning*. Motor performance is the short-term behavioral change that is achieved after instruction, coaching, and cueing. A patient might be able to demonstrate improved motor performance each time on an exercise. Motor learning occurs when there is a more permanent change in the performance based on repeated practice. This is likely when a change has occurred in the neural circuitry.

The possible consequences in failing to understand and apply knowledge of neuromuscular treatment and exercise science appropriately could mean the patient does not benefit from the treatment or that the treatment might even make the swallowing worse. An even more serious consequence is that the swallowing might get worse as a result of the treatment applied. For example, strength training is a form of active exercise. Strength training can produce fatigue, and with a disease like Parkinson's, working to the point of fatigue might reduce strength reserves (Solomon, 2006).

Conversely, there are instances in which it is appropriate to use strengthening techniques. Oral-phase dysphagia is often characterized by lingual weakness, and working on strength training is often indicated (Youmans, Youmans, & Stierwalt, 2009).

SENSORY IN SENSORIMOTOR

Swallowing is a complex sensorimotor behavior. Clinicians tend to overlook the sensory component to the compensatory (bolus modifications, increased control, postural) and rehabilitative strategies that are implemented. When sensory input is intentionally provided as part of the technique, it is with the intention to promote a motor response. For example, when using a sour stimulus bolus, the intent is to improve the timeliness of the pharyngeal response.

Whether the motor exercise is motor with a swallow or motor without a swallow, any motor behavior in and of itself provides sensory feedback to the system in the feedback–feed forward loop, by which movements are improved. For example, the Shaker exercise (motor without a swallow) does not provide any external sensory input, but the movement itself is providing sensory feedback to the peripheral and central nervous system. The Mendelsohn maneuver (motor with a swallow) also does not provide any intentional sensory input, but performing the maneuver provides sensory feedback in the loop. This sensory feedback is crucial to the client's learning to improve the movement.

Planning Treatment: Signs, Functional Impact, and Impaired Physiology

As clinicians begin working with patients with dysphagia, they tend to focus on the signs and symptoms (Figure 4.6). Signs are the characteristics observed during a bedside/clinical evaluation or during an instrumental assessment. Clinicians might observe liquid loss from the front of the mouth on a clinical exam or residue in the pyriform sinuses during an instrumental exam. A symptom is subjective, or typically what the patient reports to you that he or she is experiencing (e.g., "food feels like it is sticking," "I get choked on coffee"). As the speech–language pathologist's skills improve, the clinician "sees" the physiological problem. That is, instead of first noticing vallecular residue during a VFSS, the clinician notes the reduced tongue base movement that has resulted in the residue. The more experienced the dysphagia clinician becomes, the more the speech–language pathologist sees the impaired physiology first and understands what is causing the sign or symptom. The clinician also begins to link the sign and impaired physiology more easily to the impact it has on the functional swallow.

Trying to plan treatment based on a sign or symptom without a full understanding of the impaired physiology causing that sign or symptom can mean that SLP selects the wrong treatment strategies. One sign can have more than one cause. For example, residue in the valleculae may be related to reduced tongue-base movement or reduced pharyngeal wall squeeze (or both). Different treatment techniques are needed to address tongue base and pharyngeal walls.

Organizing Intervention Techniques for Safe and Efficient Swallow

A swallow must be both safe and efficient (Figure 4.7). A safe swallow is one in which there is no airway compromise. There is adequate and timely airway closure in the pharyngeal phase. An efficient swallow is one that clears oral and pharyngeal residue with little to no extra effort. Safety is achieved through airway closure and bolus clearance, whereas efficiency is all about bolus clearance.

Airway Closure

Airway closure can be affected by problems in coordinating movements, or impairments in the actual movements. These can be caused by neurological changes or by surgical changes in the structures of the mouth, pharynx, or larynx.

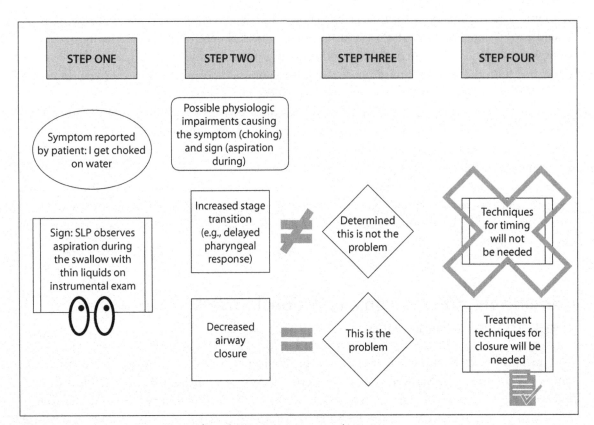

Figure 4.6 Signs and symptoms for selecting treatment techniques.

TIMING AND COORDINATION IMPAIRMENTS AFFECTING AIRWAY CLOSURE

In the pharyngeal phase, timing and coordination impairments that can affect airway closure include the following:

- Increased stage transition duration or delayed initiation of the pharyngeal response (with the bolus too low in the hypopharynx before closure occurs)

- Mistiming of the pharyngeal response (such that closure does not occur at the correct time during bolus movement, but the bolus does not dwell long enough in the pharynx to be considered a delay)

MOVEMENT IMPAIRMENTS AFFECTING AIRWAY CLOSURE CAN INCLUDE

- Poor back-of-tongue control (which can allow the bolus to enter the airway prematurely)

- Reduced closure at the level of the vocal folds (which may result in aspiration during the swallow)

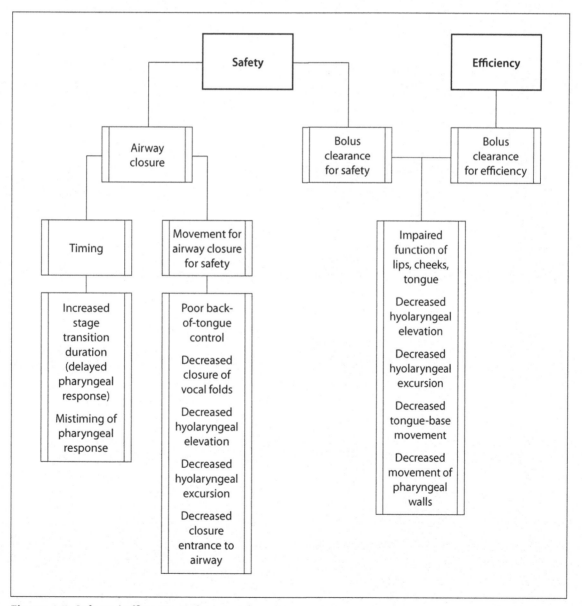

Figure 4.7 Safe and efficient oropharyngeal swallow.

- Reduced hyolaryngeal elevation or superior movement (which results in lower position of the larynx before and during the swallow, allowing for penetration and/or aspiration)

- Reduced hyolaryngeal anterior movement (which also leaves the airway exposed)

- Reduced closure at the entrance to the airway (reduced tipping of the arytenoids and folding in of the aryepiglottic folds, leaving the laryngeal vestibule exposed)

Bolus Clearance

Bolus clearance is essential for both safety and efficiency of the swallow.

ORAL MOVEMENTS FOR BOLUS CLEARANCE

All oral movements essentially serve the purpose of clearing the bolus from the oral cavity. If a bolus is not formed cohesively, it will likely leave residue. If anterior–posterior movements of the tongue are impaired, there will be residue.

EFFICIENT MOVEMENT OF PHARYNGEAL STRUCTURES FOR BOLUS CLEARANCE

Some of these same movements of structures needed for airway closure are also important to efficiently move the bolus through the pharynx so that there is no residue after the swallow that could compromise the airway:

- Reduced hyolaryngeal elevation and superior movement (which can contribute to residue in pyriform sinuses)

- Reduced hyolaryngeal anterior movement (which can contribute to residue in pyriform sinuses)

- Reduced tongue-base pressure against pharyngeal walls (which can result in residue in valleculae and/or on pharyngeal walls)

- Reduced pressure of the pharyngeal walls (which can result in residue in valleculae and on pharyngeal walls)

How to Use Treatment Techniques to Plan Treatment

Treatment strategies must be selected for oral and pharyngeal deficits. The selections are made on the basis of the impaired physiology with the intent to address a functional deficit the patient is experiencing. The reader is referred to the Chapter 4 Appendix, which delineates these techniques as compensatory and/or rehabilitative and helps the reader pair the technique with the sign observed on clinical or instrumental exam, impaired physiology intended to treat or compensate for, and intended impact on the functional swallow. The Chapter 4 Appendix should be viewed in conjunction with the next section of this chapter, which includes a comprehensive description of the treatment techniques. (Note: Table 5.2 in the Documentation chapter is organized differently, with the functional deficit listed first, then impaired physiology. That table may be easier to follow when selecting goals. See Table 4.5 for tips on when to use the Chapter 4 Appendix or Table 5.2.)

Compensatory Techniques

Some compensatory techniques may be marked in more than one category. For example, reducing sip size is a bolus modification but also gives the patient increased control of the bolus. Head tilt is postural but also gives the patient increased control. The techniques marked as rehabilitative are those designed to be rehabilitative with either some supporting evidence or a sound theoretical basis. Some rehabilitative techniques are also compensatory if they are used during PO intake. For example, the super-supraglottic swallow is rehabilitative but can be used with each swallow of food, and in those instances it is compensatory.

BOLUS MODIFICATIONS

All bolus modifications provide some sensory input. However, many bolus modifications are intended to be compensatory only to allow more control of the bolus (i.e., texture and liquid thickness changes of the bolus, or smaller bolus size). On the chart, these are marked as bolus modification and perhaps also as increased control, but the sensory input is not noted, as it is assumed.

INTENDED TO INCREASE CONTROL

Some changes to the bolus will be made with the intention that this change will give the patient more control of the bolus. For example, using a smaller bolus or a bolus of a different thickness will help the patient control the bolus in the oral cavity. Some strategies intended to increase control are not related to a bolus modification, although they may be used along with a bolus modification. For example, having the patient hold the bolus in the oral cavity and consciously prepare to swallow would be an example of a technique designed to provide increased control. It might be paired with a bolus modification of smaller size or thicker texture, but it might also be used with a normal-size bolus that has not been modified.

POSTURAL

Postural techniques are used for both the oral and pharyngeal phases. To change bolus flow, these techniques involve changing the position of the head in relationship to the neck.

Rehabilitative

These are techniques thought to have a lasting impact on the impaired physiology. They are characterized as with or without a swallow. Techniques that provide external sensory input are also indicated, as are those that utilize a device.

REHABILITATIVE: WITH A SWALLOW

These include exercises such as the supraglottic swallow or Mendelsohn maneuver. These exercises are intended to change motor behavior, perhaps a change in neural circuitry, and they follow

Table 4.5
When to Use Appendix 4.A and Table 5.2

A quick reference if you want to . . .	Use Appendix 4.A	Use Table 5.2
See what problem (sign) a technique is designed for	X	
See if a technique is compensatory or rehabilitative	X	
See the characteristics of a compensatory strategy (e.g., bolus modification, postural)	X	
See the characteristics of a rehabilitative technique (e.g., motor with or without a swallow)	X	
See what functional change is intended from using the technique	X	
See the impaired physiology related to a sign	X	X
Match a functional deficit to different physiologic causes		X
Match impaired physiology to type of problem: • Airway closure • Bolus clearance		X
Select short-term goals to address impaired physiology		X
Select treatment objectives (techniques) related to the short-term goal		X

the neuroplastic principle of specificity because a swallow is involved in the exercise. For most of these techniques, research has not demonstrated long-term, lasting effects. That is, they result in a change in behavior each time they are used but have not been demonstrated to result in a change that is maintained when the technique is no longer used. One might argue that these should be categorized, then, as compensatory, but because the intent is rehabilitation, they are marked as such.

REHABILITATIVE: WITHOUT A SWALLOW

These include exercises such as the Shaker exercise and use of the EMST (also described as a device), which are used to achieve a change in motor behavior and perhaps in neural circuitry. However, no swallow is associated with the exercises. For some of these techniques, the same caveat applies: They are intended as rehabilitative but do not have definitive evidence that they result in long-term change.

EXTERNAL SENSORY

Although, as described above, all motor movements have a sensory aspect, in the Appendix to Chapter 4, "sensory" is marked if a rehabilitative technique provides a deliberate, extrinsic sensory input (e.g., cold, carbonated), as these sensory techniques are intended to achieve a change in the motor output. They are included as "rehabilitative" though these have only short-term effects. For example, sour boluses may improve the timing of the swallow, but only when the patient is swallowing that sour stimuli. On the chart, these techniques will almost always be indicated as external sensory *and* sensorimotor with a swallow. They are described below with the rehabilitative techniques.

DEVICE

This column is marked in two situations: if a commercially available device can be used paired with the exercise listed (e.g., using sEMG with the Mendelsohn; using NMES with Effortful Swallow), or when the device is used as the exercise itself, not paired with another technique (e.g., NMES at the sensory level only; EMST). These exercises are also marked as sensorimotor with or without a swallow.

Signs, Physiology, and Function

The Chapter 4 Appendix makes it clear that one impairment in physiology may result in different signs (e.g., weakness in the lips can cause anterior bolus loss and reduced ability to close lips on a spoon). A careful review of that material also shows that one sign can have different physiologic causes (e.g., penetration can be related to impaired timing or to poor back-of-tongue control). It also demonstrates that some treatment techniques (e.g., effortful swallow) address more than one physiologic deficit (e.g., tongue-base retraction, reduced tongue-to-palate pressure).

Treatment Techniques: How to Perform, and Related Evidence

The following section of the book is organized to move from compensatory strategies (not broken down by phase) to rehabilitative strategies, first for oral and then for pharyngeal.

Treatment for problems in the oral preparatory phase are designed to get the bolus into the oral cavity, place it mid-tongue, and prepare it for transit to the back of the oral cavity, while preventing spillage over the back of the tongue or from the front of the mouth. Treatment for the oral (transit) phase should help the client move a cohesive bolus from the mid-tongue to the back of the oral cavity and over the back of the tongue. This requires intact structures and coordinated movements of the lips, jaw, tongue, and soft palate. Compensatory and rehabilitative strategies can be used to treat problems in the oral preparatory and oral (transit) phases, although because of a lack of evidence of the effectiveness of many rehabilitation exercises for oral motor movements, many times the clinician relies on compensatory strategies.

There is little empirical evidence for most of the oral, and many of the pharyngeal, rehabilitative techniques discussed here. Empirical evidence helps a clinician determine if a specific technique works. Considered a must-read on neuromuscular treatments for swallowing is a tutorial by Heather Clark (2003, 2005) that explains the different types of exercises (e.g., active, passive, stretching, physical modalities). Understanding the theoretical framework for neuromuscular treatments helps the clinician understand whether a technique should work.

Readers are also referred to a series of evidence-based systematic reviews undertaken by ASHA's National Center for Evidence-Based Practice (NCEP), which examined treatments for oropharyngeal dysphagia treatments. Some of those findings are included below, but a thorough review of all four parts is essential reading for clinicians who treat dysphagia (Frymark, Mullen, Musson, & Schooling, 2009a, 2009b; Frymark, Schooling, Mullen, & Musson, 2009; Wheeler-Hegland et al., 2009).

In the early decades of dysphagia management, each phase of the swallow was viewed as a distinct phase, with no overlap. That is, when one phase ended, the next began. More recent investigations of the swallow, though, have demonstrated that the phases overlap and are well integrated (Martin-Harris, Brodsky, Michel, Lee, & Walters, 2007). There is increasing understanding of the relationship between the oral (transit) phase and the pharyngeal phase, with recognition that the movement of the tongue initiates the pharyngeal phase. More work has been done in researching techniques for pharyngeal-phase deficits than for oral deficits.

Keeping in mind Rosenbek's (1995) admonition that lack of evidence does not necessarily mean that a treatment technique does not work, clinicians should carefully use the information that is provided on commonly used compensatory and rehabilitative strategies to address functional deficits in each phase of swallowing described here. Most of these techniques are described in a patient handout included with the Supplemental Materials (see Education Materials Patient/Family, Swallowing Exercises Instructions). A list of the exercises that can be given to the patient is also found there (Education Materials, Patient/Family, Swallowing Exercises List). References grouped by treatment technique are found in the section Efficacy References. Readers are referred to the referenced documents for full articles about a technique.

Readers are also referred to the website of the National Foundation on Swallowing Disorders (NFOSD, 2017), which provides free handouts for patients describing techniques and has videos to show how to perform some of the exercises. The NFOSD is a nonprofit patient education, support, and advocacy group.

Prerequisites for Compensatory or Rehabilitative Treatment

ORAL SENSITIVITY TRAINING

Patients who are not eating by mouth may show reduced sensitivity to material in the oral cavity. If a patient's oral cavity is very dry from mouth breathing and having no liquids, it is inappropriate to initially present food to the patient without first completing some oral sensitivity training. Be sure the patient is positioned upright, and then use a Toothette or a swab to moisten the oral cavity. Adequate saliva is essential for a patient to be able to form a good bolus. If the patient is able to complete such a maneuver, you may even have him or her swish and spit some liquid from his mouth. This sensitivity training is in addition to a regular routine of oral hygiene.

ORAL HYGIENE

Although oral hygiene is not the responsibility of the speech–language pathologist, it is an oft-neglected area of patient care. Providing oral care in health-care facilities is typically the responsibility of nursing assistants. Yet nursing tends to rate oral care as a low priority as compared to other pressing needs (Wårdh, Hallberg, Berggren, Andersson, & Sörensen, 2000). Demonstrated gaps in knowledge exist regarding oral health and the correct procedures for performing oral care (Adams, 1996; Boczko, McKeon, & Sturkie, 2009). Even when nursing assistants acknowledge that oral care is important, they still tend to perform oral care less than the optimal number of times a day and with a less-than-optimal technique (Jablonski et al., 2009).

Nursing assistants on medical floors in hospitals likely view oral care as a low priority, as has been found in other settings (e.g., skilled nursing facilities) (Wårdh et al., 2000). It is also likely that nursing assistants in an acute-care hospital lack knowledge of the relationships among oral hygiene, respiratory health, and overall health.

An interesting finding from a study of elderly nursing home residents found that intensive oral care increased cough reflex sensitivity (Watando et al., 2004). For all these reasons, and in light of the relationship between poor oral health and aspiration pneumonia, speech–language pathologists have often taken the lead in initiating or reenergizing an oral hygiene program at their facility (Harting, 2012; Swigert, 2013). See Chapter 8, Education and Advocacy, for materials to use in oral hygiene programs.

APPROPRIATE POSITIONING

During the oral intake of medicines, foods, and/or liquids, it is optimal for a patient to be seated at a 90° angle, whether in a bed or in a chair. This position is also optimal for performing rehabilitative techniques.

At bedside, use a draw sheet (a sheet placed under the patient's torso) to assist in positioning. To use the draw sheet, put the bed in a flat position and have someone stand on either side of the patient, holding on to the draw sheet. Use the sheet to pull the patient toward the head of the bed. If the patient is able, ask him or her to bend his knees and push as you pull. Raise the head of the bed to its highest point and lower the foot of the bed to its lowest point. The patient should then be sitting at a 90° angle. Pillows may need to be placed behind the patient's back and/or head to achieve the correct position. A towel roll can further help with keeping the head upright.

Similarly, for the patient seated in a chair, the 90° angle is necessary before and during feeding. If the chair has a soft or slanted back, use pillows to attain the desired angle. Being at 90° allows the patient to control material in the oral cavity with a minimal impact of gravity. This position must be maintained during and following the meal. Repositioning is frequently required during the meal.

Compensatory Strategies

Compensatory strategies are categorized into three types and are used during PO intake:

- Bolus modifications

- Strategies to give the client increased control of the bolus

- Postural changes

Bolus modifications are selected to address deficits in the oral phases as well as the pharyngeal phase. For example, a smaller bolus may be easier for the patient to manipulate in the oral cavity but may also pose less risk of residue in the pharyngeal phase. Sensory changes to the bolus may increase the client's ability to manipulate the bolus but may also change the timing of the pharyngeal phase.

Strategies to increase control also have implications for the oral and pharyngeal phases. Holding the bolus and waiting to swallow may help the client maintain the bolus in the oral cavity and thus may also improve timing and coordination of pharyngeal movements. These strategies may be cognitive in nature, such as holding the bolus for a cued swallow, or involve external support to the lips or jaw. On occasion, a postural strategy (i.e., chin down, head tilt) may also help increase control. They will be mentioned in each section (postural and increased control), and described in more detail in the postural section.

Many bolus modifications also have the effect of giving the client increased control. Changing the thickness of liquid (a bolus modification) may help the client keep the bolus from prematurely falling over the back of the tongue. Those strategies will be described below with bolus modifications, but the Chapter 4 Appendix indicates which are also considered to help the client have more control of the bolus.

Postural strategies are generally used to keep the bolus in a certain spot or direct the flow of the bolus. Most postural strategies address deficits in the oral phase or pharyngeal phase, but not in both. For example, head tilt is used for an oral-phase deficit and head turn for a pharyngeal-phase deficit. Those strategies that may address oral and/or pharyngeal deficits are described below with postural changes. See Table 5.2 for more information on when to select which strategy.

BOLUS MODIFICATIONS

Size of sip or bite. Perhaps the easiest way to modify a bolus is by controlling the size of the bolus. Some patients can self-regulate or respond to minimal cueing to take small bites and sips, which can then make the bolus easier to control to reduce anterior loss or premature spill over the back of the tongue. Smaller boluses may have a positive impact on oral phases but also have a significant impact on the pharyngeal phase, such as reducing the chance of spill of residue out of the valleculae or pyriforms. Presenting a smaller bolus can sometimes compensate for an issue with timing of the pharyngeal response, not because it changes the timing, but because the bolus is then small enough to rest in the valleculae (or sometimes even in the pyriform sinuses) during the delay and not spill into the airway. Results vary among individuals depending on the size of these pharyngeal spaces. We know that when not regulated, healthy individuals and patients take larger sips (Bennett, Van Lieshout, Pelletier, & Steele, 2009). Other patients may need external controls to regulate bolus size. Patients who are self-feeders may need stand-by assistance for cueing at each bite or sip. There are also commercially available cups and straws designed to control bolus size. Such products may allow a client to drink safely without constant cueing or supervision.

Texture changes. As the IDDSI framework points out, *texture* involves mechanical properties (e.g., hardness, cohesiveness, adhesiveness) and geometrical or shape attributes, particularly relevant regarding choking risk. Readers are referred to the IDDSI site for more details (IDDSI Framework, 2018).

The texture of foods can be altered in several ways. Food can be given a uniform texture through pureeing. These smooth purees can be runny or more pudding-like. Making foods a uniform texture can make them easier to manipulate as they maintain their cohesiveness in the oral cavity. Other foods, though not pureed, can also retain cohesiveness. When they are chewed and formed into a bolus, they tend to come together easily into a bolus and not leave particles of food across the oral cavity. The more cohesive the bolus, the easier it is to manipulate in the oral phases.

Another consideration when modifying the texture of foods is the concept of mixed consistencies. Examples of foods of mixed consistencies are those that enter the mouth as mixed, such as cereal on a spoon with milk, or vegetables that are not drained. Some foods may appear to be a single consistency, but when masticated they break into two consistencies. Sometimes this happens when the water from the food is expelled during chewing, as with citrus fruits and melons. It also happens when two different parts of the food become separated by chewing, such as the skin of peas.

Using food of increased texture may be indicated when the client needs more sensory input or when working on chewing and bolus manipulation. A client might be prescribed a simpler level of diet at meals that can be eaten safely without supervision, then more complex textures can be used during treatment sessions to develop skills.

Thickness of liquid changes. Thick liquids are prescribed for a variety of reasons. The client may have better control of a thicker liquid in the oral cavity with less resultant anterior loss or premature spill over the back of the tongue. When an instrumental exam reveals that the patient swallows thicker liquids more safely than thin, it is postulated that this is because the thicker ones maintain cohesiveness and move more slowly, giving the patient time to achieve closure of the airway. An interesting study with healthy young individuals found that they exhibited increased velocities and higher peak velocities of hyoid movement, meaning the hyoid moved faster and further, when swallowing nectar compared to thin. So perhaps it is not that the thicker boluses move more slowly, but that the thickness changes the timing of the movement of the hyoid, facilitating more timely laryngeal closure. This has yet to be studied further with patients (Nagy, Molfenter, Péladeau-Pigeon, Stokely, & Steele, 2015).

The IDDSI framework also describes different thicknesses of liquids. The inverted, overlapping pyramids make it clear that some foods are the same thickness as the moderately and extremely thick liquids. In general, the thicker the liquid, the easier it is to manipulate in the oral cavity. However, the thicker liquids may also result in more pharyngeal residue. Thickness of liquids can change based on things such as temperature, how long the liquid sits after being mixed with the thickening agent, the type of liquid thickened (e.g., juices, milk), and the manufacturer (e.g., type of modified starch, processing) (Tymchuck, 2006). Some foods may also change consistency once in the mouth and be considered more of a liquid. For example, if ice cream or sherbet are held in the oral cavity, they melt and are then of a different thickness from their original form. Popsicles, which are often stocked on patient floors, would likely be considered a thin liquid.

Temperature changes. Most food presented to patients is at room temperature. Caution is advised in checking the temperature of foods to be sure they are not too hot when working with patients with dementia, who may have lost the ability to check for temperature before taking a bite or sip. Several studies have looked at the combination of cold and taste—or cold, taste, and touch—to see if these different sensory inputs changed timing, but they found that the results were only temporary, reducing delay only on stimulated swallows (Ali, Laundl, Wallace, deCarle, & Cook, 1996; Kaatzke-McDonald, Post, & Davis, 1996; Sciortino, Liss, Case, Gerritsen, & Katz, 2003).

Taste changes. The sensation of taste (and often smell and taste, which are related) declines with aging (Kaneda et al., 2000; Morley, 2001; Stevens, Cruz, Hoffman, & Patterson, 1995). These changes can result in reduced food intake. One study demonstrated that taste sensation can be increased as a result of oral care (Ohno, Uematsu, Nozaki, & Sugimoto, 2003). Individuals with dementia also demonstrate a decline in taste and smell (Behrman, Chouliaras, & Ebmeier, 2014; Lang et al., 2006). Certain medications, surgery, and environmental exposure can also result in changes in taste. For example, patients undergoing chemotherapy often experience the sensation of an unpleasant metallic taste in the mouth. The speech–language pathologist should closely collaborate with the registered dietitian to determine how the taste of food can be altered to increase intake.

Chemesthetic changes. Chemesthesis comprises the chemically initiated sensations that occur via the touch system. Examples in the mouth include the burn of capsaicinoids in chilies, the cooling of menthol in peppermint, and the tingle of carbonation. It is physiologically distinct from taste and smell (McDonald, Bolliet, & Hayes, 2016). Chemesthetic sensations are transmitted via the trigeminal nerve (Wysocki & Wise, 2003). A discussion of chemesthetic stimuli is included in the rehabilitative pharyngeal section below.

STRATEGIES TO INCREASE CONTROL

Strategies to help the client maintain control of the bolus apply mostly to the oral phases, although keeping the bolus in the oral cavity and only initiating posterior movement of the bolus when ready can have a significant impact on aspects of the pharyngeal phase as well. For example, if providing a sip of liquid to mix with a dry food allows the patient to form a more cohesive bolus, it may mean the patient propels a more cohesive bolus into the pharynx rather than doing so in a piecemeal fashion. Another example is size of bolus presented. The smaller size not only affords better control in the oral cavity but it may mean less risk of spill from residue in valleculae or pyriform sinuses.

External support to lips or jaw. The patient may need assistive support at the lip and chin/jaw. Support to the lips is intended to reduce anterior loss. Support to the jaw, not used frequently with adults, can aid in biting and chewing. Place your finger under the chin or lower lip to help maintain closure of the mouth. For the patient with a labial droop, fingertip support may be sufficient to provide lip closure to keep the material in the oral cavity. This technique is particularly helpful for thin liquid maintenance.

For patients with more severe involvement, provide support to compensate for both labial and jaw weakness. Position the thumb along the mandible with your index finger beneath the lower lip and your middle finger beneath the patient's chin. Some patients can provide their own external support, especially if shown in a mirror how this helps.

External pressure to cheeks. Placing pressure on the affected cheek may also help a patient with oral weakness. The benefits for the patient are that the pressure decreases the amount of material falling into the weaker lateral sulcus and helps the tongue action in the formation of a cohesive bolus. The pressure can also help keep the bolus on the chewing surface.

This tactile cue also reminds the patient to check the buccal pocket or lateral sulcus for material that could have fallen there. This technique compensates for decreased muscle tone.

Pressure to the cheek on the weaker side can help keep the bolus on the chewing surface.

Placement of straw. When patients have unilateral facial weakness, they may have trouble closing the lips on the straw to form a seal. Placing the straw on the stronger side, often paired with support to the lips on the weaker side, can help the patient drink from the straw. Clinicians generally agree that drinking from a straw may place some patients at higher risk for aspiration, although no empirical evidence supports this. A straw may help some patients maintain a chin-down position while taking liquids. The straw can be pinched to control bolus size. The best way to determine if use of a straw will be a safe and effective strategy is to try it during an instrumental exam. Research has been done on straw drinking but typically with healthy individuals (Daniels et al., 2004; Daniels & Foundas, 2001; Lawless, Bender, Oman, & Pelletier, 2003).

Placement of bolus. In the case of unilateral weakness, having the client place the bolus on the stronger side should increase the likelihood of better control. In the case of a bolus requiring mastication, it should help keep the bolus on the chewing surface. If the patient has reduced tongue control, placing the bolus on the chewing surface bypasses the need for the patient to manipulate the bolus with the tongue to place it on the chewing surface. This placement on the stronger side may also reduce residue from the buccal cavity on the weaker side.

Change of utensil or modified utensil. Occupational therapists are expert in identifying the need for adaptive equipment. If you want bolus size control, you may recommend that all presentations be made from a spoon or you can put a small amount of liquid into a cup before giving it to the patient. Remember that a cup tends to cause a patient to tip his head back when taking a drink. A cut-out cup can help reduce this tendency. There are other commercially available cups to control bolus size.

Allow self-feeding. Patients with apraxia may do better when they feed themselves, as this makes it a more automatic task. In addition, for patients with dementia, allowing self-feeding as long as possible helps the patient maintain a level of independence. Self-feeding in this population can be enhanced by altering the diet to include more finger foods and providing adaptive utensils.

Added stimulation or cue. Patients with dementia may also experience agnosia, not recognizing that food has been placed in the oral cavity. They may hold the bolus despite verbal cues to chew or swallow. Sometimes providing added tactile cues by using firm downward pressure on the tongue when placing the bolus will cue initiation of manipulation of the bolus. Other times, presenting an empty spoon and touching the lips while the patient is holding the bolus may also cue initiation.

Liquid mix or wash. A liquid mix occurs when liquid is presented with a solid bolus still in the oral cavity, whereas a liquid wash occurs after the patient has swallowed the bolus and the wash is used to clear any residue. Some patients need to make sure they have swallowed several times to clear the oral cavity before any liquid is presented. Others do better if they are allowed to have a liquid to wash down the material. In particular, patients who have undergone radiation therapy may suffer from xerostomia and may need liquid mixed with each bolus to compensate for the dry mouth. For some patients, using a liquid mix or wash makes the swallow less efficient or less safe.

Clean lateral sulci and buccal cavity. If patients have residue, they can be cued to clear the residue with the tongue if they are able to lateralize the tongue. They can also be cued to clear the residue with their finger, or with liquid wash. If it is not safe for the patient to swallow thin liquids, he or she can use a wash and spit.

Three-second prep. The 3-second-prep technique is based in neuropsychological research, which indicates that getting into a mental "set" to perform an action helps initiate the action. Ask the patient to think about getting ready to swallow while you count to 3. When you get to 3, the patient should swallow. Langmore describes a similar methodology, the three-step swallow (Langmore, 2011). This strategy is designed to elicit more cortical control of the swallow response.

Multiple swallows. Some patients may need to be cued to quickly use a second dry swallow to clear residue. This may be oral residue or residue from the pyriform sinuses and valleculae that has been observed during an instrumental exam. In a study of consecutively referred patients, the number of repeat swallows on each bolus corresponded to the amount of residue in valleculae as judged by clinician (Veis, Logemann, & Colangelo, 2000).

Tip head up. A posterior head tilt is rarely recommended, but it may be helpful with patients who exhibit decreased ability to propel the bolus posteriorly to initiate a swallow, such as patients who have undergone partial or total glossectomies or laryngectomies and those with tongue scarring.

Tipping the head back allows gravity to propel the bolus posteriorly to initiate the swallow response. Use this technique only with patients who are intact cognitively and present an efficient, strong response to penetration into the airway. However, instead of providing increased control of the bolus, for some patients it results in reduced control, with the bolus falling over the back of the tongue and into the airway.

Chin down. The chin-down position may help patients who have decreased back-of-tongue control. For a patient who exhibits materials falling over the back of the tongue, a chin-down position may increase oral and pharyngeal control of the bolus. Orally, the patient gains volitional control for propulsion of the bolus. Pharyngeally, the chin-down position can compensate for mistiming as it widens the valleculae in many patients to allow for collection of material without spill to the pyriform sinuses or into the trachea. The bolus can "rest" there until the pharyngeal response initiates.

The chin-down position, or chin tuck, in those patients for whom the posture widens the valleculae, tucks the airway entrance beneath the tongue base and epiglottis, affording increased airway protection. The degree of chin tuck required to provide optimal protection and control varies from patient to patient, based on the degree of compromised functioning. The utility of this position should be assessed with an instrumental study because it can decrease the safety of the swallow in some patients related to their physiology. If the vallecular space is not widened, this posture may expose the airway and increase risk of penetration and/or aspiration.

Several studies found that chin tuck eliminated aspiration (Logemann et al., 2008; Rasley et al., 1993; Robbins, Gensler, et al., 2008). Chin tuck was also one of the strategies studied in Protocol 201, a large, randomized trial, and was found to be less effective in eliminating aspiration than thickened liquids in the patients with dementia with or without Parkinson's (Robbins et al., 2008). These are temporary anatomical changes that in some studies resulted in a safer swallow by reducing or eliminating aspiration, but there is no evidence that any physiological changes occur (Robbins, Gensler, et al., 2008).

An interesting study found that speech–language pathologists had different definitions of exactly what a chin-down or chin-tuck position meant. This inconsistency in how the position is described may account for differences in the results of studies of the technique (Okada et al., 2007).

Tilt head to stronger side. For patients who exhibit hemiparesis of the tongue and pharynx, a lateral head tilt to the patient's intact side may help. The bolus would be directed to the side of the oral cavity with greater muscle tone, which helps in oral control of the bolus.

Head rotation. Head rotation helps patients who have unilateral pharyngeal paresis or paralysis by decreasing the pharyngeal space by 50%.

On a videofluoroscopic or endoscopic evaluation, unilateral paralysis can be observed in the A-P view by looking for the variation in residue within the pyriform sinuses. If the residue is significantly asymmetrical, pharyngeal weakness or paralysis may be present. This condition can also be observed endoscopically.

A patient with pharyngeal paralysis should rotate his head all the way toward the damaged side. This technique closes the pyriform sinus on that side, increases vocal fold closure, and reduces resting tone in the cricopharyngeal muscle. The amount of pyriform sinus residue will be decreased by directing the flow of the bolus down the stronger, more intact side (Logemann, Kahrilas, Kobara, & Vakil, 1989; Ohmae, Ogura, Kitahara, Karaho, & Inouye, 1998).

Under videofluoroscopy or endoscopy, you can also try rotating the patient's head to the "good" side. Although this should not work, because it results in the bolus being directed to the weaker side of the pharynx, it has been found in some patients to result in some improvement.

Rehabilitative Techniques: Oral Phase

Consider the following exercises in light of the fact that little to no empirical evidence exists that these are actually rehabilitative. That is, it is not known if these exercises will actually result in a change in physiology.

LIPS

Closing lips around object and maintaining closure to increase strength. An easy way to have the patient practice lip closure is to tie a piece of dental floss around a Lifesaver candy (one string on each side) and put the candy inside the lips, between the lips and the front teeth, with the candy perpendicular to the floor. Pull gently on the two pieces of floss and have the patient squeeze the lips to keep the candy in place. A button can be used instead, and then only one piece of floss needs to be inserted into the middle holes on the button and both loose ends held by the clinician. This will keep the button from slipping off. However, strengthening exercises used for reduced lip closure are generally not supported by any studies demonstrating a change in function as a result of exercise. One study found improved lip strength and swallowing capacity in patients with stroke after training with a device called an oral screen (Hägg & Anniko, 2008; see also Hägglund et al., 2017).

Pucker and retract lips. Have the patient pucker the lips and then retract in a wide smile. This is a range-of-motion exercise and not a strengthening exercise.

Puff cheeks and maintain closure. Having the patient puff the cheeks and maintain a tight lip seal, particularly as the clinician tries to squeeze air out of the cheeks, may be a strength exercise for the lips.

Suck from a straw or use high-resistance straw. Although sucking from a straw requires good lip seal, it may not be building strength in the lips. Clark and Shelton saw no change in lip or cheek strength following 4 weeks of training with high-resistance straws (Clark & Shelton, 2013; Shelton, 2011).

JAW

Opening and closing against resistance. The clinician's hand can be placed under the jaw with some upward pressure, and the patient can be asked to open the jaw against the resistance. Conversely, the clinician can place a hand on the lower jaw and hold the jaw open while the patient tries to close the jaw against this resistance. The use of a swallow exercise aid was explored with healthy subjects. The device was used to provide resistance while the subject opened the jaw. The exercise was called "jaw opening against resistance" (JOAR). This same study examined chin tuck against resistance (CTAR) in healthy elderly individuals. Mean chin-tuck strength and mean jaw-opening strength increased in this population of healthy individuals (Kraaijenga et al., 2015). The techniques have not been studied in patients. A discussion of these two exercises is also included in the pharyngeal-phase rehabilitative section, as they are designed to mimic the Shaker exercise and result in change in the suprahyoid muscles, thus improving hyolaryngeal elevation.

CHEEKS

If the cheeks have normal tone, they remain tight against the gums, keeping the bolus from falling into the lateral sulci. Some of the exercises used for the lips (e.g., puffing cheeks, pucker and retract) use muscles in the cheeks as well as the lips. These exercises are also not generally supported in the literature. For example, Clark and colleagues found no change in cheek strength in healthy adults following 9 weeks of training with the Iowa Performance Instrument (IOPI; Clark, Solomon, O'Brien, Calleja, & Newcomb, 2008).

TONGUE

Exercises with the tongue have been studied more than for other oral structures and have the best evidence of oral motor exercises; moreover, evidence continues to emerge demonstrating positive effects from strengthening exercises for the tongue. Unfortunately, with few exceptions, many of these studies were performed with healthy adults. More recent studies have demonstrated that some exercises of the tongue have also resulted in improvements in certain aspects of the pharyngeal phase of the swallow, and those results will be mentioned below.

Lingual strengthening is the subject of much recent research. Many studies have demonstrated increased tongue strength, and others have demonstrated increased lingual volume, improved swallowing pressures in healthy aging (Robbins et al., 2005), increased swallowing pressures and reduced airway invasion (Robbins et al., 2007), and improved bolus control and functional dietary intake (Yeates, Molfenter, & Steele, 2008).

When utilizing tongue strength as a measure of improvement from a lingual strengthening exercise program, subjective measures may not be adequate. Inexperienced and experienced raters judged tongue strength differently, and correlations to specific functional aspects of the oral swallow differed between these rater groups (Clark, Henson, Barber, Stierwalt, & Sherrill, 2003). Several devices allow for objective measures of tongue strength and are described later in this chapter. Some common tongue exercises used by clinicians are listed here with the intended outcome of that exercise.

Press tongue tip out or up against tongue depressor. This is intended to increase strength for protrusion or elevation.

Sweep tip of tongue from front to back along the hard palate. This is intended to mimic the movement of bolus transport, although bolus transport involves sequential squeezing of the tongue against the hard palate, not pulling the tip back against the roof of the mouth.

Push blade of tongue up against tongue depressor. This is thought to increase strength for bolus propulsion.

Lateralize tip of tongue. This can be done to the corner of lips or either buccal cavity or inside of cheek. For the latter, provide resistance by placing fingers on cheek and pushing against tongue.

Push lateral border of tongue against tongue depressor. This is designed for increased strength for lateralization.

Push back of tongue against tongue depressor. This is intended to increase strength of the back of the tongue to help keep bolus in the oral cavity.

Sensory strategies for tongue. These have not typically been employed to elicit changes in the tongue, but Pelletier and Dhanaraj (2006) found that moderately sweet and highly sour and salty concentrations yielded higher lingual swallowing pressures.

SOFT PALATE

The soft palate typically rests against the back of the tongue during the oral phases to help maintain the bolus in the oral cavity. This is the position of the soft palate at rest and therefore should not need to be addressed. During the pharyngeal phase, the soft palate elevates to tightly seal off the nasopharynx and prevent nasal backflow during the swallow. Tight closure of the nasopharynx presumably helps create pharyngeal pressure to aid bolus flow. Although more integral in the pharyngeal phase, the soft palate is discussed here because it is typically considered part of the oral musculature. There are no studies of exercises for improved velopharyngeal closure for swallowing, nor are there any postures or compensations that might reduce nasal backflow. One might have the patient take smaller sips of liquid or avoid straws if large boluses and straw drinking precipitate nasal backflow.

Rehabilitative Techniques: Pharyngeal Phase

THERMAL-TACTILE APPLICATION

Thermal-tactile application (originally called thermal-tactile stimulation) was first described by Logemann (1983) and reduces the delay in the initiation of the pharyngeal response. It is typically used with patients who show a more than 2-second delay in initiating the swallow response or who aspirate during the delay. The stimulation does not cause the response to happen but heightens the awareness of that region in the mouth to increase the likelihood that a swallow will occur. This sensory technique is paired with asking the client to swallow.

Generally, a double 00 laryngeal mirror is used. Hold the mirror like a pencil so you can easily rotate it in your hand. Dip it in ice and rub it up and down five times on one of the patient's anterior faucial arches. Then dip it back into the ice quickly, rotate it so the flat head of the mirror is facing in the other direction, and rub it on the other faucial arch. Instruct the patient to swallow in order to invoke the voluntary component of the swallow.

You can pair thermal-tactile application with small amounts of liquid if the patient is allowed to have anything to drink. This technique may help elicit a swallow response. If a patient tries to close his mouth around the mirror, apply downward pressure to the jaw and give verbal cues to keep the mouth open.

Subsequent studies have only inconsistently found that the use of thermal application reduces swallow delay, and then only temporarily (Daniels et al., 2004; Rosenbek, Robbins, Fishback, & Levine, 1991; Rosenbek et al., 1998; Rosenbek, Roecker, Wood, & Robbins, 1996). That is, the gains do not hold after the therapy session is over. Several studies have looked at the combination of cold and taste, or cold, taste and touch, but also found that the results were only temporary, reducing delay on only the stimulated swallows (Cola et al., 2010; Kaatzke-McDonald et al., 1996). To date there is no evidence that thermal-tactile application effects are long lasting. Therefore, although listed in the Chapter 4 Appendix as rehabilitative, the strategy is probably best considered compensatory.

NEUROSENSORY STIMULATION

This technique is a nice alternative when a patient will not open his or her mouth to allow you to perform thermal-tactile application. Because this technique uses sensory (cold) input, it may help to improve the pharyngeal response.

Fill a finger of a glove with water, tie it off, and freeze it. (If you forget to plan ahead, you can also fill the finger of the glove with crushed ice and tie it off.) Have the patient suck on the cold finger of the glove and then swallow. This technique combines the thermal aspect of thermal-tactile application with suck-swallow. It also helps moisten the patient's mouth.

CHEMESTHETIC AND TASTE CHANGES

Chemesthetic changes are those caused by chemicals that activate other receptors associated with other senses that mediate pain, touch, and thermal reception. Different chemesthetic agents have been studied related to swallowing, including sour, sweet, carbonated, and capsaicin. These sensations are medicated by the trigeminal nerve (Green, Alvarez-Reeves, George, & Akirav, 2005). Altering taste alone (not with temperature) has been explored by several investigators (e.g., Pelletier & Dhanaraj, 2006; Logemann et al., 1995; Palmer et al., 2005).

Sour bolus. Logemann et al. (1995) found that a bolus that was 50% barium and 50% lemon juice used in individuals with dysphagia of a neurogenic nature resulted in changes in the swallow. For all patients, faster oral onset was observed, whereas in patients with stroke, decreased pharyngeal delay was seen, and in patients with other neurogenic disorders there was reduced aspiration frequency.

Some patients may benefit from presentation of a very sour bolus, like lemon juice. This technique can significantly improve the onset of the oral and/or pharyngeal phases of the swallow. For the patient who is NPO, lemon glycerin swabs provide a source of sour stimulation, though studies have not been completed to judge the impact on swallow. Note that when lemon glycerin swabs are used for oral hygiene, they are considered ineffective. In fact, the lemon reduces oral pH below the normal level and dehydrates the oral tissues. According to Trenter-Roth and Creason (1986), the acid conditions in the mouth can irritate, cause pain, and decalcify teeth, thereby increasing the risk of dental decay.

Sucrose, salt, and sour. Pelletier and Dhanaraj (2006) found that moderate sucrose, high salt, and high citric acid elicited significantly higher lingual swallowing pressures compared to pressures generated with water. High salt and citric acid elicit chemesthesis mediated by the trigeminal nerve. Therefore, the authors hypothesized that chemesthesis may play a crucial role in swallowing physiology. If true, trigeminal irritants like carbonation may be beneficial to individuals with dysphagia. Stronger muscle contractions were also observed in other studies, and this may result in more timely movement of structures, but also in better clearance of the bolus (Ding, Logemann, Larson, & Rademaker, 2003; Leow, Huckabee, Sharma, & Tooley, 2007; Miura, Morita, Koizumi, & Shingai, 2009; Palmer, McCulloch, Jaffe, & Neel, 2005). For all these sensory inputs, changes are seen only on the swallows using these inputs.

Carbonation. Bulow and colleagues showed during a therapeutic VFSS that carbonated liquid reduced penetration/aspiration and pharyngeal transit time (Bülow, Olsson, & Ekberg, 2003). There was also less pharyngeal retention. The authors explained these results in terms of the stimulating effect of carbonic acid on receptors in the faucial pillars, leading to quicker activation of the solitary tract nucleus in the medulla oblongata of the brain stem. Recent results from Miura et al. (2009) confirm these observations with healthy subjects. Michou observed change in swallowing in healthy individuals with carbonation and cold and suggested that combining the two features might be most beneficial with patients (Michou, Mastan, Ahmed, Mistry, & Hamdy, 2012). A reduction in penetration–aspiration scores was seen but no change in oral transit times, pharyngeal transit times, or initiation of pharyngeal swallow in another study (Sdravou, Walshe, & Dagdilelis, 2012). A reduction in penetration–aspiration scores was also observed with both discrete and continuous sips of carbonated beverages in patients with neurogenic dysphagia, although not every patient got better and not all changes were clinically significant (Turkington, 2017).

Capsaicin and other stimuli. Newer studies have begun to explore the effect of stimuli like capsaicin (hot pepper) on swallowing. One study from Japan used a capsaicin gel in the auditory canal and found improvement in swallowing parameters after using this stimulus (Kondo et al., 2014).

For more in-depth information about the sensory aspects of swallowing, readers are referred to two reviews: Loret (2015) and Steele and Miller (2010).

BREATH HOLD (VALSALVA MANEUVER)

The breath hold, or Valsalva, is an example of a technique that is motor without a swallow. Asking the patient to take a breath, bear down, and hold it achieves closure of the true and false vocal folds in most subjects (Donzelli & Brady, 2004). Watch carefully, as many patients think they are holding their breath but they continue to breathe. If you watch a patient's upper chest, you can usually tell when she is really holding her breath. There is no evidence this carries over to closure during swallowing, but does support that the super-supraglottic swallow, which instructs patients to hold their breath tightly, is more likely to achieve closure of both the true and false vocal folds.

SUPRAGLOTTIC SWALLOW AND SUPER-SUPRAGLOTTIC SWALLOW

The supraglottic and super-supraglottic swallow strategies are completed by having the individual take a breath, let a little out, hold the breath, swallow, and then cough or swallow again. The cough is designed to clear any residue from the airway. The difference in the super-supraglottic is that it is performed with strength (e.g., "Hold your breath as tightly as you can and swallow as hard as you can"). Although originally intended to improve closure, these strategies were also found to have some impact on timing of several events:

- Earlier and longer laryngeal closure (Logemann, Pauloski, Rademaker, & Colangelo, 1997; Ohmae, Logemann, Hanson, Kaiser, & Kahrilas, 1996)

- Higher position of hyoid bone at swallow onset (Bülow et al., 1999)

- Earlier and longer PES opening (Ohmae et al., 1996)

- Longer duration of hyolaryngeal complex movement in healthy volunteers (Ohmae et al., 1996)

- Longer duration of pharyngeal wall movement, also done with healthy volunteers (Miller & Watkin, 1997)

The changes are more successful and maintained longer with the super-supraglottic than the supraglottic maneuver. There are no studies documenting long-term improvement with these techniques. The super-supraglottic did not result in a change in manometric measures in healthy patients (Bülow et al., 1999) and had no impact on the number of misdirected swallows in a small group of patients (Bülow, Olsson, & Ekberg, 2001).

THE MENDELSOHN MANEUVER

This maneuver occurs at the height of the swallow. That is, the individual is instructed to swallow and when the larynx is at its highest point in the throat, to forcefully push the tongue against the roof of the mouth to keep the hyolaryngeal complex in that elevated position. The maneuver was also originally targeted for another change in physiology (prolong and hold the hyolaryngeal excursion) (Mendelsohn & Martin, 1993), but Lazarus and colleagues also found it to have an impact on timing in a single subject (Lazarus, Logemann, & Gibbons, 1993). In healthy volunteers, the Mendelsohn maneuver resulted in increases in both the pharyngeal peak contraction and contraction duration. If that were true in patients, it might result in an improved propulsion of bolus into the esophagus (Boden, Hallgren, & Witt Hedström, 2006).

Despite a lack of definitive answers about techniques like supraglottic, super-supraglottic, Mendelsohn, and even strategies to improve control of the bolus such as 3-second prep (see below), it seems to make sense that these could help improve overall coordination and timing of the events of the swallow. The specific directions and steps the person has to follow would seem to result in some cortical control of these movements. This cortical control uses more of the top-down principle of motor learning. In addition, the principle of using sensory feedback to improve performance of an action is at play in these step-by-step swallowing techniques.

EFFORTFUL SWALLOW

The effortful swallow reduces residue in the valleculae by increasing the pressures in the mouth and upper pharynx to push through the bolus. It also results in earlier onset of these pharyngeal pressures. The exercise can also increase the extent and duration of laryngeal elevation (Jang, Leigh, Seo, Han, & Oh, 2015). Typically, the patient is instructed, "Swallow as hard as you can." Huckabee and Steele (2006) compared the performance of healthy volunteers when the directions given varied for this exercise. One group was told to swallow with emphasis on pushing the tongue against the palate. The other group was not told to emphasize this movement. The group that put the emphasis on the tongue pushing against the palate demonstrated more pressure with the tongue and in the upper pharynx. As with all exercises, careful monitoring of the patient's behavior is essential. One subject (Garcia, Hakel, & Lazarus, 2004) developed timing issues with nasal backflow when using the effortful swallow.

CAUTION WITH USE OF BREATH-HOLDING TECHNIQUES

Clinicians should be aware that swallowing is inter-related with respiration and cardiac function, and that altering the swallow with techniques that include increased effort and/or breath holding has the potential for negative effects on patients. In normal, healthy women, using the effortful swallow indicated cardiac overload (Gomes et al., 2016). A study with patients with a history of stroke and cardiac disease found cardiac changes with the supraglottic and super-supraglottic swallow techniques and suggested that those techniques might not be appropriate for that population (Chaudhuri et al., 2002).

THREE-SECOND PREP

This is also called a three-step swallow (Langmore, 2011). This technique is based in neuropsychological research, which indicates that getting into a mental "set" to perform an action helps you initiate the action. Ask the patient to think about getting ready to swallow while you count to 3. When you get to 3, the patient should swallow. Using a technique like this, or the suck-swallow described below, should increase cortical control of the swallow.

SUCK-SWALLOW

The suck-swallow technique should also help the patient coordinate the steps of the swallow and bring it under more conscious control. The intent is to improve the overall timing of the swallow. It might also be described as a "lollipop swallow" if a lollipop is used to help initiate the movement (National Foundation on Swallowing Disorders, 2017). A sucking motion draws saliva to the back of the mouth, which may increase sensory input for the swallow. Ask the patient to pretend he or she is sucking something very thick up through a very narrow straw for 2–3 seconds. Then have the patient swallow.

TONGUE-BASE RETRACTION AND TONGUE PULLBACK

Ask the patient to pull the base of his tongue toward the back wall of the throat (posterior pharyngeal wall) with lots of effort and to hold it there for several seconds. This technique develops strength in the base of the tongue to reduce vallecular residue. If the patient instead tries to curl the tip of the tongue back, hold the tip of the tongue and ask the patient to pull back against this resistance. A piece of gauze (or in a pinch, a paper towel) can be used to hold the tongue tip.

In a study with healthy volunteers, tongue pullback without resistance did not increase activity of the submental muscles, but tongue pullback with resistance did. The authors are exploring the development of a device to hold the tongue tip and offer resistance (Slovarp, King, Off, & Liss, 2016).

PRETEND TO GARGLE

This technique increases the movement of the posterior pharyngeal wall and the base of the tongue. The patient is asked to pretend to gargle and then hold that position. It is best to try this technique under fluoroscopy to see if it will help the patient. This movement could be visualized on endoscopy.

PRETEND TO YAWN

This technique also increases the movement of the posterior pharyngeal wall and the base of the tongue. The patient is asked to yawn and then hold the position. As with the gargle, it is best to try this technique under fluoroscopy, and it probably cannot be adequately viewed on endoscopy.

TONGUE RETRACTION, GARGLE, AND YAWN COMPARED

These three techniques—tongue retraction, pretend to gargle, and pretend to yawn—were studied in 20 consecutively referred patients. The gargle task was the most successful in eliciting tongue-base retraction for the group of subjects, although not in every subject. Gargle also resulted in greater tongue-base movement than swallow more often than the other two voluntary tasks (Veis et al., 2000).

TONGUE HOLD, OR MASAKO

This technique was serendipitously discovered when the researchers observed that patients with tongue-base resection over time demonstrated an increased bulging of the posterior pharyngeal wall. They hypothesized that simulating tongue-base resection by having the client stick the tongue out of the mouth (and thus move the tongue base farther away from the posterior pharyngeal wall) would yield the same effect of increasing the forward movement of the posterior pharyngeal wall as it moves forward to meet the base of the tongue. The patient is asked to protrude the tongue slightly and hold it between the teeth while he or she swallows (Fujiu & Logemann, 1996).

This technique is done with saliva swallows, as it is difficult to control a food bolus while performing this technique, and it can have unintended consequences that should be considered. In healthy volunteers, use of the technique resulted in lower pharyngeal peak pressure and shorter pharyngeal pressure durations compared to control swallows. Further, tongue-hold swallows produced lower UES relaxation pressures while using that technique (Doeltgen, Macrae, & Huckabee, 2011; Doeltgen, Witte, Gumbley, & Huckabee, 2009). It would not be desirable to have a patient swallow a bolus with resultant lower pharyngeal pressures.

EFFORTFUL PITCH GLIDE, OR FALSETTO

Clinicians have used a technique called falsetto for years, hypothesizing that the elevation of the larynx for falsetto was similar to the elevation during swallowing. A recent study with healthy adults demonstrated the similarity between what they call effortful pitch glide and these movements for swallowing: anterior hyoid, superior hyoid, hyolaryngeal approximation, laryngeal elevation, and lateral pharyngeal wall medialization. Only superior hyoid movement was greater during swallowing. This initial study supports that, theoretically, this technique will work to improve the movements for swallowing (Miloro, Pearson, & Langmore, 2014).

Ask the patient to produce /i/ in a continuous note as he or she increases pitch until he or she reaches the falsetto, and to hold it there. Some patients may have more success with simple pitch change activities when asked to sing up the scale.

HEAD-LIFT (SHAKER) MANEUVER

The head-lift maneuver is also called the Shaker (emphasis on the second syllable) exercise. This technique is designed to increase forward movement of the hyoid bone, which actually helps the entire hyolaryngeal complex move forward. This results in the cricopharyngeus opening more widely and staying open longer, which should allow more of the bolus to enter the esophagus and thus reduce the amount of residue that would remain in the pyriform sinuses. It has been studied with normal as well as with different patient populations (Antunes & Lunet, 2012; Easterling, Grande, Kern, Sears, & Shaker, 2005; Logemann et al., 2009; Shaker et al., 2002; Shaker et al., 1997).

The exercise has two parts: sustained (isometric) and repetitive (isotonic). For each, the patient lies flat on a bed or on the floor with no pillow under his or her head. For the sustained part of the exercise, have the patient lift his head (keeping his shoulders on the surface) and look at his toes. Have the patient hold the position for 60 seconds. For the repetitive part, keep the patient in the same position. Have her raise and lower her head 30 times in a row. Patients may need to work up to this duration for the sustained part and the number of repetitions on the isotonic part.

ALTERNATIVES TO HEAD LIFT

Some clients have difficulty with this exercise due to rigidity or other neck problems. Perhaps because of this, alternative exercises have been explored to improve activation of the suprahyoid muscles and tongue strength.

The Recline Exercise (RE). This exercise was explored with healthy adults but needs more exploration. RE is performed in a seated and 45° reclined position with the head unsupported. It has both an isometric and isotonic portion similar to the head lift exercise (Mishra, Rajappa, Tipton, & Malandraki, 2015).

Tongue press. An exercise called the tongue press was also studied in healthy adults who were asked to push the tongue hard against the palate and maintain that position. The sustained posture (isometric) yielded higher muscle activity in the submental muscles (Yoshida, Groher, Crary, Mann, & Akagawa, 2007). See the literature for any newer studies on either of these techniques.

CTAR and JOAR (chin tuck against resistance and jaw opening against resistance). Yoon and colleagues first described the CTAR with healthy subjects seated upright, using a small, inflatable rubber ball placed between the chin and chest (Yoon, Khoo, & Liow, 2014). The exercise was designed to change the function of the suprahyoid muscles. Exercise with the ball showed significantly greater maximum sEMG values during the CTAR isokinetic and isometric exercises than during the equivalent Shaker exercises, and significantly greater mean sEMG values were observed for the CTAR isometric exercise than for the Shaker isometric exercise.

In a feasibility study, the CTAR was then studied along with an exercise called jaw opening against resistance and the effortful swallow in healthy elderly subjects using a device called a Swallow Exercise Aid. Mean chin-tuck strength and mean jaw-opening strength increased in this population of healthy individuals. In healthy individuals, suprahyoid muscle volume increased, which might indicate stronger function of these muscles that serve to elevate the hyoid. This has not been studied in patients, and no measure of change in swallowing function was included since the subjects were healthy elderly (Kraaijenga et al., 2015).

Exercise as Preventive

Most of the time, dysphagia therapy is used to rehabilitate or compensate for a swallowing disorder. However, exercises can also be applied prophylactically to prevent problems from developing. Preventive therapy is most often used with patients who have cancer of the head and neck and undergo radiation therapy. In fact, there is a specific name for the dysphagia that occurs after radiation therapy: radiation-associated dysphagia, or RAD.

Fibrosis of the muscle fibers is the major cause of RAD and can develop slowly over time, as the effects of the radiation therapy are cumulative. Preventive exercises are designed to combat the development of fibrosis and typically are exercises for maintaining range of motion. For example, range-of-motion exercises may be used for the jaw, lips, and tongue. Pharyngeal exercises like the Mendelsohn maneuver are also used to maintain movement of pharyngeal structures (Carnaby-Mann, Crary, Schmalfuss, & Amdur, 2012; Hutcheson et al., 2012; Hutcheson et al., 2013; Kotz et al., 2012; Langmore & Krisciunas, 2010; Paleri et al., 2014; Rosenthal, Lewin, & Eisbruch, 2006; Van der Molen et al., 2011). There is also evidence that continuing to eat during the course of the chemoradiotherapy results in better outcomes (Hutcheson et al., 2013). There is evidence that starting these exercises even before the patient presents with signs of dysphagia can be the most effective, although patient compliance is not always good (Shinn et al., 2013). Examples of the kinds of exercises that might be used in a preventive program are listed in Table 4.6

Adjunctive Devices and Tools Used in Therapy With Other Exercise

There are different types of devices and tools that can be used with some of the exercises described above. Some incorporate a swallow with the exercise (e.g., IOPI) and some do not (EMST). This is meant not to be an exhaustive list but to provide examples of the ways some of the devices are used. It is beyond the scope of this chapter to summarize the research surrounding the devices. Readers are encouraged to seek out the most current information on each device.

DEVICES TO PROVIDE BIOFEEDBACK

Surface electromyography (sEMG). Surface electromyography involves placing electrodes, usually submentally, to measure muscle activity. It is not providing any electrical input to the muscles. It appears to be particularly helpful in measuring the movements of the submental muscles during swallowing activities (e.g., Mendelsohn maneuver, effortful swallow) and nonswallowing activities (e.g., EMST, head lift). The information is typically a visual, graphic display so that the client can see the results of the activity and make changes, such as while performing the Mendelsohn maneuver, holding the larynx in an elevated position for longer time, or lifting the larynx higher than on previous attempts. Steele et al. (2012) provided a comprehensive summary of the use of sEMG in swallowing.

Table 4.6
Prophylactic Exercises During Organ Preservation Treatment

Exercise	To address
Jaw stretch	Range of motion
Slide jaw to one side and hold (then reverse)	Range of motion
Tongue out, back and each side. Hold each position several seconds	Range of motion
Gargle	Strength and movement, base of tongue and pharyngeal walls
Effortful swallow	Strength and movement, base of tongue and pharyngeal walls
Tongue hold (Masako)	Strength and movement, pharyngeal walls
Yawn and maintain that opening/stretch	Range of motion, but also movement of base of tongue and pharyngeal walls
Head lift	Movement of hyolaryngeal complex
Mendelsohn	Superior movement of larynx

Note. Many of these are demonstrated in videos on www.swallowingdisorders.org

DEVICES THAT PROVIDE SENSORY INPUT

NMES. Neuromuscular electrical stimulation also uses electrodes, but differs from sEMG in that electrical stimulation is provided to muscles involved in swallowing. The electrodes are placed at different locations on the front of the neck. At the lowest levels set on the device, only sensory input is provided. That is, the stimulation is not turned up high enough to elicit a motor response. ASHA has an FAQ on NMES (Frequently Asked Questions About Electrical Stimulation, n.d.) that readers might find helpful.

DEVICES THAT PROVIDE ELECTRICAL STIMULATION FOR A MOTOR RESPONSE

NMES. Neuromuscular electrical stimulation can also provide direct stimulation to the muscles at a level designed to elicit a motor response. The intent is to obtain more muscle movement, such as more elevation of the larynx during the swallow.

DEVICES USED WITH EXERCISES TO INCREASE AND MEASURE STRENGTH AND PROVIDE BIOFEEDBACK

The two devices described below are used most often for lingual strengthening programs. McKenna and colleagues provide a systematic review of lingual strengthening programs (McKenna, Zhang, Haines, & Kelchner, 2017).

IOPI. The Iowa Oral Performance Instrument is a small handheld device that measures and records lip and tongue strength. A small bulb is placed in the mouth, and the pressure placed on the bulb by the lips or tongue (or cheeks) is recorded.

SwallowSTRONG. This device also measures and records tongue strength. It differs from the IOPI in that instead of a single bulb, it has a cross-shaped sensor that is fitted to the individual's mouth, with a sensor at four locations. It interfaces with a tablet with a visual display for the patient to see whether targets are being met.

DEVICES USED WITH EXERCISE TO INCREASE STRENGTH OF SUBMENTAL MUSCLES

Expiratory Muscle Strength Trainer (EMST). Another exercise to increase the activity of the submental muscles uses a device called an Expiratory Muscle Strength Trainer. Although there are several respiratory training devices on the market, the one with which the research has been conducted is the EMST150 (http://www.emst150.com). The EMST150 is a pressure-threshold device, as the device requires the client to blow against a preset level of resistance to get a spring-loaded valve to open. Other devices are resistance flow devices, giving the clinician no control over the amount of force needed, nor a way to measure it. With the pressure-threshold device, the forceful blowing increases the activity of the submental muscles, resulting in an increase in hyolaryngeal excursion. It utilizes a training regimen with multiple repetitions over many treatment sessions and requires the muscles to work harder than they usually do.

The amount of pressure can be adjusted with an external dial, ranging from 0–150 cmH2O. The clinician bases the setting on the person's maximum expiratory pressure (MEP). The threshold is set at 75% of the MEP and increases as the person gets stronger. Sufficient pressure from expiratory force must surpass the spring-loaded valve; when achieved, the valve opens and air flows through the device. The pressure-released valve requires a consistent flow of air for the valve to remain open. However, if there is inadequate force during expiration, the valve will stay closed and no air will flow through the device. It is thought that this serves as biofeedback to the client.

Research with the device has been completed with patients with Parkinson's disease, ALS, and stroke with effects seen on swallowing:

- Penetration–Aspiration Scale scores improved.

- Movement of the hyolaryngeal complex increased (Pitts et al., 2009; Troche, 2015; Troche et al., 2010; Wheeler-Hegland, Rosenbek, & Sapienza, 2008).

An interesting related finding is that the device increases the strength of the cough, an important protective mechanism. For clinicians who want to begin using respiratory training with clients, the article in *ASHA Perspectives* by Michelle Troche (2015) provides information on different training protocols and more information on how to use the device.

DEVICES FOR RANGE OF MOTION

TheraBite Jaw Motion Rehab System. This handheld device is designed to maintain range of motion and prevent trismus.

Cases to Practice Planning Treatment

The Supplemental Materials contain seven case examples (SLP Resources, Case Examples: Treatment Planning) that provide a succinct history and selected findings from evaluations, comprising the signs and the underlying impaired physiology. Long-term goals have been selected as well as short-term goals and treatment objectives. A complete list of long- and short-term goals and treatment objectives for oral and pharygeal deficits is provided in the Supplemental Materials (SLP Resources, Goals and Treatment Objectives).

Chapter 4 Appendix

Treatment Techniques: Compensatory and Rehabilitative

ORAL-PHASE TECHNIQUES: Lips

Technique	Compensatory: Bolus modification	Compensatory: Increased control	Compensatory: Postural	External sensory	Sensorimotor with a swallow	Sensorimotor without a swallow	Device	What sign you observe	Impaired physiology	Intended impact of the technique on the functional swallow
Closing lips around Lifesaver™						X		Losing bolus from front of mouth	Weakness in lips	To maintain closure to keep bolus in the mouth
Closing lips around oral screen (or IOPI bulb)						X	X	Reduced ability to close lips on straw, cup, or spoon		
Pucker lips/retract						X				
Puff cheeks and maintain closure						X				To use the lips to help get bolus into the mouth
Suck from straw/high-resistance straws					X		X			
External support to lips		X								To use the lips to remove food from utensil
Reduce size of sip or bolus	X	X								
Tip head up		X	X							
Placement of straw on stronger side		X								
Modify texture of bolus	X	X								

Signs, Physiology and Function

Rehabilitative

ORAL-PHASE TECHNIQUES: Jaw

Technique	Compensatory: Bolus modification	Compensatory: Increased control	Compensatory: Postural	External sensory	Sensorimotor with a swallow	Sensorimotor without a swallow	Device	What sign you observe	Impaired physiology	Intended impact of the technique on the functional swallow
					Rehabilitative			Signs, Physiology, and Function		
Open jaw against resistance					X		X	Impaired ability to bite and chew	Weakness of jaw muscles	Enhance movement of the jaw for improved biting and chewing
Close jaw against resistance					X					
External support to the jaw		X								
Change texture of bolus	X									

ORAL-PHASE TECHNIQUES: Cheeks

Technique	Compensatory: Bolus modification	Compensatory: Increased control	Compensatory: Postural	External sensory	Sensorimotor with a swallow	Sensorimotor without a swallow	Device	What sign you observe	Impaired physiology	Intended impact of the technique on the functional swallow
Pucker/retract lips (as in exaggerated "oo" and "ee")						X		Residue in cheeks	Reduced tone in cheeks	Keep the bolus on the tongue and not falling into buccal cavities
Cheek-strengthening exercise						X	X			
Provide external pressure to the cheek to reduce pocketing		X								
Place bolus of food on the stronger side		X								
Clean the buccal cavity periodically during meal with the tongue (or finger)		X								
Rinse and clear the oral cavity after eating		X								
Change texture to more cohesive	X	X								

ORAL-PHASE TECHNIQUES: Tongue

Technique	Compensatory: Bolus modification	Compensatory: Increased control	Compensatory: Postural	External sensory	Rehabilitative: Sensorimotor with a swallow	Rehabilitative: Sensorimotor without a swallow	Device	What sign you observe	Impaired physiology	Intended impact of the technique on the functional swallow
Tongue protrusion against tongue depressor						X		Reduced ability to clean lips with tongue or lick (e.g., ice cream)	Reduced anterior movement	Improved strength and coordination of tongue for formation and manipulation of bolus in oral cavity or compensate for reduced strength and coordination
Tongue-tip elevation against pressure from tongue depressor (or against device)						X	X	Reduced ability to lift tongue tip to get bolus in place on tongue	Reduced tongue-tip elevation	
Sweep tongue tip from front to back along hard palate						X		Reduced ability to move bolus back in oral cavity	Reduced anterior-posterior movement	
Push blade of tongue against tongue depressor (or against device)						X	X			
Tip chin up		X	X							
Lateralize tongue tip to corners, sulci, or cheeks						X		Reduced ability to use tongue to clear residue in buccal cavity	Reduced ability to use tongue to clear residue in buccal cavity	
Push lateral border of tongue against tongue depressor (or up against device)						X	X			

Treatment Technique	Reduced ability to maintain bolus in oral cavity / Reduced back-of-tongue strength/control	Reduced ability to form and manipulate bolus / Reduced strength and accuracy of lingual movements	Impaired ability to chew on one side / Unilateral lingual weakness	Uncoordinated lingual movements / Swallow apraxia	Holding the bolus in oral cavity / Swallow agnosia	Residue in oral cavity after swallow / Any of the lingual deficits or agnosia that might result in residue	Rationale
Push back of tongue against tongue depressor (or against device)	X						Better control of back of tongue to keep bolus from falling over into airway
Chin tuck	X						Compensate for poor back-of-tongue control to keep bolus in oral cavity
Reduce size of sip	X						
Modify texture of food	X						
Lingual strengthening and precision with IOPI, Swallow Strong		X					Improved strength and coordination of tongue for formation and manipulation of bolus in oral cavity
Resistance Straws		X					
Tastes (sweet, sour, salty)				X			
Place bolus of food on stronger side			X				Keeping the bolus where the client can best manipulate it
Tilt head toward stronger side			X				
Allow self-feeding				X			Makes the task more automatic and natural
Downward pressure with spoon on tongue					X		Less holding and response to cues to individual to begin manipulating the bolus
Touch spoonful of food to lips					X		
Modify taste/texture					X		
Sip of liquid as a wash						X	Clear oral cavity to reduce the risk that the residue might fall into the airway
Liquid mix with bolus						X	
Cue patient for second swallow to clear						X	

PHARYNGEAL-PHASE TECHNIQUES

Technique	Compensatory: Bolus modification	Compensatory: Increased control	Compensatory: Postural	External sensory	Sensorimotor with a swallow	Sensorimotor without a swallow	Device	What sign you observe	Impaired physiology	Intended impact of the technique on the functional swallow
Chin-down posture		X	X					Penetration and/or aspiration before the swallow	Poor back-of-tongue control	To keep the bolus in the oral cavity until ready to swallow so it does not fall into the airway. And/or….
								Aspiration during the swallow	Delayed pharyngeal response / Mistiming	The chin down can sometimes widen the valleculae and tuck the airway entrance under the tongue base for added protection. The chin down sometimes works to provide a space to retain the bolus in the valleculae until airway closure is achieved. The bolus has to be of a size that can be retained.
								Aspiration of penetrated material after the swallow	Reduced laryngeal elevation / Reduced closure at the entrance to the airway	
Thermal-tactile stimulation / Neurosensory stimulation				X	X			Penetration and/or aspiration before the swallow / Aspiration during the swallow / Aspiration of penetrated material after the swallow	Delayed pharyngeal response	To increase sensitivity and awareness at the faucial pillars to enhance pharyngeal response
Sensory/chemesthetic (e.g., cold, sour, carbonated, capsaicin)	X			X	X			Pharyngeal residue		To provide increased sensory input to heighten awareness of the bolus and reduce delay/improve timing of pharyngeal response / Increase swallowing pressures

Technique	Problem	Physiological deficit	Goal
Valsalva tight-breath hold	Penetration and/or aspiration before the swallow	Reduced closure at entrance to airway	To increase closure at entrance to airway, with better movement of arytenoid cartilages
Supraglottic swallow*	Aspiration during the swallow	Reduced closure of vocal folds	To volitionally close the larynx at the level of the vocal folds to prevent the bolus from entering the airway
Super-supraglottic swallow	Penetration and/or aspiration before the swallow	Reduced closure of true and false vocal folds/tipping of arytenoids with aryepiglottic folds collapsing into space	To volitionally close not only at the level of the vocal folds but also at the entrance to the airway with arytenoid cartilages and aryepiglottic folds, to keep material from penetrating
	Aspiration of penetrated material after the swallow	Mistiming of the closure of the structures for airway protection	To improve the timing of the movements
	Aspiration of penetrated material after the swallow	Reduced laryngeal elevation	To increase the speed of initiation of the laryngeal elevation and the cough; might clear any penetrated material
Mendelsohn maneuver*	Residue in the pyriform sinuses that might be aspirated after the swallow	Reduced laryngeal elevation	To increase laryngeal elevation and length of time PES is open, to reduce residue
		Reduced anterior movement of hyolaryngeal complex	Improved bolus propulsion through pharynx
		Reduced pharyngeal peristalsis	
	Material penetrating into the upper laryngeal vestibule that might or might not remain and be aspirated	Mistiming of the closure of the structures for airway protection	Normalize overall timing of pharyngeal swallow events
	Residue in valleculae that might be aspirated after the swallow	Reduced laryngeal elevation	Elevation of larynx takes epiglottis to horizontal, which should help clear the bolus during the swallow

(continues)

PHARYNGEAL-PHASE TECHNIQUES (continued)

Signs, Physiology, and Function

Technique	Compensatory: Bolus modification	Compensatory: Increased control	Compensatory: Postural	External sensory	Rehabilitative: Sensorimotor with a swallow	Rehabilitative: Sensorimotor without a swallow	Device	What sign you observe	Impaired physiology	Intended impact of the technique on the functional swallow
Effortful swallow*		X			X		X	Residue in valleculae or on pharyngeal walls with possible aspiration after from the residue; Residue in valleculae and pyriform sinuses; Residue in pyriforms	Reduced base-of-tongue/pharyngeal wall squeeze; Reduced linguapalatal pressure; Reduced pharyngeal pressure; Reduced hyolaryngeal excursion (anterior and superior movement); Reduced duration of UES opening	Increase pressure on the bolus to clear the pharynx and eliminate or reduce residue; Increase amount and duration of laryngeal elevation to prevent residue if more bolus can enter esophagus
								Penetration	Impaired timing of hyolaryngeal excursion	Improved timing of pharyngeal response to eliminate penetration
Three-second prep		X			X			Purposeful movement of bolus over the back of the tongue into vestibule or airway	True delayed pharyngeal response or mistiming of the response	Utilize cortical control for neural preparation of the swallow
Suck-swallow gestures		X			X			Aspiration before or during the swallow	Mistiming or delayed pharyngeal response	Organize oral movements to coordinate timing of swallow response
Head rotation to weaker side (though sometimes works to the strong side)		X	X					Aspiration during the swallow; Significant pyriform sinus residue after the swallow putting patient at risk to aspirate	Reduced closure at level of vocal folds; Reduced anterior superior movement of the hyolaryngeal complex, resulting in reduction in PES opening	To help stronger vocal fold move toward weaker; Facilitate PES opening; close off the pyriform on weaker side, reducing the amount of reside that remains and might be aspirated
Different utensil		X						Poor control of the bolus in the oral cavity, especially with liquids falling over back of tongue too soon	Poor back-of-tongue control	Help the patient gain control of the bolus

Technique	Symptom / Observation	Physiological Cause	Rationale / Goal
Multiple swallows	Residue in valleculae	Reduced tongue-base/pharyngeal-wall movement	Eliminate residue that might be aspirated
	Residue in pyriform sinuses	Reduced elevation of larynx; Reduced anterio-superior movement of hyolaryngeal complex	
Oral exercises for back of tongue*	Bolus falling over back of tongue	Poor back-of-tongue control	Improve control of back of tongue so bolus remains in cohesive fashion in oral cavity until patient is ready to swallow
Sustained tongue retraction / Tongue pull-back*	Residue in valleculae	Reduced base-of-tongue to pharyngeal-wall pressure	Improve base of tongue to pharyngeal wall contact to reduce vallecular residue
Pretend to gargle	Residue in valleculae	Reduced base-of-tongue and pharyngeal-wall pressure	Improve base-of-tongue and pharyngeal-wall movement for increased pressure to reduce vallecular residue
Pretend to yawn*	Residue in valleculae	Reduced base-of-tongue and pharyngeal-wall pressure	Improve base of tongue to pharyngeal wall contact to reduce vallecular residue
Tongue hold (Masako)*	Residue in valleculae and/or on pharyngeal walls	Reduced movement of pharyngeal wall	Increase movement of pharyngeal walls to improve base of tongue to pharyngeal wall contact to reduce vallecular residue
Controlling bolus size	Penetration or aspiration of the bolus during the swallow	Mistiming of closure	Provide a bolus of the size that can be managed safely
	Aspiration during the swallow from bolus in pyriforms before pharyngeal response	Delayed pharyngeal response or mistiming of response	Provide a bolus of the size that does not overwhelm the pyriform sinuses
	Aspiration of residue after the swallow from valleculae or pyriform sinuses	Reduced superior movement of larynx and anterior-superior movement of hyolaryngeal complex resulting in pyriform residue	Provide a bolus of the size that residue after the swallow does not overwhelm the pyriform sinuses

(continues)

PHARYNGEAL-PHASE TECHNIQUES (continued)

Technique	Compensatory: Bolus modification	Compensatory: Increased control	Compensatory: Postural	Rehabilitative — External sensory	Rehabilitative — Sensorimotor with a swallow	Rehabilitative — Sensorimotor without a swallow	Device	Signs, Physiology, and Function — What sign you observe	Signs, Physiology, and Function — Impaired physiology	Signs, Physiology, and Function — Intended impact of the technique on the functional swallow
Multiple swallows		X						Residue in valleculae	Reduced tongue base/pharyngeal wall movement	Eliminate residue that might be aspirated
Effortful pitch glide/falsetto*						X		Residue in pyriform sinuses	Reduced anterior hyoid movement; Reduced laryngeal elevation; Reduced medialization of pharyngeal walls	To improve laryngeal elevation, anterior movement of hyolaryngeal complex, and pharyngeal wall movement to reduce pyriform sinus residue
Head lift (Shaker)*						X		Residue in valleculae that might be aspirated after swallow; Residue in pyriform sinuses; Reduced opening of PES	Reduced laryngeal elevation; Reduced anterior-superior movement of the hyolaryngeal complex	Elevation of larynx takes epiglottis to horizontal, which should help clear the bolus during the swallow; To improve the anterior and superior movement of the hyolaryngeal complex, reducing pyriform residue
EMST						X	X	Penetration into upper laryngeal vestibule before or during; Residue in pyriforms	Reduced closure at entrance to airway; Reduced hyolaryngeal excursion	Improve closure at entrance to airway to eliminate penetration; Improve hyolaryngeal excursion to reduce pyriform residue

Note. Exercises marked with an asterisk have videos of how to perform on the National Foundation of Swallowing Disorders website.

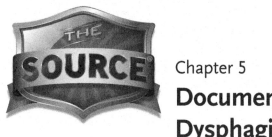

Chapter 5

Documentation of Dysphagia Treatment

Why Documentation Is Important

Documentation is the proof that what the clinician says was done was actually done. Sometimes it seems as if the clinician spends as much, or more, time documenting what was done as in providing the service. The documentation is a reflection of the quality of services provided, and to many audiences, the documents produced by the speech–language pathologist are the only basis on which the clinician's skills are judged. The speech–language pathologist spends most of the time documenting for client management reasons. Speech–language pathologists document evaluations and treatment plans. Progress notes document the client's status and progress. Discharge summaries provide the basis for the next level of care.

However, there are many other reasons besides client management that a clinician documents. Documentation serves business purposes, such as supporting reimbursement of services rendered and demonstrating productivity. Third-party payers such as Medicare and private insurers audit records to see whether services were appropriately reimbursed. Medical records are reviewed for a variety of other reasons. Facilities review records to see whether they are meeting quality benchmarks. Facilities and payers review records to determine whether services were appropriately utilized. Regulatory agencies review records to ensure compliance with laws and regulations. Records are also used as the basis for research, particularly epidemiological studies. And every piece of documentation serves as a legal document.

Each treatment setting has different demands for documentation and different formats that must be learned. It is beyond the scope of this chapter to describe all the different requirements in these settings. For that, readers are referred to books specifically written on documentation (Swigert, 2018). Instead, this chapter describes the basic rules of documenting dysphagia treatment.

Regardless of the setting, being able to efficiently and accurately record what the patient has done in treatment is essential. This documentation is one of the most important ways in which clinicians communicate with physicians, other health-care providers, case managers, and payers. It begins with an evaluation report and includes the treatment plan, progress/daily treatment notes, progress reports at certain intervals, recertifications, and discharge summaries. Evaluation reports were described in Chapters 2 and 3. The results of the clinical and instrumental exams, including all information about function derived from the clinician's observations and caregiver and client reports, are used to establish goals for treatment. This information serves as the benchmark against which to compare progress. This chapter focuses on general expectations about documentation that apply in any setting as well as on forms and formats for treatment plans, treatment and progress notes, periodic reports, and discharge summaries.

Developing Treatment Plans With a Focus on Function

The treatment planning process should be a collaborative one between clinician and client, and caregivers when indicated. Keeping the ICF framework in mind, goals need to be set that will address impairments not only at the body structure and function level but also at the level of the client's activity and participation. Short-term goals focus on the body structure and function level, whereas long-term goals focus on activity and participation. Consideration must be given to the personal and environmental factors that will affect the client's ability to achieve the established goals in the plan. These considerations can be addressed in long-term goals. For example, Long-Term Goals 6 and 7 describe the environment in which the patient can eat. Any long-term goal can be modified to mention personal factors such as food preferences. For example, an LTG could be written as follows: "Patient will be able to eat foods within liquid base containing small pieces of solids."

Clinicians often discuss treatment goals with the client and caregivers, but they may not always get a commitment from them on what they are willing to work toward. Too often, SLPs set goals they expect the patient to achieve in the therapy sessions with them, which may be focused at the level of impairment in body structure and function. For example, an SLP may be addressing impaired hyolaryngeal excursion or impaired lingual strength. These impairment goals may have little meaning to the client unless he or she understands the impact that improving these impairments will have on function, such as returning to thin liquids or being able to eat solid foods. With the changing health-care environment, SLPs should develop treatment plans with a focus on the patient working on the goals outside of the therapy session as much as possible to achieve the needed intensity and frequency of exercise.

Writing SMART Goals

One framework that is helpful in writing good goals is to use the SMART criteria. SMART criteria are commonly attributed to Peter Drucker's concept of management by objectives (Boudreaux, 2005; Bovend'Eerdt, Botell, & Wade, 2009). SMART is an acronym that stands for *specific, measurable, attainable, realistic,* and *time bound* (Figure 5.1).

SMART goals are increasingly used in health care to help patients learn to manage their own health, especially chronic conditions, but the principles can easily be applied to goals to address dysphagia.

Specific

A specific goal has a much greater chance of being accomplished than a general goal. To evaluate whether a goal is specific, assess how well it addresses the five *W* questions:

- Who: Who is involved? Almost always, this is the client. In certain cases, only the caregiver may be involved. For example, a patient with moderate dementia may not be able to actively participate in treatment, but a goal may be written for the caregiver to implement. In many cases, client and caregiver(s) are involved in the treatment.

- What: What do I want to accomplish? Keeping the focus on function, this question should be "What do the client and I agree we should work to accomplish?"

- When: Set a time frame. Much more information is addressed under "T," timebound.

- Where: Identify a location. Is this a goal to be achieved in the treatment setting? Transferred to settings outside the treatment room? Generalized to all settings?

S

Specific: Who, what, when, where, which, and why?

M

Measurable: Which metric will be used to measure progress?

A

Achievable: The goal should require the client to stretch but should be set so it is achievable.

R

Realistic: A goal may be attainable, but is it realistic that the client will work hard enough to achieve it?

T

Time bound: Must have a time frame.

Figure 5.1 SMART goals.

- Which (how): Identify requirements and constraints. Think about what will be required to achieve the goal and what might impede progress. Recall the personal and environmental factors of the ICF framework. Which of those will work to facilitate or impede? What specific steps need to be taken to achieve the goal?

- Why: the specific reasons, purpose, or benefits of accomplishing the goal. This really helps to keep the focus on function. Clients want to know why we are working on a specific task.

WRITING A SMART GOAL THAT IS SPECIFIC

A general goal would be "Client's swallowing skills will improve." A specific goal would be "Client's swallowing skills will improve through increased ability to use the effortful swallow during meals in the dining room so that he can swallow mechanical soft foods with less oral and pharyngeal residue on 90% of trials with no cues within 4 weeks."

Who?	The client
What?	Wants to eat mechanical soft foods rather than pureed
When?	Within a month
Where?	In the dining room
Which/how?	Will need support of family members. Will need cueing by staff. May need picture cues in the environment.
Why?	So that the client can eat in the dining room with other residents without the help of an aide.

CUEING TO MAKE IT MORE SPECIFIC

SLPs sometimes use the levels of cueing that physical and occupational therapists use: minimal, moderate, or maximum assist. These do not really apply to dysphagia therapy, though. How, for example, would one provide maximum assist to a patient as she performs the effortful swallow? Instead, it is more appropriate to describe the type of cues, such as verbal, visual, and tactile. The frequency of cueing can also be included (Henley, 2017).

Measurable

There must be tangible criteria for measuring progress toward the attainment of each goal set. This applies to both long- and short-term goals. In addition, terms must be operationally defined. For example, if a goal uses words like *efficiently*, *accurately*, or *quickly*, these must be defined. If not, how would one know when the goal was achieved?

To determine whether a goal is measurable, ask questions such as, How much? How many? How will one know when it is accomplished?

MEASURABLE LONG-TERM GOALS

Long-term goals sometimes pose the biggest challenge for making them measurable. Consider these long-terms goals and decide whether it would be easy to know when the patient had achieved them. Some probing questions are listed after each goal:

- Patient will eat optimal diet. *What is optimal?*

- Patient will advance diet as far as possible. *How far is it possible for the patient to go?*

- Patient will eat foods she likes. *What are the desired foods?*

- Patient will safely consume thin liquids. *How will it be determined to be safe? No coughing? No pneumonia? No upper respiratory infection? Confirmed by an instrumental exam?*

MEASURABLE SHORT-TERM GOALS

Short-term goals, in particular, are written with a percentage accuracy or number of times a response needs in order to be considered accurate. The goals often need to indicate type of cueing required. If that information is omitted, it will make success difficult to measure.

Attainable

An attainable goal (sometimes also called actionable or achievable) is based on an accurate prognosis. Consider a patient with advanced dementia who cannot follow commands and takes only pureed foods and some sips of liquid. A long-term goal for the patient to return to a regular diet is not an attainable goal. In contrast, a long-term goal for the patient to take some soft finger foods may be attainable. If the clinician has discussed prognosis with the caregiver, and the caregiver understands and accepts the prognosis, it is more likely that attainable goals will be set.

USING ASHA'S NATIONAL OUTCOMES MEASUREMENT SYSTEM (NOMS)
TO WRITE ATTAINABLE GOALS

The ASHA NOMS Adult Component has a new feature that gives clinicians access to real-time national benchmarking data to help SLPs establish an attainable goal. When the patient's information is entered into the NOMS system and the Functional Communication Measure (FCM) rating is given, the SLP can select "View National Goal Setting." This data indicates what percentage of patients nationally who have started at the same FCM level and were treated in the same setting achieved each FCM level by discharge. The NOMS system also includes a reporting feature that allows clinicians to receive more detailed information, such as how many sessions or what length of time it took on average for patients with similar characteristics (e.g., medical diagnosis, severity level) to reach that level at the facility compared to patients receiving treatment nationally (National Outcomes Measurement System, 2016).

Realistic

A realistic goal is one that is attainable but also one the patient is willing to work toward. Setting a realistic goal requires significant discussion with the client and caregivers. Not only must the prognosis be considered, but the level of commitment of client and caregivers also has an impact. Perhaps a client can swallow thin liquids safely with head rotation and multiple swallows in no larger than teaspoon amounts. This could be an attainable goal, but is it realistic to think the client will do that on every sip of liquid throughout a meal?

Time Bound

Establish a time frame. Depending on the setting, short-term goals are for a period of weeks or months. Long-term goals are usually set for the time frame the client is expected to be at that level of care. For example, in an acute-care hospital, the long term might be at time of discharge in 4–5 days, whereas in an outpatient setting the long-term goal might be 1–2 months.

In outpatient settings, short-term goals are likely updated and changed periodically as dictated by the payer. Medicare, for example, requires that the treatment plan (a *certification*, in Medicare terms) be updated and signed again by the physician. The period covered during each certification varies by setting. Even at points not required by a third-party payer, the clinician may want to update the treatment plan. It might be determined that one of the goals was too challenging, or that a goal has already been achieved. In other instances, the clinician may want to add goals and treatment objectives. If an update required by a third-party payer is imminent, make those changes at that time. If there are no requirements for periodic updating of the treatment plan, the clinician can make those changes at any time (Swigert, 2018).

Developing a Treatment Plan

In settings in which services are provided to clients with Medicare as the payment source, the treatment plan is called a certification and requires a physician's signature on the plan. The plan must be updated periodically, at different times depending on the setting, and signed again. This is referred to as recertification.

The treatment plan can be documented in various ways depending on the setting in which the services are provided. Most health-care settings utilize an electronic health record (EHR). Each EHR differs in how the information is entered and what a printout looks like. Inpatient settings not on an EHR may have specific forms to be used for the treatment plan or certification. A useful format in outpatient settings includes spaces for all required information in a table format, which can also be used for the goals. (See the Supplemental Materials, SLP Resources, Treatment Plan Examples, for an easy-to-use treatment plan format.) This same form can then be used as updates (recertifications) and for the discharge summary.

Regardless of the format, the treatment plan should contain the following:

- Client identifying information

- Diagnoses

- Date the plan was established

- Period of time the plan will cover

- Type (e.g., individual, group), amount (e.g., number of times in a day), frequency (e.g., number of times in a week), and duration of services (e.g., period of time, number of weeks or months)

- Long-term goal(s)

- Short-term goal(s)

- Treatment objectives (or short-term goals with objectives embedded)

- Signature, date, and professional designation of the person who established the plan (CMS, 2012)

Long-Term Goals

Typically, long-term goals are also for the length of time the patient will be in that level of care. What level of skill and function do clinician and client agree is realistic and attainable by the time the client moves to the next level of care? Clinicians should not use terms like *optimal diet* or *least restrictive diet*. Those are moving targets, and one would never know for sure when one of them was achieved. Examples of long-term goals are found in the Supplemental Materials (SLP Resources, Goals and Treatment Objectives). The speech–language pathologist will need to individualize long-term goals to include all SMART criteria and to focus on functions important to that client. In dysphagia, long-term goals can be harder to measure. Ideally, a patient with a pharyngeal dysphagia could undergo a repeat instrumental exam to determine whether the physiological deficits had been resolved. Realistically, however, the long-term goal may need to be worded on the basis of observing the patient consuming the diet without complications, defined by the SLP.

Short-Term Goals

If the clinician is following the SMART guidelines, short-term goals will be written in functional terms, which includes telling not just the what but also the why. A functional goal tells why the client is working on something. It should be written in terms that someone who is not an SLP can understand. For example:

> Not functional: "Client will improve tongue strength."

> Functional: "Patient will improve tongue strength so he can clear a bolus of food from the mouth with one swallow."

Write short-term goals as the smaller steps needed to reach the long-term goal. There may be multiple short-terms goals for each long-term goal.

Treatment Objectives

Short-term goals can be broken into more measurable steps called treatment objectives. One short-term goal might have several treatment objectives. Treatment objectives are the steps to achieve the short-term goal and are often equivalent to therapeutic activities. Which activities will be used to achieve the goal? Treatment objectives answer the *how* question: How will the clinician help the patient reach the short-term goal?

For example, the short-term goal "Within 2 weeks, client will increase closure at the entrance to the airway with occasional visual cues on 90% of trials to contribute to keep food from entering the airway" might have the following (and more) measurable treatment objectives:

- Client will perform super-supraglottic swallow with visual cues on 90% of trials with small sips of thin liquid.

- Client will control bolus size to 1 teaspoon on all bites of pureed food with no cues 95% of trials.

- Client will perform effortful swallow with teaspoon amounts of pureed food on 90% of trials with occasional verbal cues.

COMBINING SHORT-TERM GOALS AND TREATMENT OBJECTIVES

If the charting system does not accommodate both short-term goals and treatment objectives, the short-term goal and treatment objective can be combined. For example: "Within 2 weeks, client will increase closure at the entrance to the airway with occasional visual cues on 90% of trials to contribute to keep food from entering the airway by performing super-supraglottic swallow on 90% of small sips of liquid."

Selecting Long-Term and Short-Term Goals and Treatment Objectives

The Goals and Treatment Objectives, in the Supplemental Materials, provides examples of long-term goals as well as an extensive list of short-term goals and related treatment objectives. When using the materials to establish treatment plans, the SLP should be aware of how the information has been organized, as reflected in Tables 5.1 and 5.2. Table 5.1 is the list of long-term goals and Table 5.2, the master list of the functional deficits addressed by short-term goals. The Goals and Treatment Objectives in the Supplemental Materials and these tables should be used together with the Chapter 4 Appendix, which provides detailed information about each of the treatment techniques.

In Table 5.2, the first column is the number of the goal, the second column lists the description of the functional problem (e.g., anterior loss is *AL*), and the term or terms in the fourth column indicate the impaired physiology determined during the assessment to be causing the functional deficit (e.g., reduced lip closure is *lc*). The abbreviations in the right-most column indicate the same relationship between functional disorder and physiological cause. In both the oral and pharyngeal phases, some functional deficits have more than one possible physiological cause. For example, difficulty with bolus formation or propulsion might be caused by decreased lingual movement, or motor planning or agnosia. Aspiration before the swallow might be due to a problem with control of the back of the tongue or a timing issue. Some of the pharyngeal goals are still more detailed. For example, aspiration after might come from material in the pyriform sinuses or from penetrated material in the laryngeal vestibule. The location of the residue is indicated in the third column and in the middle of each abbreviation (e.g., AA/*LV*/vc). For the goals unrelated to specific pharyngeal residue, there is no abbreviation in the middle but, instead, are two slashes (e.g., //, such as in AL // lc).

Table 5.1

Examples of Long-Term Goals

1	Patient will safely consume _____ diet with _____ liquids without complications such as aspiration pneumonia.
2	Patient will maintain adequate nutrition and hydration through oral diet.
3	Patient will be able to complete a meal in fewer than _____ minutes.
4	Patient will maintain nutrition/hydration via alternative means.
5	Patient's quality of life will be enhanced through eating and drinking small amounts of food and liquid.
6	Patient will be able to eat targeted foods and liquids without signs of discomfort (e.g., palliative goal).
7	Patient will be able to eat meals with family and friends in controlled environment.
8	Patient will be able to eat meals with others in public places.

Table 5.2

Master List of Functional Deficits Addressed by Short-Term Goals

Goal	Functional deficit	Residue location	Physiologic deficit	Safety	Efficiency	Abbreviation for short-term goal and treatment objective
1	Anterior loss		Lip closure		X	AL/lc
2	Anterior loss		Jaw closure		X	AL/jc
3	Bolus formation and propulsion		Tongue movement	X	X	BPF/tm
4	Bolus formation and propulsion		Motor planning or agnosia	X	X	BPF/mp,a
5	Bolus formation and propulsion		Tone in cheeks		X	BPF/tc
6	Aspiration before the swallow		Tongue control	X		AB/tc
7	Aspiration before the swallow		Timing	X		AB/t
8	Aspiration during the swallow		Laryngeal closure	X		AD/lc
9	Aspiration during the swallow		Timing	X		AD/t
10	Aspiration after the swallow	Pyriform sinuses	Laryngeal elevation and/or hyolaryngeal excursion	X	X	AA/P/le,hle
11	Aspiration after the swallow	Laryngeal vestibule	Laryngeal elevation	X	X	AA/LV/le
12	Aspiration after the swallow	Laryngeal vestibule	Vestibular closure	X	X	AA/LV/vc
13	Aspiration after the swallow	Laryngeal vestibule	Timing	X	X	AA/LV/t
14	Aspiration after the swallow	Pharyngeal residue	Tongue base	X	X	AA/PR/tb
15	Aspiration after the swallow	Pharyngeal residue	Pharyngeal walls	X	X	AA/PR/pw
16	Multiple deficits related to reduced ROM (e.g., oral residue, reduced jaw opening or movement for biting and chewing, pharyngeal residue, aspiration)	Multiple locations	Reduced range of motion of oral and pharyngeal structures; exercises are often prescribed as preventive	X	X	OPROM

Note. Before using abbreviations, check with your facility to determine whether they are acceptable. Notes on terms used: *Pharyngeal residue* indicates residue high in pharynx (e.g., valleculae, on tongue base, on pharyngeal walls). If it is not this general term for where the residue is, then the specific terms *valleculae* and *pyriforms* will be used. The term *timing* is used to indicate increased stage transition duration (what used to be described as pharyngeal delay or delay in pharyngeal response) or mistiming of the movement of the structures. *Vestibular closure* means closure at the entrance to the airway. *Laryngeal closure* refers to closure at the level of the vocal folds. *Hyolaryngeal excursion* refers to the anterior movement of the hyoid but also to the superior movement (and larynx moves with it to a large extent).

Each functional deficit could have more than one physiological deficit causing it. Therefore, separate short-term goals are written for each physiological cause, highlighting again how important it is to plan treatment based on physiology, not on the functional result of the impairment. For example, aspiration after the swallow from pharyngeal residue might be caused by reduced tongue-base movement or reduced pharyngeal wall movement. Although many of the techniques would apply to both physiological deficits (e.g., effortful swallow addresses both), some address only deficit (e.g., tongue hold more directly addresses pharyngeal wall movement) (Figure 5.2).

Table 5.2 also indicates whether the functional deficit is related to the efficiency of the swallow, the safety of the swallow, or both (columns 5 and 6). This information can be used to further refine how the short-term goal is written. For example, aspiration after the swallow from pyriform sinus residue is obviously a safety issue. The goal could state: "Patient will improve the safety of the swallow by increasing laryngeal elevation to reduce the amount of pyriform sinus residue that might fall into the airway." Residue in the pyriform sinuses is also an efficiency issue because the bolus is not cleared on the first swallow. The goal might be tweaked to state: "Patient will improve the efficiency of the swallow by increasing laryngeal elevation to reduce the amount of pyriform sinus residue that requires multiple swallows to clear." Some payers like to see additional information, particularly about safety of the swallow.

CHOOSING "ASPIRATION" GOALS WHEN THE PATIENT IS NOT ASPIRATING

Short-Term Goals 6–15 relate to aspiration before, during, or after the swallow. Sometimes a patient does not aspirate but appears to be at high risk of doing so. In that case, these short-term goals

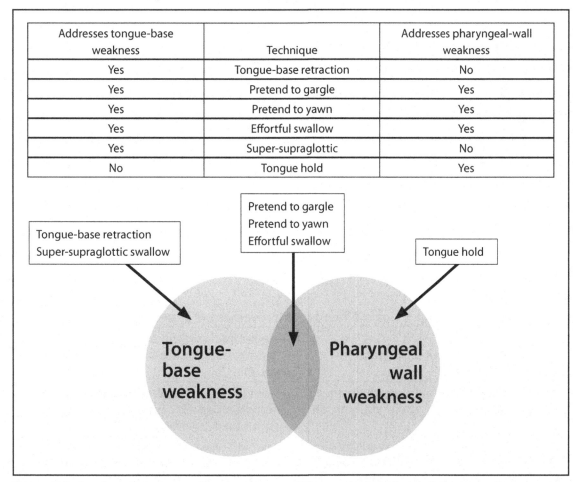

Addresses tongue-base weakness	Technique	Addresses pharyngeal-wall weakness
Yes	Tongue-base retraction	No
Yes	Pretend to gargle	Yes
Yes	Pretend to yawn	Yes
Yes	Effortful swallow	Yes
Yes	Super-supraglottic	No
No	Tongue hold	Yes

Figure 5.2 Overlap of treatment objectives to treat different physiological deficits.

would be appropriate. Penetration alone is not a reason to restrict a patient's diet. However, even if the patient does not aspirate the penetrated material, the SLP might want to improve laryngeal vestibular closure to reduce the amount of penetration. Each of these goals has several alternative wordings from which to choose in order to indicate whether the aspiration is actually occurring or whether the goal has been chosen to reduce the risk of aspiration.

SETTING GOALS WHEN NO IMPROVEMENT IS EXPECTED

For some clients with a chronic or progressive condition, no improvement is expected. Medicare requirements had historically held that for services to be reimbursed, there had to be an expectation that improvement would be made, often referenced as the "improvement standard." In 2013, in a case called *Jimmo v. Sebelius*, a federal court held that Medicare could not deny services because the client showed no functional progress in cases of degenerative or progressive disorders, such as ALS, MS, or Parkinson's disease. The court stated that Medicare had to cover services to maintain skills and prevent deterioration (ASHA, 2016; *Jimmo vs. Sebelius Settlement Agreement Fact Sheet*, 2014).

Note that these still need to be skilled services. Medicare will not cover services designed to "practice" or "drill," as such activities can be completed by caregivers. In the case of degenerative and progressive disorders, it may be very appropriate for the speech–language pathologist to periodically reassess, intervene, and modify maintenance programs to address the client's current level of swallow function.

For the client with a chronic disorder who is not functioning at an optimal level, the focus of a short course of treatment might be on teaching compensatory strategies and helping client and caregiver learn ways to improve both the safety and the efficiency of the swallow. The same is true for a client with a progressive disorder for which intermittent courses of treatment are indicated at various stages of the disease (Swigert, 2018).

When no improvement is expected, the goals are worded to reflect not an expected improvement in skill but rather improved use of compensations and adaptations. Goals might also be written for a change in caregiver behaviors, such as cueing. For example, instead of the goal "Client will improve laryngeal elevation to reduce pyriform sinus residue that might fall into the airway," a goal might read "Client will compensate for reduced laryngeal elevation with pyriform sinus residue by taking only controlled bolus size sips" or "Caregiver will cue multiple swallows to clear pyriform sinus residue that results from reduced laryngeal elevation."

Rewording goals for compensation only. If only compensation treatment objectives are appropriate for a patient (e.g., no potential for improved physiology, inability to participate in treatment), then the functional short-term goal should be reworded. As they are written in the Goals

Table 5.3
Editing Goals When No Improvement Is Expected

Functional short-term goals when improvement is expected	Reworded functional short-term goals if only compensation objectives are appropriate because no improvement is expected
• Patient will increase elevation of the larynx to reduce the amount of food remaining in the pyriform sinuses that falls into the airway after the swallow.	• Patient will compensate for decreased laryngeal elevation to reduce the amount of food remaining in the pyriform sinuses that falls into the airway after the swallow.
• Patient will increase closure at the entrance to the airway to keep food from entering the top of the larynx and falling into the airway after the swallow.	• Patient will compensate for decreased closure at the entrance to the airway to keep food from entering the top of the larynx and falling into the airway after the swallow.

and Treatment Objectives in the Supplemental Materials, the short-term goals presume working toward improved function. Examples for rewording are provided in Table 5.3.

WORDING TREATMENT OBJECTIVES WITH OR WITHOUT FOOD/LIQUID

The goals for sensorimotor techniques with a swallow are worded in a way that involves food. Therefore, if the goal is selected as a treatment technique without food, the treatment objective would need to be reworded. For example, Treatment Objective AA/LV/le-4: "Patient will use effortful swallow for _____ consistencies on _____ of _____ trials" would be worded that way if used with, for example, a bolus of pudding.

If, however, it is not safe for the patient to swallow food, the treatment objective might be reworded as follows: "Patient will use effortful swallow for saliva swallows with/without cues on 7 of 10 trials."

If the patient is using compensatory strategies during meals, the speech–language pathologist might indicate whether the patient is to use the technique with certain foods only, for part of the meal, or for the entire meal. Also the kind of cues needed should be indicated.

TREATMENT OBJECTIVES

Each short-term goal has multiple treatment objectives. These are equivalent to the treatment techniques used in therapy. The initials after each treatment objective indicate whether the technique is intended to be rehabilitative (though for many, strong evidence does not exist to demonstrate long-lasting effects), compensatory, or both. If compensatory, the description also includes the type of compensatory strategy: postural (P), designed to increase control (IC), and bolus modification (B) (Table 5.4).

Treatment objective used as rehabilitative and compensatory. When choosing a technique that is both compensatory and rehabilitative, indicate on the treatment plan in which way, or ways, it is intended to be used. For example, Short-Term Goal 8 is to be used if the patient is aspirating during the swallow because of reduced closure of the vocal folds. Treatment Objective AD//lc-2 is use of the supraglottic swallow. The speech–language pathologist might select that technique for the patient to use during meals as compensation. However, the speech–language pathologist might not want the patient to use it during meals if she is unable to remember to follow the directions or may become fatigued. In that case, AD//lc-2 might be selected only as a rehabilitative technique. Another patient might use the technique during meals and therapeutically as both compensation and rehabilitation.

How and when to use the technique. Each treatment objective can be described in terms of when and how often the patient is to use the technique and with how much cueing. For instance, if the effortful swallow is to be used as a compensation during meals, the objective might read: "Patient will use effortful swallow during liquid swallows 100% of the time with consistent verbal cues given by clinician."

Table 5.4
Understanding the Types of Treatment Objectives

C	Compensatory techniques compensate for a deficit; further defined as to the type of compensation
C/BM	Compensation by bolus modification
C/IC	Compensation to give increased control
C/P	Compensation that is postural
R	Rehabilitative treatment techniques to improve function
C/R	Compensatory techniques that also act as rehabilitative to return of function

Making the objectives measurable. To provide precise measurement capabilities, include target percentages, frequency of cueing, and situations in which the technique is to be used. This strategy enables the clinician to document accomplishments of small steps toward achieving the functional short-term goal.

Treatment objective related to more than one short-term goal. One treatment objective may seem related to more than one short-term goal. For example, the Mendelsohn maneuver is a technique to improve elevation and timing. It can be listed under each short-term goal. When completing the exercise, accuracy can be reported under each short-term goal.

Treatment Notes and Progress Notes and Reports

Treatment Notes

The terms *treatment note, progress note,* and *daily notes* are often used interchangeably. These notes are typically written each time the client is seen, but in some inpatient settings they may be written once a week with supporting documentation for each date or visit reflected in that weekly note. If notes are written weekly, it is important to have a chart to document the number of visits or units completed on each date. Examples of treatment notes can be found in the Supplemental Materials (SLP Resources, Treatment Notes Examples). Whether per visit or once a week, the treatment note must summarize what has happened in treatment and also particularly highlight the client's progress toward goals that occurred during that period. Although Medicare does not specify a frequency for note documentation, it would expect the documentation to support the progress claimed if Medicare were to conduct an audit. Medicare does require that the following information be documented for each visit:

- Date of service

- Procedure(s) performed (including the CPT code)

- Length of time involved with each procedure (which would be crucial only if a timed CPT code was used; otherwise length of the session generally is equal to the amount of time spent with the patient in that session)

- Signature and professional identification of the provider of the procedure(s) (*Medicare Benefit Policy Manual,* 2016)

If writing a progress note for each visit, in addition to the information listed above, the note should also contain much more detailed information to demonstrate skilled service and significant progress.

Medicare can deny payment based on one specific session or an entire group of sessions. If the progress note is written for a week and the documentation is not sufficient to show significant improvement, the entire week of sessions may be denied.

The treatment note documentation can take a variety of formats, including SOAP notes, various charts or graphs, or standardized forms. The SOAP format is typically used for writing treatment notes. This format helps to organize the information into sections on subjective data, objective data, data analysis, and plan for next steps. The treatment notes are also where the speech–language pathologist demonstrates that the services being provided are medically necessary, meeting the standards of *reasonable, necessary, specific, effective,* and *skilled.*

SOAP FORMAT

The well-recognized SOAP note format is not required, but it can be helpful because it forces the SLP to analyze a patient's performance. SOAP stands for *subjective, objective, analysis, plan.*

Subjective. Include initial observations of the patient or anything the family has said about how the patient is doing, for example, "Mrs. P. was choking on her coffee" or "The patient reports a nurse gave her pills without crushing them and she had difficulty swallowing them."

Objective. Include any objective data taken during the session. Objective data should be collected on treatment objectives and include percentages and the patient's response to the clinician's analysis and feedback.

Analysis. Summarize and put in functional terms exactly what happened during each session. Instead of concentrating directly on the treatment objectives, talk about how progress on the treatment objectives moved the patient closer to achieving the functional goals. Use comparative statements like "better than the session yesterday" or "increased percentage of ability to perform exercises."

Plan. Explain what is planned for the next session. Avoid "Continue per treatment plan" as this provides no direction for next steps. It is better to include suggestions that are more specific. If the speech–language pathologist noted in the session that the patient does better with a new compensatory technique than had been initially determined, the plan might be to include this compensatory technique in future sessions. This part of the note can also mention exercises the client is to practice between sessions or specific activities to be addressed in the next session. The *P* of the SOAP process should be specific enough that another SLP could cover the session if the treating clinician is not available.

Electronic Health Records and Point-of-Care Documentation

Electronic Health Records

Most health-care settings now use some form of electronic documentation. These are called electronic health records (EHRs) or electronic medical records (EMRs). Depending on the design of the system, it may or may not be easy to demonstrate that all Medicare documentation guidelines are being met. These records should be designed so that most documentation is point-and-click, with choices available from dropdown menus. There should be little need for the SLP to annotate (enter lengthy, typed information). However, if the system was not designed with all documentation requirements in mind, the clinician may be forced to do just that. EHRs should be constructed to make it easy to do the following:

- Document skilled care. A list of statements documenting skilled care can be included in a dropdown menu.

- Select long- and short-term functional goals. These goals can be organized according to physiological deficits.

- Document client progress. It should be easy to document progress in treatment sessions and in periodic updates. If constructed well, the goals can be pulled up for each session and progress documented by each goal.

- Summarize care in a discharge summary. The latest level of success on each goal can pull from the last progress note to the discharge summary.

Point-of-Care (POC) Documentation

"See one, chart one" refers to charting after each patient. Point-of-care documentation takes that a step further to "see one, chart *with* one." POC documentation is done while the provider is with the client and is a growing practice in health care. It is typically done when an EHR is used, but it can also be done in a paper charting system. Charting should be considered something that the clinician does as a part of the service provided, not something extra done after the service is completed. If done correctly, point-of-care documentation can increase collaboration between clinician and client. It is also a more accurate way to chart than trying to remember all that happened at the end of the session or, worse yet, after seeing three or four clients and then charting all the visits at once. The goal is to be able to log off or close the paper chart when the treatment session is over, or to have only a minute or two still needed to flesh out narrative sections.

Documenting during treatment takes practice and is easier with some clients and in some settings than others. The clinician should explain to the client and caregivers that notes will be taken throughout the session. It is likely the client has already experienced POC documentation at the physician's or dentist's office. The speech–language pathologist can use a standard phrase to introduce the client and his or her caregivers to this type of documentation. For example:

- "I'll be making notes throughout the session to be sure I capture everything we do."

- "I'll stop here and there during the session to record information on how you are doing." This method is particularly helpful when the SLP has on gloves working on particular exercises and does not want to take the gloves off between each exercise to record performance levels.

- "It's important that I record how you are doing, so I'll be taking notes as we go."

- "I'll be sure to let you know how things are going as I take some notes during the session."

Documenting to Demonstrate Skilled Care

Treatment for dysphagia should be given only if the skilled services of a speech–language pathologist are required. Medicare indicates that skilled therapy services may be necessary to improve a patient's current condition, to maintain the patient's current condition, or to prevent or slow further deterioration of the condition.

Just because the service was provided by a speech–language pathologist does not make it skilled. If the service could be self-administered (e.g., client practices a swallowing exercise she already knows how to perform), or safely and effectively provided by an unskilled person, without the direct or general supervision of the speech–language pathologist (e.g., client's spouse provides cues to slow down and use multiple swallows), then it is not considered skilled, even if the speech–language pathologist performs these tasks. Medicare also indicates that just because there is not a competent person without specific skills to practice with the client, the service is not skilled if the speech–language pathologist instead "practices" with the client (*Medicare Benefit Policy Manual*, 2016).

Demonstrating Skilled Care in Progress Notes

The ASHA website provides detailed information on how the speech–language pathologist can demonstrate skilled services in the progress notes. See example statements in Table 5.5.

The documentation of skilled treatment activities should show that the activities:

- Followed a hierarchy of complexity

- Were focused on achieving the target skills for a functional goal

- Were modified on the basis of the speech–language pathologist's expert observation to maintain patient motivation and facilitate success by:

  ◆ Increasing or decreasing the complexity of treatment task

  ◆ Increasing or decreasing the amount or type of cuing needed

Table 5.5
Example Statements to Show Skilled Care

Demonstrated and explained: _____ .
Provided feedback on client's performance: _____ .
Analyzed client's response, and on the basis of analysis:
• Modified instructions given to client
• Increased difficulty of task by:
• Reduced difficulty of task by:
• Provided _____ cues to enhance client's performance
Added new goals to increase challenge
Discontinued goal because _____ .
Provided training and instruction to ( ) in home exercise
Evaluated family member's ability to _____ .

- ◆ Increasing or decreasing the criteria for successful performance (e.g., accuracy, number of repetitions, response latency)
- ◆ Introducing new tasks to evaluate the patient's ability to generalize skill

ASSESSING RESPONSES, EXPLAINING RATIONALE, AND MAKING MODIFICATIONS

If behaviors were practiced with the client, this practice should be combined with explaining the rationale and expected results and/or providing reinforcement. The patient's responses should be continually assessed to modify intervention as needed.

DOCUMENTATION THAT WOULD NOT DEMONSTRATE SKILLED CARE

The ASHA website describes documentation that would indicate the services were *unskilled*:

- Report on performance during activities without describing modification, feedback, or caregiver training provided during the session.
- Repeat the same activities as in previous sessions without noting modifications or observations that would alter future sessions, length of treatment, or plan of care (e.g., "continue per plan of care," as above).
- Report on activity without connecting the task to the long- or short-term functional goals.
- Observe caregivers without providing education or feedback and/or without modifying plan. (ASHA, 2016).

Periodic Reports and Recertifications

In most settings, a written summary is required periodically to document progress and ask for approval for reimbursement for more treatment sessions. These reports should indicate changes in functional behavior from the time of the initial evaluation or the most recent summary. The frequency with which these reports need to be completed is dictated by the setting and by the payer. For example, in outpatient settings, for a patient with Medicare B, it is every 90 days.

Keep in mind the requirements Medicare has for documentation and how to incorporate them into periodic progress notes. These are important points to include in these notes:

- Number of treatments completed and dates of treatment
- Statement of positive expectation

- Techniques for achieving short-term goals
- Statement regarding short-term-goal achievement or progress
- Any changes expected within the course of the next term of treatment

Document changes in functional behaviors that have improved the patient's ability to function within his or her environment. In the area of dysphagia, a functional swallow is a swallow that sustains nutrition orally. How this goal is achieved is not the issue. The desired outcome for Medicare reimbursement is that the functional goal *is* achieved.

These are examples of functional behavior statements:

- "The patient is able to eat soft foods without any choking behavior."
- "The patient is able to maintain food in her mouth without losing any out of the front."
- "The patient is able to eat a meal in significantly less time than at evaluation."

MEDICARE PART B RECERTIFICATIONS

Summary reports for Medicare patients are also called *recertifications*. With a recertification, the physician is asked to state that more services are needed. Each recertification should be signed by the physician. An example of a progress report or recertification is provided in the Supplemental Materials (SLP Resources, Recertification Example).

TENTH-VISIT PROGRESS

These notes or reports are required by the Medicare Part B program at a minimum every 10th treatment session as part of the functional outcomes reporting requirement, commonly called G-codes. These reports and the plan of care are used by medical reviewers and auditors to determine whether the services were medically necessary and skilled. The 10th-visit progress note and the daily visit/treatment note can be one and the same, but if so, then the note needs to clearly distinguish which information is the daily treatment note and which is the 10th visit.

The progress reports must contain the following:

- Who performed the treatment
- Assessment of improvement or the extent of progress made toward therapy goals, including objective measurements. Objective measurements include standardized patient assessment tools, outcome measurement tools, or measurable data that capture function.
- Information about need for continuing treatment and any revisions to the treatment plan
- Changes to the long- or short-term goals
- Functional outcomes reporting
- Current status
- Goal status
- The corresponding G-codes and severity modifier for the primary area (Services, 2016)

These progress reports are the most logical place to report on the closure of one G-code (functional area) and the opening of another G-code (functional area). The progress report does not have to be done on the 10th visit. It can be done before that but must be done at least by the 10th visit. Two examples of 10th-visit progress reports are included in the Supplemental Materials (SLP Resources, Progress Report Examples).

MEDICARE DEFINITION OF TERMS

Several terms are important to understand when documenting progress on a patient covered by Medicare. These concepts are important for any payer.

Significant Progress. Medicare states that significant progress should be made for intervention services to continue. This should be kept in mind when writing either a recertification or a 10th-visit progress note. By definition, *significant progress* means a generally measurable and substantial increase in the patient's present level of swallowing, independence, and competence compared to her levels when treatment began. Progress must be substantial and efficient in relation to how long the progress took. For example:

> Insufficient statement: "The patient's oral swallowing skills have significantly improved."

> Better statement: "Because of improved oral motor control, the patient is able to swallow liquids thickened to nectar consistency."

> Even better statement: "Improved tongue control has resulted in improved oral swallow. Previously, liquids needed to be thickened to a pudding consistency to be swallowed safely, but now less thickener is needed and the patient can swallow liquids of nectar consistency. Continued treatments to improve tongue strength and coordination should allow the patient to progress toward swallowing thin liquids (e.g., water, juice, coffee) without aspiration."

When treatment techniques are rehabilitative and the patient is NPO, the significance of progress may be questioned. For example, if a patient has been using tongue hold and effortful swallow to reduce vallecular residue, and on repeat instrumental exam the patient now has slightly less residue but still aspirates and needs to remain NPO, is this significant progress? Would a Medicare reviewer who sees that the patient is still unable to consume PO intake understand that this is significant progress? Document why the change in amount of residue is a significant factor and why further progress is expected. Also discuss how continued progress will help the patient reach a functional goal: "The patient initially had severe residue in valleculae with aspiration after the swallow. Following therapy to improve tongue base and pharyngeal wall movement, the patient has less residue. With continued decrease in residue, the patient should be able to begin to eat orally."

Positive expectation. The periodic report (recertification or 10th visit note) must show a positive expectation for continued treatments that require skilled services. Which abilities has the patient shown to indicate the intervention is going to be of continued help?

For example, baseline information indicated that the patient was initially able to perform the supraglottic swallow on 20% of trials, but the patient has shown excellent response to learning the supraglottic swallow and can now perform it 100% of the time. Further, the note might state that it is expected with continued intervention that she will be able to use this technique to safely swallow thin liquid boluses of any size without cues. This information uses a comparative statement to show the progress and expectation for continued improvement. The note also uses the client's previously learned skills to show what she may be able to accomplish.

If the patient has made significant improvement but has not reached a level of independence, the note should be worded to make it clear that skilled services are still needed. A note might say, "The patient is able to maintain adequate airway closure during swallow within structured therapeutic settings, but needs further intervention to reach independence with use of the technique." This statement indicates that the expectation is to move the patient to the point where she can do so independently.

Discharge Summaries

Knowing When to Discharge

SLPs are often faced with the decision of when to end therapy. Guidelines for termination of direct skilled intervention services can include the following:

- The physician orders the service discontinued.
- The patient reaches a plateau in progress.
- The patient achieves her treatment goals.
- The patient no longer needs skilled therapy services.
- The patient is discharged from the facility or clinic.

Unfortunately, services are also sometimes discontinued because the patient's payer will no longer pay for the service and the patient is unable to pay. For example, in long-term care, the patient may no longer qualify for one of the rehabilitation categories under Part A—PPS. The patient may also have reached the cap on the limit of dollars that can be spent for that service. The speech–language pathologist must then make sure other caregivers know the techniques needed to keep the patient eating safely.

Gather Client and Caregiver Input to Include in Discharge Summary

The clinician should explain what the objective data mean to the client, particularly in terms of functional gains. If there are remaining problems to be addressed and goals that were not met, these should be discussed and a prognosis given for continued improvement. At the conclusion of intervention, the client's and caregiver's impression of what was accomplished during the intervention should be sought. If the treatment plan and intervention have focused on function, then it should be relatively easy for the client and caregiver to report on changes they notice in day-to-day activities. The speech–language pathologist is seeking their input not necessarily on how they think the client did on specific treatment activities (e.g., using effortful swallow, remembering to use a compensatory strategy), but instead on the impact the improvements have had in daily life (e.g., eating more types of foods, willing to eat in the dining room with other residents). Gathering information on their view of the client's current status compared to when intervention started and perhaps as compared to baseline can make the discharge summary more meaningful to anyone who reads it.

What Else Should Be Included in a Discharge Summary?

Discharge summaries should include the baseline information reported in initial functional goals and statements to show the progress the patient has made toward achieving those functional goals. The discharge summary should provide a succinct but complete picture of what occurred during the course of intervention, including things such as the following:

- Client's and caregiver's view of what was accomplished in treatment
- Objective data (testing or measures of success on goals)
- Treatment methodologies used
- Impact the intervention had on function
- Remaining problems or challenges
- Reason for discharge
- Plans for further intervention or evaluations/consults

Any personal or environmental factors that had an impact on the client's performance in treatment and the impact the treatment has had on impairment, activity, and participation should also be summarized. An example of a discharge summary is included in the Supplemental Materials (SLP Resources, Discharge Summary Example).

Establishing a Maintenance Program

Many times, at the conclusion of treatment, there are things the speech–language pathologist wants the client to continue to practice and address in order to maintain the skill. Perhaps the client just needs to carry over the skill into more settings. The client might need to complete activities designed to progress further or to keep the client's skills from deteriorating. For patients with Medicare Part B, the speech–language pathologist may establish a functional maintenance program and provide instruction on how to carry out the program. After that instruction has taken place, the skilled services of the speech–language pathologist are no longer needed (*Medicare Benefit Policy Manual*, 2016).

Regardless of the format or specifics of the home program, the fact that one was designed at all should be documented in the chart. The discharge summary is a good place to do this. If a detailed written maintenance program was given, a copy of that program should be placed in the chart.

In some instances, the home program might refer the client to a website for video examples of exercises. The National Foundation on Swallowing Disorders, a consumer advocacy organization, has clips of various dysphagia exercises that the client can watch for practice (National Foundation on Swallowing Disorders, 2017).

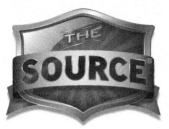

Chapter 6
Special Considerations in Critical Care

What is so different about evaluating and treating patients with dysphagia while they are in a critical care or intensive care unit? These patients are critically ill compared to patients on a medical floor, at home, or in a skilled nursing facility. The fact that they are critically ill has implications for how we evaluate and treat them. Patients who are critically ill may experience more significant responses to changes in their environment. For instance, moving a patient in bed to achieve a good position for feeding may result in a significant change in his respiratory rate and/or blood pressure. Patients' conditions may fluctuate widely from day to day or within a day. Therefore, recommendations made one day may be inappropriate the next if the patient's status has changed. Frequent monitoring is necessary to ensure that recommendations made to facilitate safety of swallowing are not now putting the patient at risk of aspiration. If the patient is post-surgical, she may experience rapid improvement in her condition. This situation also requires careful monitoring so you can change recommendations as soon as it is appropriate.

It is not unusual for an SLP and other rehab professionals to be consulted within hours of the patient's admission to a critical care unit, particularly for a patient who has suffered a cerebrovascular accident (CVA). In the current health-care environment, the minute the patient arrives at the hospital, the emphasis is on planning for discharge to the next level of care. For patients to be discharged sooner to another level of care, rehabilitation services must begin as soon as possible. In addition, there is recognition that early initiation of dysphagia services can prevent costly complications, such as aspiration pneumonia.

Working in the intensive care requires that you have knowledge of a variety of instruments, devices, and monitors. You must be able to read the monitors and understand when a change is significant enough to require the attention of the nurse or respiratory therapist. It is also important to gather other history pertaining to the patient's critically ill status and make adjustments in the bedside or clinical evaluation of swallowing as needed. For example, other techniques (e.g., suctioning) are possible with patients who have tracheostomies.

Multiple Factors Contribute to ICU-Related Dysphagia

With an increasing number of patients surviving critical illness, there is an urgent need to more fully address the long-term consequences of intensive care for survivors and their families. An interdisciplinary stakeholders' group regarding critical care identified five areas of gaps in research, and one area was problems related to the larynx, voice, and swallowing after extubation and their connection to long-term impairments (Needham et al., 2012). Discussion of the need for speech–language pathology intervention for establishing a means for and facilitation of communication is beyond the scope of this book. There is, of course, a great need for identification and management of swallowing disorders. There are many interrelated factors that can contribute to ICU-related dysphagia (Figure 6.1). Several examples are described below.

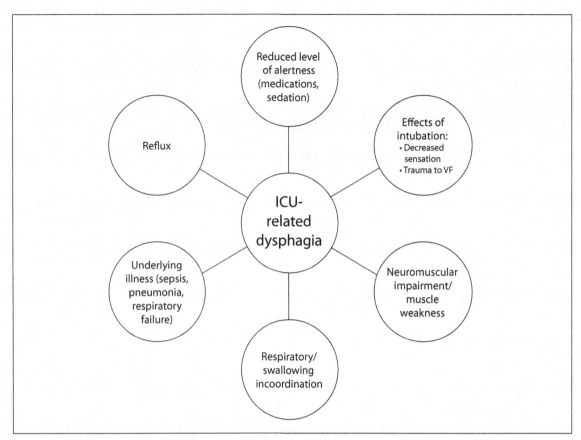

Figure 6.1 Factors that contribute to ICU-related dysphagia.

Underlying Disease

Of primary note is the underlying disease that caused the patient to be admitted to an intensive care unit. SLPs should learn all they can about the diseases common in their critical care patient population.

SEPSIS

Sepsis is a potentially life-threatening complication of infection. People in the intensive care unit are especially vulnerable to developing infections, which can then lead to sepsis. While any type of infection—bacterial, viral, or fungal—can lead to sepsis, the most likely varieties include the following:

- Pneumonia
- Abdominal infection
- Kidney infection
- Bloodstream infection (bacteremia)

Risk factors for developing sepsis include advanced age, weakened immune system, and invasive devices (e.g., catheters, intubation tubes). Mortality rate for sepsis is 50% (Dellinger et al., 2004).

PNEUMONIA

Patients in ICU can develop any type of pneumonia (viral or bacterial from numerous sources), but the most common type is ventilator-associated pneumonia (VAP). VAP is the most common nosocomial infection in patients receiving mechanical ventilation, and it is a hospital-acquired bacterial pneumonia that occurs 48 hours or more after tracheal intubation (Hunter, 2006). It can be classified as early-onset or late-onset pneumonia. Early-onset pneumonia occurs within 4 days of intubation and mechanical ventilation, and it is generally caused by antibiotic-sensitive bacteria, meaning the infection can likely be treated with antibiotics. Late-onset pneumonia develops after 4 days and is commonly caused by multidrug-resistant pathogens (Klompas, 2007). It is typically caused by microaspiration of contaminated oral secretions. These contaminated secretions pool above the cuff of the trachea or tracheostomy tube and then work their way into to the airway via folds in the wall of the cuff (Zolfaghari & Wyncoll, 2011).

Several interventions are in standard use in ICUs to prevent the development of VAP. One addresses the microorganisms at their source: the oral cavity. Aggressive oral hygiene is performed, usually every several hours. This is done not with toothpaste but with an antiseptic called ch-lorhexidine. This is used to clean the oral cavity in combination with mechanical cleaning (i.e., brushing) of all oral surfaces (Barnes, 2014; Munro, Grap, Jones, McClish, & Sessler, 2009). The other intervention addresses the pooling of secretions above the cuff. Modified endotracheal tubes have a subglottal port immediately above the cuff that is connected to continuous suction to remove those secretions (Figure 6.2). Some manufacturers have also changed the material that the tube or cuff is constructed of (to keep the biofilm from clinging) or have coated the tube with antibacterial material (Deem & Treggiari, 2010).

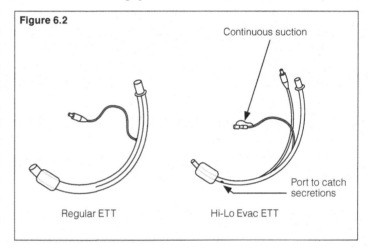

Figure 6.2

Muscle Wasting and Weakness

Pneumonia alone, without the development of sepsis, can render a patient weak and affect swallowing. Patients with acute respiratory failure will also exhibit weakness and likely compromised respiratory–swallow coordination. Patients who are bedridden become weak. Patients lose about 2%–4% of muscle mass a day during their illness (Mendez-Tellez & Needham, 2012). In a study on larger skeletal muscles, it was found that muscle wasting occurred early and rapidly during the first week of critical illness and was more severe among those with multiple-organ failure compared with single-organ failure (Puthucheary et al., 2013). It is logical to assume that similar muscle wasting would occur in the muscles involved in swallowing.

Reflux

Reflux and subsequent aspiration of gastric contents in patients who are tube fed is common. This is a major risk factor for pneumonia. Furthermore, it leads to greater use of hospital resources. For example, length of stay in the intensive care unit and need for ventilator support were significantly greater for patients with pneumonia. One study found that the most significant independent risk factors for pneumonia were aspiration, use of paralytic agents, and a high sedation level (Metheny et al., 2006).

Effects of Intubation on Swallowing

Many patients in intensive care have been intubated. During the period of intubation, if the patient is alert, the speech–language pathologist can assess and provide intervention to establish a method of communication. Once the patient is extubated, the physician is eager for him or her to return to eating by mouth. Any period of intubation places the patient at increased risk of aspiration.

Surgery patients who experience no complications are typically extubated within hours after surgery. Patients who have undergone a coronary artery bypass graft are typically weaned within 6 hours. A short period of intubation does not necessarily have a negative effect on swallowing skills. Of course there are exceptions, and each case must be carefully analyzed.

Dysphagia frequency after intubation has been reported to be between 3% and 62%, increasing in frequency with the length of intubation (Skoretz, Flowers, & Martino, 2010). Studies have shown that the severity and presence of dysphagia, specifically including aspiration, can be independently predicted by a greater length of intubation, with incidence increasing with length of intubation (Barker, Martino, Reichardt, Hickey, & Ralph-Edwards, 2009; Kim, Park, Park, & Song, 2015; Scheel, Pisegna, McNally, Noordzij, & Langmore, 2016; Skoretz et al., 2010).

There is little information in the literature about the exact length of time a patient has to be intubated before you can expect problems or how long after the extubation before swallowing function recovers. A study by de Larminat, Montravers, Dureuil, and Desmonts (1995) concluded that a marked impairment in the sensitivity of the swallowing response may be seen as quickly as after 24 hours of intubation. Most studies cite "prolonged intubation," which is sometimes not defined in the articles but is generally considered greater than 48 hours (Ajemian, Nirmul, Anderson, Zirlen, & Kwasnik, 2001; Barquist, Brown, Cohn, Lundy, & Jackowski, 2001; Brown et al., 2011).

Elpern, Scott, Petro, and Ries (1994) found that swallowing disorders were common in their group of 83 subjects who received long-term mechanical ventilation. Fifty percent aspirated during modified barium swallow studies; of those, 77% were silently aspirating. The authors also found that advanced age increased the risk of aspiration.

Leder, Cohn, and Moller (1998) studied 20 consecutive trauma patients who were translaryngeally intubated for at least 48 hours. They used the FEES approximately 24 hours after extubation. They found aspiration in 45% of the patients; of those, 44% were silently aspirating. Therefore, silent aspiration occurred in 20% of the patients studied. Eighty-nine percent of aspirating subjects resumed an oral diet from 2 to 10 days following extubation. Prolonged intubation and multiple intubations increased the risk of aspiration (Leder, Cohn, & Moller, 1998).

This article speaks to the importance of a dysphagia evaluation with the implied benefit of preventing complications. When you are asked to evaluate a patient at bedside who has just been extubated, often the best recommendation you can give is for the patient to remain NPO with NG feedings for a few days. This recommendation is especially warranted when you listen to the patient's voice and it is very breathy, indicating probable edema or reduced movement of folds. This study also speaks to the importance of instrumental assessment of these patients after extubation.

INJURY TO OROPHARYNX AND LARYNX RELATED TO INTUBATION

Laryngeal injuries are common after intubation. It is thought that movement of the endotracheal tube causes abrasion of the mucosa and pressure necrosis. Colice, Stukel, and Dain (1989) reported information about the kind of damage that can be caused by prolonged intubation, called *translaryngeal intubation*. The typical pattern of laryngeal damage was described in the report as mucosal ulcerations along the posterior-medial aspects of both vocal folds. There were also varying degrees of laryngeal edema in 94% of patients. No relationship was found between laryngeal pathology and the development of adverse laryngeal effects. In a study of patients who had been intubated for more than 4 days, it was reported that 9% of the patients had a normal-appearing larynx at extubation, 78% had laryngeal healing by 8 weeks, and 7% developed a laryngeal granuloma (Colice, 1992). These studies did not assess swallowing function or safety.

Edema of the vocal folds and larynx would understandably have an impact on safe swallowing. Tissues that are edematous are not able to move as well as they should. Edema occurs frequently but is not the only injury found. In a study of 136 patients extubated after more than 24 hours of intubation, endoscopic exam within 6 hours of extubation revealed that laryngeal injury occurred in 73% of patients. These injuries were associated with length of intubation and lack of use of myorelaxant drugs at intubation (Tadié et al., 2010). It is not just the larynx that may be affected by intubation. Sensorimotor function of the tongue is reduced following oral endotracheal intubation (Su et al., 2015). Table 6.1 describes injuries to the oropharynx and larynx following extubation.

Recovery of Swallowing Function in Patients With Dysphagia in Intensive Care

The speech–language pathologist working with patients in intensive care units applies all knowledge and skills that are used with patients in other settings. However, there are specific factors to keep in mind when working with patients who are critically ill.

Swallowing Problems Do Not Necessarily Resolve Spontaneously

Perhaps it appears that patients who are critically ill are just that—too ill to participate in treatment. However, the alternative is to place the patient at greater risk for lingering problems after discharge from intensive care. In fact, evidence suggests that patients who are elderly are in particular at risk for persistent swallowing problems after a stay in intensive care. After 2 weeks, 13% of elderly patients (older than age 65) in one study continued to have swallowing problems (El-Solh, Okada, Bhat, & Pietrantoni, 2003).

In patients with neurological impairment who are critically ill, longer duration of mechanical ventilation is independently associated with postextubation dysphagia, and the development of post-extubation dysphagia is independently associated with a longer hospital length of stay after the initial clinical swallow evaluation (CSE) (Macht et al., 2013).

A longitudinal 5-year study of adults who had recuperated from adult respiratory distress syndrome (ARDS) revealed that each 1-day increase in ICU length of stay (LOS) is independently associated with a 4% reduction in the probability of recovery (Brodsky et al., 2017). Brodsky et al. (2017) had previously reported that during the first 6 days of intubation, the duration of oral endotracheal intubation in patients with ARDS was independently associated with patient-reported dysphagia symptoms at hospital discharge.

Table 6.1
Injuries After Intubation

Type of injury	Related to
Vocal fold edema	Had longer term of intubation than those without edema
	Associated with emergency intubation
	Height-to-ETT-size ratio
Abnormal vocal fold mobility	Traumatic intubation
	Height-to-size-ETT-ratio
	Higher number of intubations
	Longer duration of intubation
Ulceration	Longer duration of intubation
Granulation	Longer duration of intubation
Sensorimotor function of tongue reduced	Independent of age, gender, tobacco use; related to intubation

Note. Adapted from Tadié et al. (2010); Su et al. (2015).

Early Intervention Is Important in Critical Care

It is a generally accepted principle in the care of patients in intensive care units that early preventative forms of physical and cognitive rehabilitation and engaging the critically ill person in activity helps with recovery of the cardiopulmonary system, prevents muscle deterioration, and reduces delirium (O'Mahony, Murthy, Akunne, & Young, 2011). Just as early mobility by physical and occupational therapy (PT/OT) has shown positive outcomes in ICU patients (Adler & Malone, 2012), it follows that early treatment to restore swallowing function is indicated. The same principles of exercise rehabilitation apply (Burkhead, 2009). A recent study showed that early implementation of a swallow rehabilitation program is feasible for patients on mechanical ventilation (Rodrigues et al., 2015).

Screening Dysphagia in Critical Care

One of the most efficient ways to identify patients in critical care who may need an assessment for dysphagia is to implement a formal dysphagia screening program. Identify which patients in intensive care should be screened. It may be that all patients in certain designated critical care units warrant a screening (e.g., neurological unit), whereas others may not be at such high risk (e.g., short-term postsurgical ICU). It may be that any patient who has been intubated, or at least intubated 48 hours or longer, should be screened.

Determining when after extubation the screening should occur warrants consideration. Immediately after extubation may not be the best time to have the nurse administer a screening. If the patient has an alternative source of nutrition (e.g., NG tube), it is often advantageous to have the nurse administer the screening when the patient becomes consistently alert and appears to be managing secretions. This would likely give the patient the best chance to pass the screening. See Chapter 2 for detailed information about screening.

Clinical Swallow Assessment in Critical Care

When reviewing the chart and gathering information from the nurse, some things require particular attention before assessing critically ill patients. Ask the nurse if this is a good time to evaluate the patient. Patients in intensive care require extensive nursing care, and some nursing procedures cannot wait while your assessment or treatments are done. In addition, these patients may have fluctuating periods of alertness, and you want to complete the evaluation when the patient is alert. In particular, postsurgical patients may be given pain medications that alter their level of alertness. Ask the nurse if there are any positioning restrictions for the patient (e.g., patients with temporary renal catheters in the groin may not be able to sit up). If the patient has a tracheostomy, determine whether the patient's cuff is typically inflated all the time or whether it can be deflated. Do you need to reinflate the cuff after your evaluation? In general, it is preferable to complete the evaluation with the cuff deflated to allow for maximum movement of the larynx.

Clinical Assessment of Patients With Tracheostomies

A prospective, descriptive study of 25 consecutively referred patients who were tracheostomized was conducted to see how accurate the results of a clinical swallow exam were. The positive predictive value of aspiration or penetration was 91%; that is, when a patient failed a clinical assessment, there was a very high probability the patient would also fail on fiberoptic endoscopic evaluation of swallowing (FEES). However, the negative predictive value was only 64%; that is, more than one-third of patients who pass a clinical assessment later fail a FEES. So more than a third of patients who pass the clinical assessment are at risk of penetration, aspiration, or failed decannulation (Hales, Drinnan, & Wilson, 2008).

ASSESSING A PATIENT WITH A TRACHEOSTOMY

If a patient is on a ventilator, you should coordinate your assessment with the respiratory therapist to manage the vent settings if you plan to make any adjustments, such as deflating the cuff or placing a one-way speaking valve. The respiratory therapist can also help you take baseline information from the ventilator (e.g., respiratory rate) to determine whether the patient's respiration changes during your evaluation.

Physiological changes with tracheostomy or ventilator. Patients who have a tracheostomy and are on the ventilator experience changes in physiology. These include the following:

- Decreased airflow through the hypopharynx and oropharynx
- Reduced pharyngeal and glottis sensation
- Reduced sense of smell
- Reduced sense of taste
- Difficulty managing secretions
- Decreased vocal fold closure
- Decreased subglottic pressure
- Decreased spontaneous swallowing
- Miscoordination of breathing or swallowing timing (on ventilator) (Goldsmith, 2000; Leder, Joe, Ross, Coelho, & Mendes, 2005)

Cuffs on tracheostomy tubes. The purpose of a cuff on the tracheostomy tube is to provide a closed loop when the patient is on a ventilator. With the cuff inflated, all the air from the ventilator reaches the lungs, and the air expelled from the lungs returns to the ventilator so that inhalation and exhalation values can be measured and monitored by the ventilator. Respiratory therapists and pulmonologists may insist that the cuff stay inflated if the patient is on the ventilator, since it creates a closed-loop system for the ventilator.

Once the patient is weaned from the ventilator, the physician determines whether the cuff needs to remain inflated. The cuff may be left inflated if the patient is not managing secretions and the physician's intent is for most of the secretions to remain above the cuff.

The cuff on a tracheostomy tube is in the trachea, well below the vocal folds. Therefore, its purpose is not to prevent aspiration; if food or liquid reaches the cuff, it has already been aspirated (the definition of aspiration is food or liquid entering the airway below the folds). Elpern, Jacobs, and Bone (1987) used a blue-dye procedure to assess aspiration in patients and concluded that inflated cuffs did not prevent aspiration. In fact, the authors found that aspiration occurred with greater frequency when cuffs were inflated to occlusion than when cuff leaks were present (meaning that the cuff was not filled to tightly fit the trachea) (Elpern et al., 1987).

Tracheostomy cuffs and swallowing. Patients who have been intubated translaryngeally and cannot be successfully weaned from the ventilator have to have a tracheostomy placed. This procedure is usually done if the weaning cannot be accomplished within 7–10 days after intubation. When a tracheostomy is first placed on a patient in critical care, it is almost always one with a cuff. This is always done if the patient is on a ventilator, and even if weaned from the ventilator, a cuffed tracheostomy is used so that if the patient needs to go back on the ventilator, he or she has the appropriate type of tracheostomy.

So when studies are done to determine the effect the tracheostomy tube can have on swallowing function, these studies are really analyzing the effect of a tracheostomy tube with a cuff.

There is no definitive research to demonstrate that placement of a tracheostomy tube impairs hyolaryngeal movement, and no definitive research to demonstrate that a tracheostomy tube cuff impinges on the esophagus to cause "spillover" aspiration. The studies reported here all have some limitations.

Bonanno (1971) demonstrated that the negative effects observed in patients with a tracheostomy who exhibited dysphagia were limited laryngeal elevation and limited anterior rotation of the larynx. The tracheostomy tube appears to act as an anchor, securing the larynx to the neck and prohibiting movement. Bonanno described this as a "direct inhibition of the hyomandibular complex. This occurs as a result of the tracheostomy tube anchoring the trachea to the strap muscles and skin of the neck" so that the "usual function of the suprahyoid musculature is thereby checkreined and the laryngeal excursion is diminished" (p. 33).

Others have reported that there may also be some loss of protective reflexes and uncoordinated laryngeal closure as a result of the tracheostomy tube. Shaker et al. (1995) reported on a small study comparing six typical volunteers and six patients with tracheostomy. The authors found that although the vocal folds closed completely during swallowing, the duration of the closure was significantly shorter for those patients with tracheostomies compared with the closure duration of normal volunteers. In addition, the timing of apnea related to vocal fold closure was also altered in patients with tracheostomies.

The presence of a tracheostomy tube does not necessarily result in dysphagia, yet the incidence of aspiration associated with tracheostomy tubes has been reported to be between 65% and 87% (Bone, Davis, Zuidema, & Cameron, 1974; Cameron, Reynolds, & Zuidema, 1973). Patients who have first had a translaryngeal intubation followed by tracheostomy seem to be at particular risk for dysphagia.

DeVita and Spierer-Rundback (1990) studied 11 patients after prolonged translaryngeal intubation (mean duration 19.9 days), 10 of whom then received a tracheostomy. All patients received a modified barium swallow study. The authors found that all of the patients had at least one problem from a list of 11, with a mean of six defects per patient. The most common defects were delayed triggering of the swallow (seen in all patients) and pharyngeal pooling of contrast material. The patients had no evidence of neurological dysfunction. The authors concluded that prolonged oral intubation with subsequent tracheostomy may cause severe dysphagia. Interestingly, five of the patients received a repeat study after the tracheostomy tube was removed and continued to show some deficits, although the problems were mild. The authors concluded that the deficits may be due to muscle atrophy, with resultant weakness and miscoordination of the swallow response.

Tolep, Getch, and Criner (1996) reported that patients requiring prolonged mechanical ventilation have a high incidence of swallowing abnormalities, whether or not they have an accompanying neuromuscular disorder. They studied 35 patients who received oral intubation first and then tracheostomies. Findings on the MBS studies were abnormal in 83% of the patients (85% in patients with neuromuscular disorders and 80% in patients without). The authors also examined the patients with laryngoscopy and confirmed others' findings that the abnormalities seen included decreased sensation of the vocal folds, pooled secretions above the folds, limited movement of the vocal folds, and edema of the arytenoids.

Suiter, McCullough, and Powell (2003) examined the effects of cuff deflation on swallow function in 14 individuals who were not on mechanical ventilation. Participants completed a videofluoroscopic swallow study (VFSS) with and without the tracheostomy cuff inflated. All participants aspirated thin liquids during the cuff-inflated condition. Swallows were analyzed for seven swallow-duration measures, and although differences were found in some of the measures, the changes did not appear to affect overall swallow safety, as oropharyngeal residue and penetration or aspiration were not significantly affected by cuff deflation.

In a large retrospective study of patients with a variety of medical conditions, reduced laryngeal elevation and silent aspiration were significantly higher in the cuff-inflated than -deflated condition (Ding & Logemann, 2005). It was not possible to assess swallow physiology in the same subject in both cuff-inflated and cuff-deflated conditions. Only by doing this can the effect of cuff-inflation status on swallow physiology be determined.

Two studies compared swallowing function with trach in and trach out. Leder et al. (2005) compared three conditions in patients with head and neck cancer: trach tube present, trach tube removed and tracheostoma covered by gauze sponge, and trach tube removed and tracheostoma left open and uncovered. They found that aspiration status was not affected by tracheostomy or decannulation. Therefore, clinician impressions of increased aspiration or risk of aspiration with tracheostomy tube were not supported. Instead, the authors suggest that the patient's comorbidities predispose aspiration and that the aspiration or risk is due to the critical illness that necessitated the tracheotomy in the first place.

Another study that looked at patients' swallowing pre- and post–tracheostomy removal found that for most patients, removal of the tracheostomy tube made no difference in the incidence of aspiration and/or laryngeal penetration. Results of this study do not support the clinical notion that the patient's swallowing function will improve once the tracheostomy tube has been removed (Donzelli, Brady, Wesling, & Theisen, 2005).

Another consideration regarding these two studies is the timing of the swallowing assessment after trach tube removal. Perhaps the patients needed a few days after trach removal to recover from the effects of the tracheostomy tube.

Tracheostomy tube occlusion/use of one-way speaking valves. Evidence is contradictory as to whether patients aspirate less when the tracheostomy tube is occluded or when wearing a one-way speaking valve. Given the choice, it is preferable to assess swallowing while the patient is wearing the valve so he or she can communicate during the evaluation and you can judge vocal quality.

Patients can also phonate if the tracheostomy tube is occluded, which can be done with a gloved finger or a plug designed to fit into the trach tube. At the beginning of exhalation, use a finger to occlude the tube and allow the patient to phonate. Take your finger away from the tracheostomy during inhalation and when the patient is not talking. A physician's order is generally required before the tracheostomy tube can be plugged. Oxygen delivered at the tracheostomy will need to be switched to a nasal cannula, but brief periods of occluding the tracheostomy with a finger are usually tolerated well by the patient, as oxygen is blocked only temporarily. Some patients can be taught to occlude their tracheostomies lightly with their own fingers so they are able to speak on exhalation. Be sure their hands are clean, or let them wear gloves, as the tracheostomy area should be kept clean.

Eibling and Diez Gross (1996) reviewed the evidence supporting the role of subglottic pressure rise in swallowing efficiency. They explained the interdependence of subglottic air pressure and the glottic closure reflex. They stated that when subglottic air pressure builds up, stretch receptors are activated. This signals the respiratory muscles so they do not inhale during this period of swallowing. The authors hypothesized that if subglottic air pressure cannot be built up because of the tracheostomy tube, then inhibition of inspiration may also be affected. They reported on 11 patients who were known to aspirate during the modified barium swallow (MBS) and who were evaluated with and without the Passy-Muir valve. The authors found significant decrease or elimination of aspiration with the Passy-Muir valve on. They postulated that restoration of normal subglottic pressures by the Passy-Muir valve was key to clinical improvement.

Two separate studies demonstrated that occlusion of the tracheostomy tube had no effect on the prevalence of aspiration and found no trends related to bolus consistency, type of tube, or presence versus absence of a nasogastric tube (Leder, Ross, Burrell, & Sasaki, 1998; Leder, Tarro, & Burrell, 1996). Leder (1999) also found that incidence of aspiration was not affected by the use of a one-way tracheostomy speaking valve and concluded that the valve provided mostly nondeglutitive benefits.

Elpern, Okonek, Bacon, Gerstung, and Skrzynski (2000) completed VFSS with and without a speaking valve in place in 15 patients with tracheostomy tubes. During the valve-off condition, seven participants aspirated thin liquids during at least one presentation. Aspiration was eliminated in five participants when the speaking valve was placed.

Gross, Mahlmann, and Grayhack (2003) completed VFSS with four patients with tracheostomy tubes under two conditions: open tracheostomy tube or speaking valve (Passy-Muir, Irvine, CA). Results indicated that bolus transit times and pharyngeal activity duration times were reduced for all four participants when the speaking valve was placed. Scores on an 8-point penetration–aspiration scale were reduced (improved) for three of four participants when the valve was placed.

Suiter et al. (2003) examined the effects of one-way speaking valve (Passy-Muir, Irvine, CA) placement on swallow physiology. Eighteen patients with tracheostomy were examined using VFSS. Fourteen patients had cuffed tracheostomy tubes and completed VFSS under three conditions: cuff inflated, cuff deflated, and speaking valve in place. Four participants had cuffless tracheostomy tubes and completed VFSS under two conditions: cuffless and speaking valve in place. Swallows were analyzed for presence of penetration or aspiration, severity of penetration or aspiration based on an 8-point scale (Rosenbek, Robbins, Roecker, Coyle, & Wood, 1996), seven swallow duration measures, hyolaryngeal excursion, and amount of oropharyngeal residue. Results for the comparison of inflated cuff and speaking valve indicated that valve placement significantly reduced (improved) scores on the Penetration–Aspiration Scale. No significant changes in swallow duration measures or hyolaryngeal excursion were noted when the valve was in place. One-way valve placement actually increased the amount of residue on the tongue base, on the posterior pharyngeal wall, and at the cricopharyngeus. It is not clear why penetration-aspiration scores reduced.

Another study assessed swallowing in three conditions: (a) tracheotomy tube open with no inner cannula, (2), tracheotomy tube with Blom valve, and (c) tracheotomy tube with Passy-Muir valve. These authors found that the presence of a one-way tracheotomy tube speaking valve did not significantly alter two important components of normal pharyngeal swallow biomechanics: hyoid bone and laryngeal movements. Aspiration status was similarly unaffected by valve use. The authors concluded that the data do not support placement of a one-way tracheotomy tube speaking valve to reduce prandial aspiration (Srinet et al., 2015).

In performing an instrumental examination of swallowing, consider performing the assessment with and without a speaking valve (or occlusion of the tracheostomy) to see whether the patient exhibits any differences in swallowing.

Suctioning. Patients with tracheostomy tubes may require suctioning to help clear secretions from the airway. It is a good idea for the patient to be suctioned before you begin your assessment, as this will clear the patient's airway and reduce the work of breathing.

If you need to obtain approval at your institution to suction, the following documents from ASHA (http://www.asha.org) may be helpful in explaining that this is within our scope:

- *Code of Ethics*—ASHA's (2016) Code of Ethics states: "Individuals who hold the Certificate of Clinical Competence shall engage in only those aspects of the professions that are within the scope of their professional practice and competence, considering their certification status, education, training, and experience. This statement can be used to explain why the speech–language pathology department will work with the Respiratory Therapy Department to develop education and training regarding suctioning and to assure competence in the procedure" (ASHA, 2016).

- *Position Statement on Multiskilled Personnel* (1997)—This document states that "cross-training of clinical skills is not appropriate at the professional level of practice" but "cross-training of basic patient care skills . . . is a reasonable option." Suctioning is listed as an example of a basic patient care skill (*Multiskilled Personnel Position Statement*, 1997).

It is advisable to work with the respiratory therapist (RT) or critical care nursing staff to learn about the procedure. You will want to practice in simulation and then perform a number of procedures with the RT or critical care nurse. There is no prescribed number of times to practice. You may be ready to have your competency checked after four or five practice runs, or you may feel more comfortable after 10 or 12 practice runs. When you feel as though you have mastered the procedure, have the RT or nurse check each step to ensure that you are competent to perform independently. If you do not perform the procedure frequently, you may want to have your competency rechecked periodically. The Supplemental Materials contains a form that can help you do this (see Education Materials Staff, Suctioning Competency Validation Tool).

Modified Evans Blue-Dye Test (MEBDT). This author does not recommend the use of the MEBDT technique for screening or assessment of dysphagia and aspiration. However, when patients with tracheostomies are evaluated at bedside, some SLPs continue to use suctioning to see whether the patient has aspirated any food or liquid. Relying on suctioning to prove or disprove aspiration is quite risky, so it is important to understand the development of this procedure and its limitations.

Use of the MEBDT to determine the occurrence of aspiration in patients with tracheostomies has been documented (Cameron et al., 1973; Elpern et al., 1987; Higgins & Maclean, 1997; Spray, Zuidema, & Cameron, 1976). Cameron et al. (1973) reported that when four drops of a 1% solution of blue dye were placed on patients' tongues every 4 hours for 48 hours, 69% of patients aspirated. Other studies have shown that aspiration may also occur in healthy individuals, particularly during sleep, which means that this procedure may have false positives (Huxley, Viroslav, Gray, & Pierce, 1978).

Thompson-Henry and Braddock (1995) used a modified form of the MEBDT. They mixed blue food coloring with 3–6 cc of thin liquid and semisolid food. This test was negative for all five patients studied; however, the FEES or MBS studies conducted 4–22 days later revealed aspiration for all five patients. The authors questioned the use of the MEBDT and concluded that "caution may be warranted when using this diagnostic approach as the primary indicator of a patient's swallow function" (Thompson-Henry & Braddock, 1995, p. 174).

Tippett and Siebens (1996) indicate that the Thompson-Henry and Braddock study contains several design flaws, including unspecified subject-selection criteria, unspecified cuff status during the FEES and MBS, and the influence of time intervals between the MEBDT and the FEES or the MBS. Tippett and Siebens reinforced Thompson-Henry and Braddock in stating that "caution may be warranted" and that false negative readings are conceivable when using the MEBDT.

Leder (1996) also points out problems with the methodology of the Thompson-Henry and Braddock (1996) study. He noted that a "prospective and randomized or consecutive study using an MBS or a FEES for an objective assessment of aspiration immediately followed by a MEBDT is needed to demonstrate the efficacy and sensitivity of the MEBDT in assessing aspiration" (Leder et al., 1996, p. 81). Brady, Hildner, and Hutchins (1999) reported on such a study in which 20 consecutive simultaneous MEBDT and MBS studies were completed on patients with tracheostomies. Overall, the MEBDT showed a 50% false-negative error rate. The MEBDT identified aspiration in 100% of patients who aspirated more than trace amounts (greater than 10% of bolus) but did not identify aspiration of trace amounts. The study did not report the relationship (if any) between occurrences of aspiration and coughing.

In a study of simultaneous MEBDT and FEES, aspiration was present in 53% of the studies as documented by the FEES. The MEBDT showed an overall 50% false-negative error rate for the detection of aspiration as compared with the FEES. The MEBDT identified aspiration in 67% of patients who aspirated more than trace amounts but failed to identify aspiration of trace amounts. The results of the current investigation suggest that the MEBDT should be viewed at best as only a screening tool for the presence of gross amounts of aspiration in patients with a tracheostomy (Donzelli, Brady, Wesling, & Craney, 2001).

In a more recent study using the MEBDT, the researchers found high levels of sensitivity (Belafsky, Blumenfeld, LePage, & Nahrstedt, 2003). For the entire cohort of patients, it was 82%. They attribute the difference in their findings to the consistencies presented and the protocol used as compared to other studies. Each person in their investigation received three separate trials of 45 mL of ice chips over three consecutive 15-mL swallows as defined in their protocol. Each trial was separated by at least 1 hour. The specificity of the MEBDT using this protocol was only 33% for individuals not receiving mechanical ventilation and 40% for individuals receiving mechanical ventilation. This means there are many false positives, resulting in patients being referred for instrumental assessment unnecessarily.

With a different methodology, another group of researchers used VFSS and MEBDT ratings and found that sensitivity was 80% and specificity 62%; that is, the MEBDT did not correctly identify approximately 20% of tracheostomized patients who were aspirating and at least 38% of tracheostomized patients who were not aspirating (O'Neil-Pirozzi, Lisiecki, Jack Momose, Connors, & Milliner, 2003).

Therefore, given the contradictory findings of high false negatives in one study and high false positives in another, clinicians should be wary of relying on this technique. The MEBDT is not likely to reliably indicate whether a patient is aspirating, and it certainly cannot reveal which techniques can be used to prevent aspiration. That is the value of an instrumental assessment.

Instrumental Assessments for Patients in the Intensive Care Unit

Patients in intensive care units (ICUs), particularly those with a history of intubation or tracheostomy, are at a higher risk for aspiration and will most likely need an instrumental assessment of their swallowing. The timing of the assessment is important. A patient who has just been extubated, is nearly aphonic, and is less than optimally alert when consulted is not a good candidate for an instrumental exam. You may want to encourage the patient to continue tube feedings for several days until he or she is a better candidate, as opposed to completing an instrumental assessment immediately only to have the patient fail miserably and need another study in a few days. Of course, an instrumental assessment will provide you with the information needed to plan appropriate treatment. If the physician insists that the patient begin eating by mouth (perhaps the patient is not tolerating tube feeding), then proceed with the instrumental assessment.

If you have access to both the VFSS and the FEES, compare the two techniques to determine which is more appropriate for the patient in the ICU (see Chapter 3). Because the VFSS study requires transport to the Radiology Department, the patient's nurse (and possibly respiratory therapist, if the patient is on a ventilator) will need to accompany the patient. It is possible to complete a VFSS at bedside if the facility has an available C-arm fluoroscopy unit that can be taken to the bedside, but some of those units do not allow video recording of the study. The FEES can be done at bedside and repeated easily as the patient shows improvement and requires updated recommendations. Another advantage to performing a FEES at bedside is that the nurse and any physician present can observe the study as it takes place.

Instruments and Devices

One of the biggest differences with providing services in intensive care versus on a standard medical floor is the amount of instrumentation in use. Instruments and devices may simply monitor a body function or may actually perform that function for the patient.

Oxygen Saturation and Pulse Oximetry

Obtain baseline information on heart rate and oxygen saturation. Fragile patients in intensive care may react negatively to being moved in the bed and to physical exertion (e.g., eating). Any cardiopulmonary adaptations should be noted. Changes in oxygen saturation levels noted on the pulse oximeter may signal a variety of things. For example, oxygen saturation levels may drop when the patient coughs. See Chapter 2 on the use of pulse oximetry to make assumptions about aspiration.

Ventilators

Ventilators are medical devices used to maintain a stable respiratory rate and act as the primary respiratory pump when patients are not able to breathe adequately on their own. A ventilator controls things such as depth of breath, called *tidal volume* (Vt); percentage of oxygen inhaled (FiO_2); and respiratory rate (breaths per minute, BPM). Ventilation is the process of moving inhaled gases in and out of the lung tissue. Respiration is the actual exchange of gases between the gas inhaled and the carbon dioxide produced during cellular metabolism. The carbon dioxide is removed during exhalation.

Patients are placed on mechanical ventilation for several reasons, including the following:

- Periods of apnea secondary to drug overdose

- Acute or impending respiratory failure

- A surgical procedure that requires mechanical ventilation until the symptoms or side effects are resolved

CLASSIFICATIONS OF VENTILATORS

Manual resuscitator. This is the most basic type of ventilator: It is simply a latex-free "bag" that, when squeezed, administers a volume to the patient via a sealed mask or an artificial airway. A manual resuscitator does not deliver volume or oxygen at a precise setting. It is used in an emergency situation or before intubation.

Positive pressure ventilator. This type of ventilator creates a pressure gradient between the ambient pressure in the patient's lungs and the ventilator tubing. The gradient allows gas to flow easily into the airways and then into the lung tissue. After the volume or pressure has been delivered, the chest is allowed to recoil normally, creating exhalation. The patient must be orally or nasally intubated or have a tracheostomy in order to use positive pressure ventilation.

MODES OF VENTILATION

There are different modes of ventilation that provide varying levels of support to the patient. These are reflected in Figure 6.3.

Assist control. In the assist control modality on a mechanical ventilator, all breaths delivered to the patient are mechanical. That is, all the breaths have a prescribed, preset tidal volume. In this mode, the patient can initiate spontaneous efforts and will receive an "assisted" breath from the ventilator, but it will be at the preset volume. The term *assist control* should not be confused with the term *control mode*. Control mode is used is if there is no spontaneous effort due to a medication-induced coma for medical reasons.

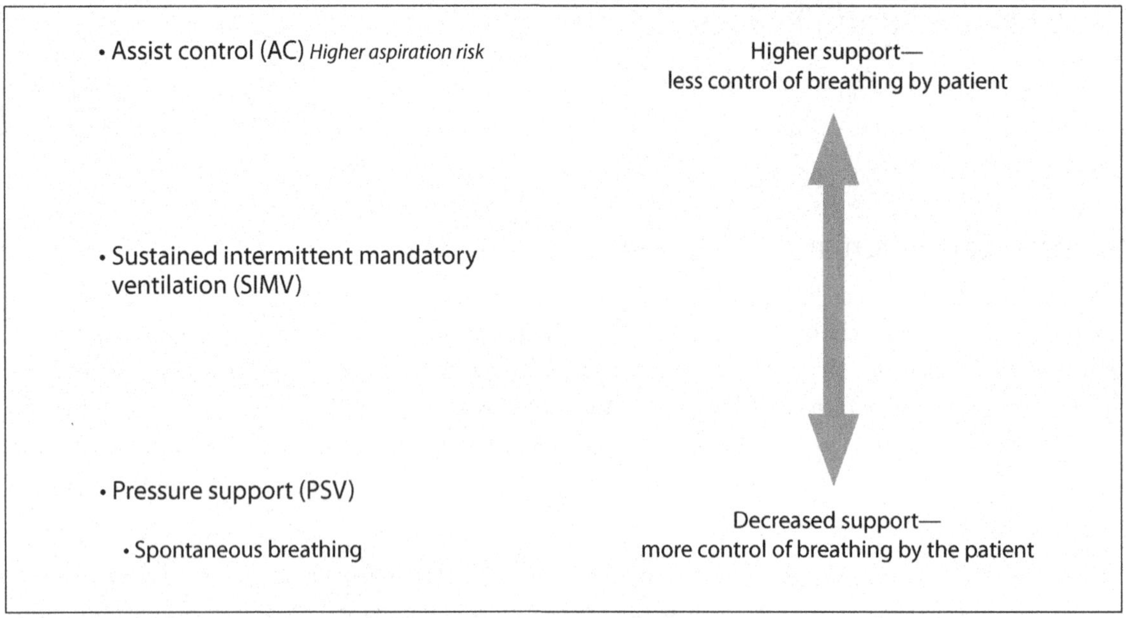

Figure 6.3 Common modes of ventilation.

Synchronized intermittent mandatory ventilation (SIMV). SIMV is very similar to assist control. The main difference is that if the patient initiates a spontaneous breath, there may be an "augmented assist" via pressure, volume, and/or flow if prescribed by the physician. If no assist is needed, the patient may determine his or her own tidal volume. However, there is usually some type of augmentation because resistance to breathing through an endotracheal tube may be too great, making the work of breathing difficult for the patient. Imagine pinching your nose, pursing your lips around a straw, and trying to inhale through the straw to get an idea of resistance to breathing.

Spontaneous/Spontaneous CPAP. The term *spontaneous continuous positive airway pressure (CPAP)* has caused much confusion, so the newer generation of microprocessor ventilators just uses the term *spontaneous*. *CPAP* is now more commonly used in reference to mask ventilation, as in the treatment of obstructive sleep apnea. The spontaneous mode allows for total independent breathing with no assist or augmented assists unless prescribed by a physician. The augmented assists are used to make the patient as comfortable as possible while allowing the endotracheal tube to "feel" as though it is not there as it relates to breathing effort. If not for these augmented assists, it would be very difficult to breathe through a small tube.

Augmented assists function only in SIMV or spontaneous modes. The following modes promote spontaneous breathing by the patient.

AUGMENTED ASSIST MODES USED TO PROMOTE SPONTANEOUS BREATHING BY THE PATIENT

Pressure support. Pressure support provides a small pressure that helps the patient during inspiration and is similar to assist control in that it is delivered each time the patient initiates a breath. The difference is that it uses a preset pressure instead of a volume. The pressure prescribed is usually lower because the patient's ability to breathe spontaneously has improved.

Volume support. With volume support the ventilator tries to adjust pressure many times a second, which allows for the patient to inhale to a target volume but only when in spontaneous mode.

Tubing compensation. This mode requires the user to program information into the microprocessor, such as type of airway, resistance to inspiration, and length. From these values, the ventilator will adjust the breath delivery many times a second to achieve the lowest assistance possible. Many proponents of this mode state that it is like breathing through the nose instead of having an artificial airway in place.

Bilevel assist. This mode is for patients who are breathing spontaneously but need increased oxygenation because they cannot tolerate low percentages of oxygen. The patient breathes spontaneously, then at a prescribed time breathes spontaneously at a high PEEP, usually for 2 seconds or so. PEEP is *positive end expiratory pressure*, indicating that a certain level of pressure is maintained in the alveoli. Spontaneous breathing then continues at a lower PEEP, usually for 1–2 seconds. This procedure is done for alveolar recruitment and is not recommended for critically ill patients.

SETTINGS FOR VENTILATORS

It is helpful to understand some of the settings on a ventilator. Ask the respiratory therapist to show you where these values are displayed on the ventilator.

Tidal volume. The amount of gas delivered to the patient's lung tissue during the inspiratory phase of the breathing cycle.

Respiratory rate. The number of breaths preset on the ventilator to be delivered in a minute.

Inspiratory flow rate/peak flow. The speed that the flow enters the patient's airway (usually set a little higher to ease any anxiety patient may feel).

Inspiratory time. The amount of time it takes to deliver the preset volume or pressure to the patient's lung tissue.

I:E ratios. The relationship between inhalation time and the time allowed for elastic recoil of the chest wall (usually 1:2 is sufficient, but patients with an obstructive lung disease or a bronchospastic component will need a long I:E ratio, essentially providing more time to exhale).

Sensitivity. A setting that can be adjusted several times a day to allow the patient to trigger or initiate a breath from the ventilator with less work of breathing, which can decrease anxiety. This setting may be in pressure mode or flow mode, depending on preference and the patient's response. If the ventilator is too sensitive, then the ventilator may autocycle, giving breaths without the patient initiating them and causing a high respiratory rate.

ALARMS ON VENTILATORS

Ventilators have several alarms, but two basic alarms will help you monitor how the patient is reacting to your treatment (e.g., Is the high-pressure alarm going off because the patient is coughing?).

High-pressure alarm. This alarm indicates that it is taking too much pressure for the ventilator to deliver a breath. It can be triggered by a number of things, such as secretions in the tracheostomy tube or a change in lung function. Since one of the causes is secretions in the tube, the alarm may be indicating that the patient needs to be suctioned. This alarm also goes off when the patient coughs or when too much water has accumulated in the tubing to the ventilator.

Low-pressure alarm. The ventilator expects a certain amount of pressure in the tubing coming back from the patient when the patient exhales. If the ventilator does not detect this pressure, the low-pressure alarm goes off. The alarm usually means the patient is disconnected from the ventilator. Other things that could cause the alarm to go off are a leaking or deflated cuff, a loosely fitted endotracheal cuff, or use of a one-way speaking valve (the cuff is deflated). The respiratory therapist will work with you to turn off the low-pressure alarm during use of the speaking valve.

Noninvasive Ventilation

All the modes of ventilation described above are invasive. That is, the patient has to be intubated or have a tracheostomy to use such a ventilator. Noninvasive ventilation can be applied without an endotracheal tube or trach tube.

BIPAP (BILEVEL POSITIVE AIRWAY PRESSURE)

A patient is not intubated or tracheotomized in order to use BiPAP. Rather, ventilation is supplied via face or nasal mask. BiPAP is used for respiratory failure and sleep apnea. The primary settings are composed of two different pressure gradients, thus the use of *bi* in the name.

The first pressure gradient is called inspiratory peak airway pressure (IPAP) or pressure support. This function operates only in the inspiratory phase of the breathing cycle. As the pressure is increased, the inhaled volume usually increases, unless there is an underlying problem with chest wall deformity or similar issue.

End positive airway pressure (EPAP), or positive end expiratory pressure (PEEP), is the residual pressure gradient left in the lungs after exhalation and continues to remain in place throughout the breathing cycle. The setting, EPAP or PEEP, serves to increase oxygen delivery to tissue and increases the patient's lung compliance, just as stretching out a balloon before blowing it up makes the process of blowing up the balloon easier.

CPAP

Continuous positive airway pressure (CPAP) may be used alone to treat atelectasis and is extremely useful in the treatment of obstructive sleep apnea. In this modality, the patient receives continuous pressure that does not change for inhaling and exhaling. The pressure actually splits open the hypopharynx, allowing for free air movement. CPAP may be used with a face or nasal mask (Figure 6.4).

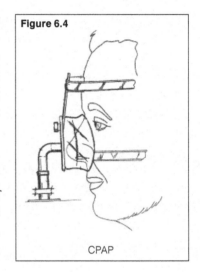

Figure 6.4

CPAP

Oxygen Devices

Patients who do not need assistance in maintaining ventilation of air into the lungs may still need supplemental oxygen, which may be delivered in various ways. Oxygen-delivery methods were described in Chapter 1. Devices that may be encountered more typically in critical care settings are described here.

HIGH-FLOW NASAL CANNULA

High-flow nasal cannula (HFNC) oxygen therapy comprises an air–oxygen blender, humidifier, heated circuit, and nasal cannula. It delivers heated and humidified medical gas at up to 60 L/min of flow. HFNC is designed to reduce anatomical dead space and provide PEEP effect, a constant fraction of inspired oxygen, and good humidification (Nishimura, 2015; Ward, 2013). In the only published study at this time analyzing swallowing in adults in critical care who were using HFNC, the medical staff determined for which patients it was thought to be safe to begin PO. Patients then underwent the Yale Swallow Protocol; those who passed went on to safe alimentation, and those who failed were referred for FEES. The authors concluded that patients on HFNC should be referred using the same criteria as patients who do not require HFNC, as it is not the use of HFNC but rather patient-specific characteristics related to swallowing readiness and their underlying medical conditions that affect readiness for oral alimentation status (Leder, Siner, Bizzarro, McGinley, & Lefton-Greif, 2016).

NON-REBREATHER

A non–rebreather is a mask that allows for delivery of a higher percentage of oxygen to the patient than either a nasal cannula (a maximum of 44% oxygen) or an oxygen mask (up to 65% oxygen) (Figure 6.5). As a patient breathes in, not all the air reaches the lungs to be exchanged. Some of it is trapped in the upper airway, called anatomical dead space. The exhaled gas is unaltered and is still the original composition that was inhaled. The non-rebreather captures the exhaled gas (trapped in the upper airway) so that it can be inhaled on the next inspiration.

T-PIECE

The T-piece (Figure 6.6) attaches to the tracheostomy tube, or ET tube, and to a source of oxygen. This device allows the oxygen to flow by the airway. The other end of the T is left open for oxygen to pass through.

TRACH COLLAR

Patients receive the oxygen from a tracheostomy collar (Figure 6.7) at the tracheotomy site.

Blood Gases

Laboratory results can provide information about a patient's condition. A laboratory result particularly important in critical care to shed light on cardiopulmonary health is the arterial blood gas (ABG). This test is typically performed by the respiratory therapist. A small sample of blood is obtained from an artery (unlike most blood draws, which are from a vein). The ABG can reveal the amount of oxygen and carbon dioxide, and can show pH imbalance, which can cause confusion or difficulty breathing. These values indicate how well the lungs move oxygen into the blood and remove carbon dioxide from the body. They can also indicate certain medical conditions, such as kidney or heart failure, drug overdose, or uncontrolled diabetes. As with all laboratory test results found in a medical record, the normal ranges will be reported and any high or low values will be flagged (Table 6.2).

Monitors

Patients in intensive care are usually attached to several kinds of monitors or to a monitor that measures several functions at once. There are many different types of monitors, so ask the critical care nurse to explain the specific monitors used at your facility. The two basic bodily functions typically monitored are as follows.

CARDIAC MONITORS

Cardiac monitors display heart rate as well as other cardiac rhythms. The normal heart rate for an adult is 60–80 beats per minute. Patients may experience increased heart rate whenever they are engaged in physical activity, such as being positioned in the bed. However, an extremely fast heart rate (100–120 bpm) is called tachycardia. An extremely slow heart rate (40–50 bpm) is called bradycardia. The monitors are usually set to give off an alarm if a patient's heart rate is too fast or too slow. If the alarm is not set, the nurse can tell you the appropriate range for the patient's heart rate.

Figure 6.5

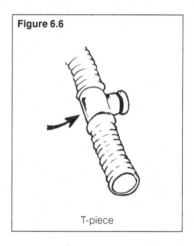

non-rebreather

Figure 6.6

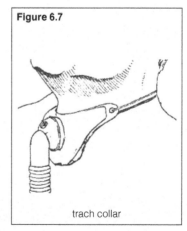

T-piece

Figure 6.7

trach collar

Table 6.2
Blood Gas Values

Acid or base	What it measures	Reference range	What abnormal values might mean	High values	Low values
pH	Number of hydrogen ions in blood	7.35 to 7.45	May indicate conditions such as COPD, asthma, pregnancy, diabetic ketoacidosis (DKA), lung disease, liver disease, or drug use	If the pH level is above 7.45, patient may have alkalosis, which could indicate stimulation of the central nervous system, lung disease, severe anemia, or drug use.	If the pH level is below 7.35, patient has more acidic blood from conditions such as airway obstruction, COPD, asthma, sleep–disordered breathing, or neuromuscular impairment.
HCO_3 Bicarbonate	Kidneys produce bicarbonate to maintain pH balance	22 to 26 milliequivalents per liter (mEq/L)	Disruption of bicarbonate levels may indicate conditions such as respiratory failure, anorexia, and liver failure	An HCO_3 level above 26 mEq/L indicates metabolic alkalosis. This may be the result of dehydration, vomiting, and anorexia.	HCO_3 level below 22 mEq/L indicates metabolic acidosis and may be the result of conditions including diarrhea, liver failure, and kidney disease.
$PaCO_2$ Partial pressure of carbon dioxide	The amount of carbon dioxide in the blood	35 and 45 mmHg	Disrupted levels may indicate shock, kidney failure, or chronic vomiting	Respiratory acidosis is present if the $PaCO_2$ number is above 45 mmHg, which means there is too much carbon dioxide in the blood, and can be a sign of chronic vomiting, low blood potassium, COPD, or pneumonia.	Respiratory alkalosis is present if the $PaCO_2$ number is below 35 mmHg, which means there is too little carbon dioxide in the blood and can signal kidney failure, shock, diabetic ketoacidosis, hyperventilation, pain, or anxiety.
PaO_2 Partial pressure of oxygen	How well oxygen flows from lungs into blood	80 to 100 mmHg	Higher or lower levels may indicate conditions such as anemia, carbon monoxide poisoning, or sickle cell disease		Indicates hypoxemia
SaO_2 saturation	How well hemoglobin carries oxygen to the red blood cells (a true measure, not an estimated value such as obtained from a pulse oximeter, which gives an SpO_2)	94%–100%			Anemia Asthma Congenital heart defects COPD or emphysema Strained abdominal muscles Collapsed lung Pulmonary edema or embolism Sleep apnea

Note. Adapted and compiled from Lian (2010); Pruitt (2010).

PULSE OXIMETER/OXYGEN SATURATION

The amount of oxygen that saturates hemoglobin is measured by a device called a pulse oximeter. A small, infrared sensor device is placed on a body part rich in capillaries, such as a finger, toe, or ear lobe. The sensor provides an estimation of arterial oxygen saturation (SpO_2). For a true measure of oxygen saturation, a measure of arterial blood gas is needed (SaO_2). The pulse oximeter also measures the patient's pulse rate (heart rate). Typically, the patient should be at 90% or greater on saturation; however, patients with COPD retain carbon dioxide, and their typical saturation level may be lower. The pulse oximeter has an alarm that signals when the patient's saturation level drops below the desired amount.

Manometer

A tracheal cuff manometer (Figure 6.8) is used to measure the amount of pressure in the trach cuff. If a cuff is overinflated, too much pressure is exerted on the tracheal walls, which can cause erosion of the tissue and result in a fistula. The cuff manometer indicates the safe range for pressure. When reinflating a cuff, use a manometer. You might think that you could just look at the syringe, note how much air you took out of the cuff, and then return the same amount. This does not work: The amount of pressure changes when the patient moves, and the trachea expands each time the patient inhales. Several factors may have changed since you removed the air, which necessitates using the manometer to measure the amount of pressure needed.

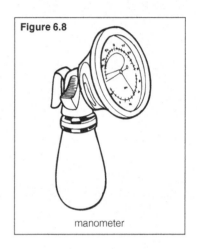

Figure 6.8

manometer

Endotracheal Intubation Tubes (ETT) and Tracheostomy Tubes

For a patient to be placed on a ventilator, an artificial airway has to be established. When a patient will have surgery or initially needs to be ventilated, the first choice is typically an endotracheal or, less often, a nasotracheal tube. Patients typically do not receive a tracheotomy until it is apparent that the need for ventilation is going to be long term.

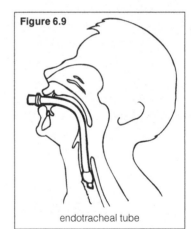

Figure 6.9

endotracheal tube

ENDOTRACHEAL TUBE (ETT)

The ETT, also called an orotracheal tube, is placed with a laryngoscope so that the vocal folds can be viewed (Figure 6.9). This method is used most frequently.

High–low tube. A variation on the ETT is a tube designed with a suction port right above the cuff. This subglottic suction port is connected to continuous suction to remove the secretions that rest on the cuff. These are designed to reduce the occurrence of ventilator-associated pneumonia. They are typically called hi–lo tubes or hi–lo evac tubes (Lorente, Lecuona, Jiménez, Mora, & Sierra, 2007; see Figure 6.2).

NASOTRACHEAL TUBE

This tube is placed in the naris through the nasopharynx and then through the pharynx and larynx into the airway (Figure 6.10). This route may be selected if there are problems in the oral cavity. Going through the nasopharynx eliminates the possibility of the patient biting on the tubing. These types of tubes are not typically placed in an acute-care hospital but may be placed by EMTs in the field. The nasotracheal tube is then often replaced with an endotracheal tube.

Endotracheal and nasotracheal tubes are both held in place by a cuff inflated with air. Patients are not able to eat with either type of tube.

TRACHEOSTOMY TUBE

When a patient undergoes a tracheotomy, a tracheostomy tube is placed (Figure 6.11). The tracheotomy is performed under general anesthetic. A surgical incision is made, usually between the second and third tracheal rings if the incision is made horizontally or through the second, third, and fourth tracheal rings if a vertical incision is made. (The vertical incision is thought to allow for more movement of the larynx). A tracheostomy tube is then placed through the incision. This tube has a cuff on it if the patient is to be placed on a ventilator.

The two main types of tracheostomy tubes are plastic and metal. Plastic tubes are less expensive than metal tubes and are disposable. Plastic tubes are used if the patient is to be mechanically ventilated because the plastic tubes have a universal 15 mm hub and cuff. Metal tubes, usually made of stainless steel or sterling silver, usually do not have a cuff and do not have the universal hub. However, metal tubes are easier to clean and they lie flat against the neck.

Tubes come in different sizes, and the one used depends on the estimated size of the trachea of the individual receiving the tracheotomy.

Regardless of the brand of trach tube, there are several basic parts to a tube. The flange, outer cannula, and universal hub are found on all tubes. The other parts may or may not be included.

Outer flange. This part rests on the patient's neck and keeps the tube from falling through the tracheostomy. The flange is tied around the patient's neck (Figure 6.12).

Outer cannula. This is the main part of the tracheostomy tube. It goes into the airway.

Inner cannula. This is a smaller tube that can be inserted into the outer cannula. An inner cannula makes it easier to clean the tracheostomy tube, as only this part has to be removed (Figure 6.13).

Obturator. This fits inside the outer cannula and has a smooth, rounded tip on it that sticks out through the outer cannula. The obturator makes insertion easier but must be taken out as soon as insertion is complete as it blocks the airway (Figure 6.14).

Universal hub. Regardless of the size of the tracheostomy tube, a 15-mm hub extends from the tube. This universally sized hub attaches to the ventilator tubing or to a speaking valve (Figure 6.13).

Cuff. This surrounds the lower part of the outer cannula and is connected to a small tube that travels to the hub and beyond. It ends in a cuff pilot or pilot balloon. Air is typically inserted into the cuff pilot via a syringe. The air travels through the tubing and into the cuff to inflate it. Some

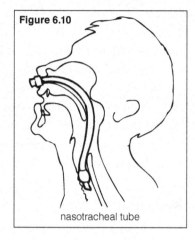

Figure 6.10

nasotracheal tube

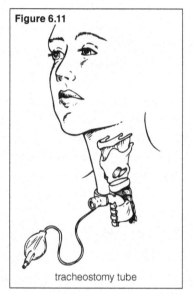

Figure 6.11

tracheostomy tube

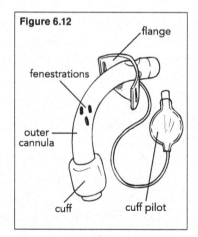

Figure 6.12

flange

fenestrations

outer cannula

cuff

cuff pilot

tracheostomy tubes have foam cuffs, rather than balloon cuffs, that fill with air. Foam cuffs do not deflate, so they cannot be used with speaking valves (see Figure 6.12).

Cuffs are necessary on tubes used with patients on ventilators to create a closed system, allowing all the air pushed in by the ventilator to reach the lungs. With a cuff, none of the air escapes into the upper airway through the larynx. The cuff is well below the vocal folds.

Fenestrations. Some tracheostomy tubes have a hole or multiple holes in the outer cannula. When the inner cannula is removed, these fenestrations allow for air to travel through the vocal folds above while the cuff is still inflated. If the patient blocks the end of the tracheostomy tube, he or she can talk. When the inner cannula is in place, the fenestrations are blocked (see Figure 6.12).

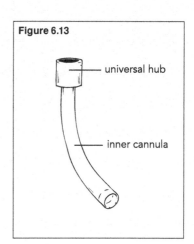

Figure 6.13

universal hub

inner cannula

Suction Kits or Catheters

Patients with endotracheal tubes and with tracheostomies need to be suctioned if they cannot clear the secretions in their airways by coughing. If they are on a ventilator, they cannot clear their own secretions because they cannot cough the secretions out. The secretions are caught below the cuff on the ETT or trach tube.

Suctioning is a sterile process and you must wear sterile gloves when suctioning a patient. The suction catheter is attached to the tubing in the wall that is attached to the suction machine. The catheter is placed into the tracheostomy tube, and just as the catheter is pulled out of the airway, the port is covered to create suction.

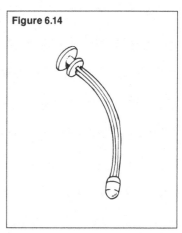

Figure 6.14

Lines and Drains

Patients in critical care units may have multiple lines and drains. When positioning patients for dysphagia evaluations, the speech–language pathologist should be careful not to disturb or dislodge these lines and drains. Examples follow.

DEEP LINE FOR TOTAL PARENTERAL NUTRITION (TPN)

Patients who have a nonfunctioning gut will receive nutrition directly into the bloodstream via a central venous line inserted surgically. This is called total parenteral nutrition (TPN). The word *enteral* refers to the gut, so *parenteral* indicates bypassing the gut. Examples of types of patients who might have a nonfunctioning gastrointestinal system include those with severe, persistent diarrhea; motility disorders of the intestinal tract; and lymphoma or colorectal cancer. This is not designed to be a long-term solution, because to keep the GI tract functioning, some food and liquid needs to be processed in the gut.

CENTRAL VENOUS CATHETERS

In addition to supplying TPN, central venous catheters are used to supply medicines (e.g., chemotherapy), fluids, and blood products, usually over a period of several weeks. Central venous catheters are typically inserted into the arm or chest. They empty out in or near the heart. These are very different from a standard IV, which is inserted into a vein near the surface of the skin. Central venous catheters are also called central lines and are attached to a port. They can also be used to take blood samples. Risk of infection is a serious delayed complication from a central line, and sterile procedures are used when inserting the line.

DRAINAGE TUBES AFTER SURGERY

Surgical drains are used after a variety of types of surgery to prevent the accumulation of fluid (e.g., blood, pus, infected fluids). For example, after open-heart surgery, a chest drainage tube is likely to be in place.

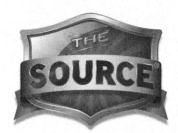

Chapter 7
Ethics and Decision Making in Dysphagia Management: Palliative and Hospice Care

Speech–language pathologists involved in dysphagia management find themselves faced with situations that require careful assessment. The situations require knowledge of professional and medical ethics to guide decision making and to serve as a resource to patients and their families.

For instance, assessment may reveal that a patient is aspirating all consistencies and compensatory strategies cannot eliminate the aspiration:

- Is tube feeding appropriate?
- What are the patient's wishes?
- Are patient and family in agreement?
- What is the physician's view of the situation?
- What is the likelihood that the patient's swallowing skills will improve?
- How does prognosis affect your recommendation?
- What do you do if you disagree with the patient's decision?
- Can you decline to provide services to the patient?

ASHA Code of Ethics

The Code of Ethics of the American Speech-Language-Hearing Association provides guidance for a variety of situations. SLPs are encouraged to familiarize themselves with all aspects of the Code of Ethics, but several principles and rules are highlighted here.

Principle of Ethics I states "Individuals shall honor their responsibility to hold paramount the welfare of persons they serve professionally" (p. 4).

Two specific rules of ethics give some guidance when dealing with ethical decisions:

Rule H: Individuals shall obtain informed consent from the persons they serve about the nature and possible risks and effects of services provided, technology employed, and products dispensed. This obligation also includes informing persons served about possible effects of not engaging in treatment or not following clinical recommendations. If diminished decision-making ability of persons served is suspected, individuals should seek appropriate authorization for services, such as authorization from a spouse, other family member, or legally authorized or appointed representative.

Rule L: Individuals may make a reasonable statement of prognosis, but they shall not guarantee—directly or by implication—the results of any treatment or procedure. (p. 5)

Principle of Ethics II states "Individuals shall honor their responsibility to achieve and maintain the highest level of professional competence and performance" (p. 6). Most of the rules provide helpful information about not providing services unless you are competent to do so, but Rule F may help if you are asked to place patients on your caseload who are not candidates for treatment.

The ASHA Code of Ethics (2016) states: "Rule F: Individuals in administrative or supervisory roles shall not require or permit their professional staff to provide services or conduct clinical activities that compromise the staff member's independent and objective professional judgment."

Ethics in Society

The clinicians' responsibility is to make patient-centered, value-driven ethical decisions rather than drawing strictly or solely from law or religion. Laws include legislative statutes, administrative agency rules, and court decisions. These can vary in different states and locations and are enforceable only in those locations. Of course, laws have to be followed, but ethics incorporates broad values and beliefs of what is correct or right. There is, of course, a lot of overlap between legal and ethical decision making. Both use case-based reasoning to try to achieve consistency, although bioethics consultations are more flexible than law.

In multicultural societies, in which no single religion prevails, a value-based approach to ethical issues is necessary, although many bioethical decision-making methods and ideals originate from religion. The clinician must be aware of the patient's religious beliefs as well as how the clinician's own religious and spiritual beliefs can affect interaction and decision making. Most religions have a golden rule, to treat others as one wishes to be treated. Problems can arise when trying to apply religion-based rules to very specific bioethics situations (Beauchamp & Childress, 2009). Because of that, several generally accepted secular principles have emerged and are used in biomedical ethics. These include autonomy, nonmaleficence, beneficence, and justice.

Principles of Biomedical Ethics

As part of applied ethics, biomedical ethics uses ethical principles and decision making to solve actual or anticipated dilemmas in medicine and biology (Figure 7.1). The field of biomedical ethics provides guidance about principles that guide decision making in our culture. A brief summary of some of the major principles is provided here, drawn from the text *Principles of Biomedical Ethics* by Beauchamp and Childress (2009).

Respect for Autonomy

Patients have the right to make independent choices about their care. For patients to make autonomous choices, they should be free from controlling interference and influence from others and free from limitations, such as not understanding the situation and choices. Such limitations would prevent the patient from making an independent choice. For a person to make autonomous decisions, two conditions must exist:

- Liberty—freedom from controlling forces
- Agency—capacity for intentional action

Patients with cognitive deficits have diminished autonomy as a result. The condition of agency does not then exist. Often patients with dysphagia have had strokes with concomitant aphasia, or they may have other diseases with reduced cognition, such as dementia, which makes it difficult for them to make independent choices. When that is the case, patients should be involved to the extent that they are able to participate, and family member(s) must be relied on to assist in decision making. Beauchamp and Childress (2009) call these individuals "surrogate decision makers." Several important court cases have involved decisions made by surrogate decision makers concerning continuing tube feeding (e.g., Karen Ann Quinlan, Nancy Cruzan, Mary Sue DeGrella, Claire Conroy, Paul Brophy, Terri Schiavo).

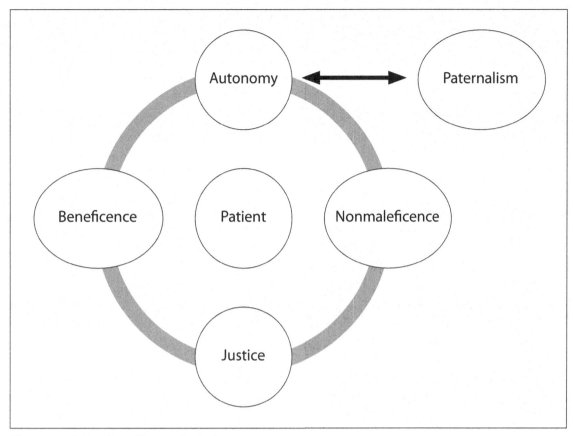

Figure 7.1 Principles of biomedical ethics.

The SLP's evaluation of cognitive and communication skills provides crucial information about the patient's ability to participate in decision making, described as decision-making capacity. A person with decision-making capacity can understand his or her medical condition and recommendations for treatment, as well as the consequences of treatment or no treatment. The person can make and communicate a choice as well as describe a rationale for the choice. Competence, however, is a legal distinction, and a person can be deemed "incompetent" only in a court of law (Wagner, 2008). Medical professionals must not assume that patients and family members cannot make complex decisions about their health. Health professionals must provide enough information and education to the patient and family to allow them to make an informed decision rather than deferring the decision to a physician, nurse, or other medical professional.

INFORMED CONSENT

The Institute for Health Quality and Ethics summarizes the American Medical Association definition of informed consent as follows:

- More than getting a patient to sign a written consent form

- A process of communication between patient and provider

- Disclosing and discussing the following:

    ◆ The patient's diagnosis, if known

    ◆ The nature and purpose of a proposed treatment or procedure

    ◆ The risks and benefits of a proposed treatment or procedure

    ◆ Alternatives

- Risks and benefits of the alternative treatment or procedure
- Risks and benefits of not receiving or undergoing a treatment or procedure

The patient should also be given the opportunity to ask questions and discuss the recommendation. Informed consent should not involve anything that could be perceived as coercion (Manson & O'Neill, 2007).

Beauchamp and Childress (2009) hold that respect for autonomy provides the justification for the policies and practices of informed consent. Informed consent in the medical field also implies authorization for the procedure or treatment. For a patient, or the patient's surrogate, to offer informed consent, he or she must have all necessary information about the situation. When the speech–language pathologist discusses a procedure or recommendation with the patient and caregivers, consider that the patient brings a lifetime of experience that has molded values and tolerance for risk taking. The clinician should present the information factually and ideally presents the patient with several choices. Presenting only one choice could be perceived as exerting influence. Presenting the information is only one part of obtaining informed consent. In fact, Beauchamp and Childress (2009) describe seven elements of informed consent (Figure 7.2).

Verbal or written consent. Typically, health-care institutions have the patient sign a written consent for "high risk" or "invasive" procedures, such as surgeries or certain diagnostic tests. It is not common for patients to have to sign a written consent for instrumental swallowing studies (e.g., FEES, VFSS). However, the speech–language pathologist should consult with the risk department at the facility when instituting new procedures that might need more than implied (verbal) consent.

Waivers. A waiver is a form a person signs giving up a right. Sometimes long-term-care facilities ask patients to sign a waiver if they disagree with a recommendation and will not follow it. For example, if it was recommended that a patient take only thickened liquids, but the patient has decided to continue to drink thin liquids, the patient might be asked to sign a waiver. These documents reportedly hold no legal weight; instead, asking the patient to sign such a document might be viewed as coercion.

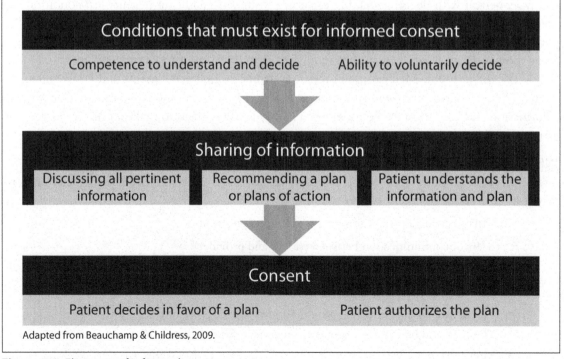

Adapted from Beauchamp & Childress, 2009.

Figure 7.2 Elements of informed consent.

PERSON-CENTERED CARE

A concept closely aligned with autonomy is person-centered care. Person-centered care is a philosophy that encourages both older adults and their caregivers to express choice and practice self-determination in meaningful ways at every level of daily life. Values that are essential to this philosophy include choice, dignity, respect, self-determination, and purposeful living. The National Nursing Home Quality Improvement Campaign defines person-centered care as follows:

> "Person-centered care promotes choice, purpose and meaning in daily life. Person-centered care means that nursing home residents are supported in achieving the level of physical, mental, and psychosocial well-being that is individually practicable. This goal honors the importance of keeping the person at the center of the care planning and decision-making process." (Person-Centered Care, 2017)

This philosophy should be honored when helping the person and their caregivers make decisions about eating and drinking.

The Pioneer Network is a group of professionals and organizations in long-term care formed to advocate for person-directed care that wanted to see a culture change in elderly nursing care. The idea behind the long-term-care culture change movement is to move from institutionalized models to more person-centered models of geriatric nursing care that promote things like flexible schedules, more choice, and self-determination (Resource Library, 2017). One of the initiatives of the Pioneer Network was the development of new dining practice standards. These standards were endorsed by ASHA and many other organizations. Although the dining standards focus on encouraging regular diets, they also recognize the importance of collaboration of appropriate professionals in determining the residents' needs. The standards mention several probes from the Centers for Medicare and Medicaid Services (CMS) interpretive guidance that highlight the importance of interprofessional collaboration:

> Was interdisciplinary expertise utilized to develop a plan to improve the resident's functional abilities?
>
> a. For example, did an occupational therapist design needed adaptive equipment or a speech therapist provide techniques to improve swallowing ability?
>
> b. Do the dietitian and speech therapist (*sic*) determine, for example, the optimum textures and consistency for the resident's food that provide both a nutritionally adequate diet and effectively use oropharyngeal capabilities of the resident? (Dining Practice Standards, 2011, pp. 5–6)

Speech–language pathologists working in long-term care should familiarize themselves with the dining standards, foster the collaboration, and participate in facility initiatives regarding dining. Patients on dysphagia diets deserve the same respect for choice and self-determination as persons on a regular diet.

The person-centered philosophy meshes well with the ICF format (see Chapter 4) encouraging clinicians to look not just at impairment but also at activity and participation and the personal and environmental factors that influence the person. It also interconnects with the principle of autonomy described above.

Nonmaleficence

This principle asserts a primary principle of medical ethics: "Above all, do no harm." Nonmaleficence means that one should not cause harm or impose risk of harm. It is closely tied to the next principle discussed, beneficence. Some ethicists consider the two to be one principle.

Several concepts that provide guidance that is more specific about doing no harm are related to patients with dysphagia. One is the discussion of a distinction between withholding (i.e., never beginning) and withdrawing (i.e., stopping once it is started) life-sustaining medical treatment. Court cases historically involved withholding or withdrawing things like mechanical ventilation (Luce & White, 2009). Some argue that withholding is not maleficence, but withdrawing is. Family members may question the difference in removing a feeding tube once it is placed and never putting a tube in to begin with. Family members may view the decision to withdraw treatment as making them responsible for the ensuing result, particularly the patient's death. They may view differently their decision not to start treatment to begin with. Moral ethicists argue that there is no distinction (Beauchamp & Childress, 2009).

Another concept addresses the difference between sustenance technologies and medical technologies. This concept directly relates to dysphagia regarding withdrawing artificial feeding versus withdrawing other life-sustaining technology (e.g., ventilator). In two early cases, *Quinlan* and *Brophy*, courts declared that medically administered nutrition and hydration were not significantly different from other life-support techniques. This view is increasingly upheld by courts.

Also related to not doing harm is the issue of whether you should make a recommendation for PO intake for a patient after a clinical swallow evaluation reveals significant signs of pharyngeal dysphagia if you cannot obtain an instrumental examination, which would allow you to plan appropriate treatment. The principle of nonmaleficence would indicate that feeding a patient at risk for aspiration without all necessary information would indeed be placing him at risk for harm.

Another situation might occur when an instrumental exam has confirmed which consistencies the patient can safely take without aspiration, but the patient declines to follow the recommendation for a restricted diet. Should the speech–language pathologist then use the consistencies found to be aspirated during treatment (e.g., use thin liquids during practice of supraglottic swallow if the patient was found to aspirate thin liquids)? The best way to "do no harm" would be to use consistencies found to be safely swallowed when working with the patient. However, the speech–language pathologist might also offer suggestions on ways the patient might reduce the amount or frequency of aspiration when taking thin liquids.

One might think that diet recommendations involving a restrictive diet are always offered if one is following the principle of nonmaleficence. For example, recommending a diet of thickened liquids and smooth, pureed foods might yield the intended benefit of reducing the risk of aspiration. However, if the patient will not eat enough of that diet, there may be an unintended consequence of malnutrition or dehydration. The speech–language pathologist should always try to consider the unanticipated consequences of all recommendations.

Beneficence

The principle of beneficence requires clinicians not only to avoid harming patients but also to provide positive benefits to them as well. Beauchamp and Childress (2009) define *beneficence* as an "action done for the benefit of others." It implies an obligation to help others. Simply following standard practice in the management of dysphagia leads SLPs to act in a beneficent way. For example, fully assessing swallowing function to identify impaired physiology and recommending ways for the patient to eat and drink safely is beneficent.

Prevention and education activities might be viewed as beneficent. For example, an SLP observing a nursing assistant feeding a patient (not on the SLP's caseload) too quickly and with the patient in an unsafe position, acting in a beneficent manner, would suggest changes in the feeding techniques to the nursing assistant. This assistance would provide a positive benefit to the patient. Providing general in-services to the staff on appropriate feeding techniques to reduce the risk of aspiration might also be viewed as beneficent acts because positive benefit to all patients in the facility might be the result.

PATERNALISM

Paternalism in the strictest sense indicates that parents make decisions for children because they have information and understanding the child does not have, and it implies that the parent acts in the child's best interests. Paternalism applied to medicine indicates that medical professionals have information and understanding that the patient does not have and are therefore making decisions for the patient, but with the patient's best interests at heart. Paternalism creates a conflict between beneficence and autonomy. Sometimes professionals must exercise paternalism to provide benefit to the patient or to avoid doing harm to the patient.

In medicine, an example of paternalism is a physician choosing not to fully disclose a medical diagnosis to a patient, given the belief that the patient will not be able to handle the information and might harm himself. Paternalism involves overriding the patient's right to make autonomous decisions. A common example in dysphagia is a patient who has had a right-hemisphere CVA declaring that he certainly can remember to take small sips and leave his chin down when taking thin liquids and therefore does not need supervision to do so. The SLP knows that the patient cannot consistently follow this precaution because of impulsivity, and so makes the paternalistic decision that he can have thin liquids but only with supervision. This paternalistic decision is a beneficent one.

Clinicians should avoid falling into the trap of acting in a paternalistic way when the patient or surrogate is fully capable of making an autonomous decision. Sometimes patients, but most often family members, will ask the speech–language pathologist, "What would you do if it were your mother or father?" Instead of immediately acting in a paternalistic way, the clinician should instead remember the elements of informed consent and provide the information needed for the caregiver to make an informed decision. A good way to respond to such a question is to reply, "I don't think I would know exactly what to do until I was in the situation, but what I would want to know is . . ." and then the clinician supplies the information the family member will need to make a decision.

Justice

The final principle is that of justice, which refers to fairness. There is much discussion at the present time about justice, or fairness, related to access to health care. Studies have demonstrated differences in access to care depending on age, race, gender, and ability to pay (Nelson, Stith, & Smedley, 2002; Oliver & Mossialos, 2004). The current debate over national health-care reform centers on providing access to health care for all Americans and how health care should be funded. The concept of justice and access to care is pertinent to the provision of dysphagia services, as patients in most settings now have their access to care limited by prospective payment methods and caps on services. Realistically, this means that the speech–language pathologist must take responsibility for monitoring the patient's and the health-care systems' limited resources when managing patient care. For example, when recommending an instrumental procedure, consider the likelihood that the results will influence the plan of care, particularly in the case of a patient in palliative or hospice care. Determining how long to keep a patient on the caseload is another example of monitoring resources.

Understanding Patients' Rights

The Patient Self Determination Act (Omnibus Budget Reconciliation Act of 1990) requires all hospitals and nursing homes receiving federal Medicare or Medicaid funding to inform patients of their rights to provide advance directives like living wills, health-care surrogates, and durable power of attorney (La Puma, Orentlicher, & Moss, 1991).

Advance Directive

An advance directive (also called a living will) is a legal, written statement of medical choices or the way the patient wants medical choices to be determined. This statement is written before the need for such decisions. Anyone age 18 or older who is of sound mind may write an advance directive. It goes into effect only when the patient can no longer decide for him- or herself or can no longer tell others of the decision. A patient cannot be required to have an advance directive.

Laws about living wills may vary from state to state, but typically a living will directive includes one or more, or all, of the following:

- Directions that life-prolonging treatment not be provided or, once started, be stopped. (Life-prolonging treatment is generally considered to be medical care used to keep a vital body function going after it fails because of illness or injury.)

- Directions that food (nutrition) and water (hydration) not be provided through artificial means (e.g., tubes) or, once started, be stopped.

- A choice of one or more persons to act as your surrogate(s) and make decisions for you

Because state laws vary, it is important to understand laws related to the state(s) in which you practice. CaringInfo.org (2017) provides free advance directives and instructions for each state that can be opened as a PDF.

Health-Care Surrogate

A health-care surrogate is a person appointed in the living will or in another written document to make medical decisions when the patient is unable to speak for him- or herself. Surrogates must be fully informed of the risks of, benefits of, and alternatives to a proposed procedure or treatment. Surrogates should base their decisions on the patient's previously expressed values and goals (substituted judgment). However, patients often do not discuss their health-care values and goals with their surrogate. In these situations, surrogates must make decisions based on what they regard as most appropriate for the patient's clinical condition, quality of life, and other factors (best interest of the patient).

Durable Power of Attorney

The durable power of attorney is an advance directive that lets individuals name someone (known as attorney-in-fact) to make medical decisions for them if they are unable to speak for themselves. It is similar to having a health-care surrogate, but an attorney-in-fact might also be given the power to make decisions about personal and financial affairs.

Palliative and Hospice Care

Regardless of the setting in which the speech–language pathologist manages patients with dysphagia, they are likely to encounter patients in palliative and hospice care. It is often those patients who present challenging situations that require that the speech–language pathologist and the health-care team apply principles of biomedical ethics.

There is sometimes confusion over the terms *palliative care* and *hospice*. Palliative care implies management of symptoms in acute and chronic illness as well as at end of life. It is intended to improve quality of life for patients and their families. Hospice embeds these same principles of palliative management of symptoms, but only at the end of life. Both terms may be used to describe a philosophy of care but also how and where services are provided, as described in Table 7.1.

The major difference in service delivery in palliative and hospice care is that hospice care, as defined in the Medicare benefit, is limited to patients not expected to live more than 6 months.

The World Health Organization describes palliative care guidelines as a philosophy of care, and the philosophy applies to patients in palliative or hospice care. These guidelines, or philosophical beliefs, are outlined in Table 7.2. The speech–language pathologist can use these guidelines when determining whether to evaluate and treat and when making recommendations.

Palliative and Hospice Care and Dysphagia Management

When a patient has acute onset of a dysphagia, the recommendations made focus on the rehabilitation techniques that are expected to help the patient regain skills for safe swallowing as well as the use of compensatory strategies for safe PO. A conservative approach to diet recommendations is usually taken in addition to an aggressive approach to treatment. Such conservative measures may also be employed if the patient has a chronic dysphagia but is not at the end of life.

When a patient is at the end of life, the decisions about whether and what the patient should eat and drink should be made in consultation with the patient (to the extent possible), family, and

Table 7.1
Palliative and Hospice Care

Question	Palliative care	Hospice care
Who can receive this care?	Anyone with a serious illness, regardless of life expectancy, can receive palliative care.	Someone with a serious illness and a life expectancy measured in months (<6 months), not years
What kind of illnesses are covered?	Illness need not be incurable: Care may be provided during early illness to manage pain, or anytime associated treatments cause significant physical or emotional distress.	Any terminal illness with life expectancy less than 6 months (e.g., cancer, dementia, end-stage renal disease, end-stage COPD)
Can patients continue to receive treatments to cure the illness?	Patients may receive palliative care and curative care at same time. For example, patient might continue with chemotherapy for cancer and receive palliative management of associated pain.	Treatments and medicines aimed at relieving symptoms are provided by hospice. Emphasis on management of symptoms (comfort) and provision of social, emotional, and spiritual support.

Curative treatments for terminal dx not given, but therapeutic care that might improve immediate quality of life may be considered (e.g., antibiotics for painful infection). The goal is comfort, not cure. |
| How long can these services continue? | This will depend on patient's care needs and coverage through Medicare, Medicaid, or private insurance | As long as the patient meets Medicare's criterion of an illness with a life expectancy of less than 6 months |
| Which organization provides these services? | Hospitals

Hospices

Nursing facilities

Health-care clinics | Hospice organizations

Hospice programs based at hospital

Other health-care organizations |
| Where are services provided? | Home

Assisted living facility

Nursing facility

Hospital | Usually, wherever the patient resides (e.g., home, assisted living facility, nursing facility, hospital). Some hospices have facilities where people can live (e.g., hospice residence) or receive care for short-term reasons (e.g., acute pain, symptom management). |

Note. Adapted from CaringInfo (2017); Get Palliative Care (2017); Palliative Care FAQ (2017).

Table 7.2

WHO Palliative Care Guidelines Applied to Dysphagia Management

WHO definition or guideline	Applying this to dysphagia management in palliative and hospice care
Provides relief from pain and other distressing symptoms	Coughing and choking when eating can be distressing. Consider this when making diet recommendations and recommendations for compensatory strategies. Optimize ability to eat and drink comfortably, and modify recommendations as condition changes. Identify and address other signs of discomfort such as xerostomia and odynophagia, or gastrointestinal symptoms.
Affirms life and regards dying as a normal process	Recognize that diseases like advanced dementia are terminal illnesses and the recommendations for nutrition and hydration should be adjusted accordingly
Intends to neither hasten or postpone death	Recommending placement of a PEG at the end of life might postpone death
Integrates the psychological and spiritual aspects of patient care	Consider the patient's and caregiver's psychological and spiritual needs in discussions about dysphagia management
Offers a support system to help patients live as actively as possible until death	When making recommendations about eating, move beyond the impairment level to making recommendations about participation
Offers a support system to help the family cope during the patients, illness and in their own bereavement	Be willing and able to discuss what the patient is going through. Share information about resources available to them. Support and educate family members about patient's declining abilities to eat and drink as disease progresses.
Uses a team approach to address the needs of patients and their families	The speech-language pathologist should be involved not only in hospice care but also in palliative care when dysphagia (and communication) are issues
Will enhance quality of life, and may positively influence the course of illness	Make recommendations for eating not based solely on impairment, but based on patient's ability to participate and enjoy eating. Consider as well things family members can do to interact with their loved one during meals. Promote positive feeding interactions for the family.
Is applicable early in the course of illness, in conjunction with other therapies that are intended to prolong life	Work with other members of the palliative care team to help them understand the services the SLP can offer.

Note. Adapted from WHO Palliative Care Definition (2017); Monteleoni and Clark (2004); Pollens (2012); Vitale, Berkman, Monteleoni, and Ahronheim (2011).

medical professionals on the hospice care team. For example, the conservative approach to keeping a patient with a recent stroke from acquiring pneumonia in the first few weeks after a stroke might include a very restrictive diet and postural modifications. With a patient at the end of life, the goal might not be to prevent or reduce the risk of aspiration pneumonia but to allow the patient to eat and drink things that can be consumed without causing the patient discomfort (e.g., severe coughing or choking). Recommendations might include some positioning changes or changes in how the foods are presented (e.g., smaller bites, different temperature of foods) to promote comfort when eating.

Patients in palliative care who present with dysphagia fall somewhere between the more conservative approach used with acute-onset dysphagia and the much less conservative approach to recommendations given at end of life. Careful consultation with the patient, caregivers, and palliative care team should guide decisions and recommendations.

Palliative Care and Dysphagia Evaluations

When the physician consults the speech–language pathologist for a patient in palliative care, it is helpful for the speech–language pathologist to know exactly what the physician wants to know and how aggressive the patient, family, and physician want to be. For example, is an instrumental exam indicated? How conservative should the diet recommendations be? These same questions need to be answered when evaluating a patient with dementia. An order set like the one in Figure 7.3 can cue the physician to provide all necessary information for the speech–language pathologist.

Dementia and Dysphagia

The most common patient population with dysphagia that SLPs encounter in palliative situations and at the end of life is individuals with dementia. There are an estimated 5.5 million Americans living with Alzheimer's, and 5.3 million of those are older than the age of 65 (Alzheimer's, 2015). There are no specific figures on the number of individuals with Alzheimer's who have swallowing problems, and it is estimated that up to half of patients with dementia who are institutionalized have dysphagia.

The characteristics of dysphagia typically differ in the different stages of the disease. In the early stages, the patient experiences mild cognitive impairment and may not be aware of or may deny the symptoms. Patients may forget to eat or lose track of schedules and skip meals. This can affect nutrition and hydration. In the middle stages of the disease, they may experience motor restlessness and continued cognitive deficits and need help for tasks like preparing meals and adequate oral care. They may be easily distracted and have a hard time staying focused on the task of eating.

In the advanced or late and end stages of the disease, patients typically lose the ability to feed themselves. They will likely present with oral acceptance and oral preparatory deficits. They may present with oral apraxia or an agnosia, which is not recognizing food in the mouth. The cognitive deficits complicate attempts to help patients eat. Sensory pathways are disturbed, impairing their senses of smell and taste. If the patient loses the ability to sense hot or cold, safety may be an issue. For example, the patient may drink liquids that are too hot. Decreased sense of smell and taste affects appetite and adequate intake. Patients may refuse certain (or all) foods and liquids. They will become less and less alert in end stages, making it challenging to find times during the day when they are awake long enough to be fed. Reduced oral intake is expected in advanced dementia not only due to these eating problems but also as a result of the physiological consequences of the disease. Perhaps because of a lower basal metabolic rate and inactivity, patients with advanced dementia have lower caloric needs (Hoffer, 2006).

Consult SLP for palliative care to evaluate for dysphagia and to facilitate communication.
May perform instrumental exam (MBS or FEES) as indicated.
PHYSICIAN: PLEASE SPECIFY PRIMARY GOAL OF CARE RELATED TO SWALLOWING:
☐ Diet and feeding plan may be established by patient/family/caregiver in collaboration with SLP.
☐ Maintain PO diet most comfortable to the patient. End of life feeding, aspiration risk acceptable.
☐ Conservative diet recommendations to minimize aspiration risk.
☐ Tube feeding is not indicated.
☐ Tube feeding may be considered
☐ Short term (NG)
☐ Long term (PEG/PEJ)

Figure 7.3 Order set for Dysphagia Evaluation for Palliative Care.

Of course it is not just cognitive and oral-phase deficits that present in mid- and late-stage dementia. Patients may also have significant pharyngeal-phase deficits. Common problems include delayed pharyngeal response and inefficient pharyngeal clearance.

Although many SLPs work with patients with dementia near the end of life, a survey of SLPs concerning dysphagia and end of life found that only 42% of SLP respondents felt moderately or well prepared to manage dysphagia. Only 22% of respondents recognized that tube feeding is unlikely to reduce the risk of aspiration pneumonia, whereas a slight majority understood that tube feeding would not likely prevent an uncomfortable death, improve functional status, or enhance quality of life (QOL). The majority were willing to consider recommending oral feeding despite the high risk of aspiration (Vitale, Berkman, Monteleoni, & Ahronheim, 2011).

CSE AND/OR INSTRUMENTAL

Patients with advancing dementia may be referred to the speech–language pathologist, particularly in the long-term-care setting, for assessment of swallowing problems. The clinical swallow examination can follow the same format as established in Chapter 2, but the patient may not be able to complete all tasks. Of particular importance when completing a clinical assessment of a patient with dementia is assessing the following:

- the patient's ability to respond to cues
- the patient's ability to comprehend directions
- functional skills during a meal to observe:
  - pace of self-feeding (or pace of the feeder)
  - response to different types of boluses
  - response to use of utensils (e.g., cup vs. straw)
  - length of time a meal takes

If the patient presents with signs of pharyngeal dysphagia, before recommending an instrumental study, the SLP must consider whether the results of the instrumental would in any way change the recommendations or course of management. For example, if the instrumental exam reveals the patient is aspirating all consistencies and this cannot be eliminated (with postural, diet, or other compensatory strategies), would it change the patient's plan of care? If the patient is noticeably distressed during the meal, with episodes of coughing or choking, then the instrumental might yield important information about what diet textures result in less coughing or how to present foods and liquids to reduce these episodes. If the patient or surrogate has indicated that changes to a regular diet are unacceptable, can anything be learned from an instrumental? Perhaps the clinician can determine strategies for the family to implement with a regular diet to make the patient more comfortable when eating and drinking. If, however, the patient shows no signs of distress and the caregivers have indicated they will not implement dietary changes, an instrumental may not provide useful information.

Utilizing the WHO guidelines for palliation (see Table 7.2) can help the clinician consider the appropriateness of recommending an instrumental study. The principles of biomedical ethics and the patient's wishes expressed in an advance directive should also guide decision making.

Documenting results of instrumental exams for palliative diets. When completing an instrumental exam on a patient in palliative or hospice care, sharing the results with the physician is not as clear-cut as it is with an acute-onset dysphagia from which the patient is expected to recover. Provide enough information to the physician so that he or she can discuss with the patient and family and determine appropriate action regarding oral or nonoral nutrition. Figure 7.4 provides examples of how a summary of an instrumental exam might be worded.

TUBE FEEDING AND ADVANCED DEMENTIA/END OF LIFE

Another decision in which speech–language pathologists are involved with regard to patients who have advanced dementia is whether a PEG tube should be inserted when the patient is not eating and drinking enough to maintain nutrition and hydration. There is convincing evidence that placing a PEG in patients with advanced dementia results in neither prolonged life nor increased comfort. An excellent article concerning the use of PEG (not just in advanced dementia) by Plonk (2005) is recommended reading. The speech–language pathologist should consider the following information and share such references with families as they make decisions about end-of-life care.

- There are numerous burdens and complications associated with tube feeding (Table 7.3).

- Factors indicating the patient is not a good candidate for successful PEG placement include many reasons a PEG is placed (e.g., previous aspiration, NPO more than 7 days, hospitalized, bedridden, confusion) (Plonk, 2005).

- No evidence that tube feeding in patients with advanced dementia prolongs survival, prevents aspiration pneumonia, reduces risk of pressure sores or infections, improves function, or provides comfort (Finucane, Christmas, & Travis, 1999).

- 50% mortality at 6 months for hospitalized patients with advanced dementia who had PEG (Meier, Ahronheim, Morris, Baskin-Lyons, & Morrison, 2001).

- Patients with dementia had worse prognoses than other patients receiving PEG (Sanders et al., 2000).

- PEGs in advanced dementia cases associated with significant increases in complication rates, restraint use, and emergency department visits (Li, 2002; Odom, Barone, Docimo, Bull, & Jorgensson, 2003).

- Aspiration pneumonia is the most common cause of death after PEG placement (James, Kapur, & Hawthorne, 1998).

- Feeding tubes (NG and PEG) increase the risk of pneumonia, possibly because of GERD and/or oropharyngeal colonization (Finucane & Bynum, 1996; Langmore et al., 1998).

- The use of feeding tubes, when compared with attempts at hand feeding, does not prolong survival for patients with advanced dementia (Candy, Sampson, & Jones, 2009).

Dementia as suspected cause

If dysphagia is new and related to recent onset of change in condition, consider short-term alternative means of nutrition/hydration (e.g., NG) and aggressive dysphagia therapy by speech–language pathologist.

However, if dysphagia is due to gradual deterioration of dementia, then patient, family and physician should discuss appropriate method for nutrition/hydration. Patient is aspirating _____ .

There is no evidence that tube feeding will prevent aspiration and therefore is typically contraindicated for patients in palliative care. If the patient is to continue to eat/drink by mouth, then to reduce (but not eliminate) the risk of aspiration, consider _____ diet and _____ liquids.

Other information that can be added: *Because patient coughs or chokes with thin liquids, thickened liquids are recommended to make the patient more comfortable.*

Because patient is very fatigued, pureed food is recommended so that patient does not fatigue during meal.

Other palliative when dementia not etiology

Results of MBS/FEES indicate that patient is aspirating (or at risk to aspirate) all textures, and the aspiration could not be eliminated with postural or other compensatory techniques.

However, we have been asked to provide recommendations for a palliative diet as patient wants to continue to eat/drink by mouth. Therefore, to reduce (but not eliminate) the risk of aspiration, consider _____ diet and _____ liquids.

Figure 7.4 Summarizing results of Instrumental Exam for Palliative Diet.

- High–calorie supplements and other oral feeding options can help individuals with dementia gain weight as an alternative to tube feeding (Hanson, Ersek, Gilliam, & Carey, 2011).

Economics and PEG. There are economic issues surrounding the use of PEG. Feeding patients in nursing homes with severe dementia costs nursing facilities significantly less per day than feeding them by hand (Mitchell, Buchanan, Littlehale, & Hamel, 2004).

Ethical issues and PEG. The issues discussed earlier in this chapter reflect many of the ethical issues surrounding PEG use. Others are addressed in the case studies found at the end of the chapter.

Making the Most of Self-Feeding

For as long as the patient is able to self-feed, this should be promoted. Many of the following suggestions also apply to the dining environment and food presentations once the patient becomes dependent for feeding (Alzheimer's Facts and Figures, 2017; Amella, 2004; Easterling & Robbins, 2008):

- Provide eyeglasses, hearing aids, and dentures.
- Minimize distractions in the environment.
- Provide a consistent environment and seating arrangement in the dining room.
- Reduce the amount of time the individual has to wait to receive food once seated in the dining room.
- Avoid interruptions.
- Provide verbal encouragement to self-feed.
- Use hand-over-hand or hand-under-hand to encourage self-feeding as needed.
- Remove condiments from the tray.
- Eliminate nonfood items from the table (e.g., centerpieces).
- Keep dessert out of sight during the meal.
- Include foods that are spicy, sweet, and sour to increase sensory input.
- Make foods visually appealing.
- Use color contrasts between foods.
- The plates or bowls should be a contrasting color from the background (e.g., tray, placemat) to compensate for changes in vision and depth perception.
- Use a damp washcloth under the plate to keep it from sliding.

Table 7.3
Complications Associated With Tube Feeding

Pain at site of tube	Diarrhea	Aspiration
Tissue damage at site of tube	Nausea	Peritonitis
Local bleeding	Fluid overload	Vomiting
Hematoma	Tube malfunction	Pneumonia
Loss of dignity	GI bleeding	GERD
Loss of social interaction	Restraint use	Gastric perforation

Note. Adapted from Plonk (2005).

- Make sure the room is well lit.
- Offer foods that can be eaten without utensils (e.g., finger foods)
- Do not serve overly hot foods, as patients lose the ability to judge temperature.
- Use utensils to promote independence (e.g., mugs or cups with lids, straws that bend, glasses filled half full).
- Plan for several smaller meals throughout the day.
- Consider food supplements and high-calorie foods.

CAREFUL HAND FEEDING

When the patient becomes dependent for feeding, he or she will need to be fed by caregivers or family. Keep in mind the tips provided above, but consider these suggestions when training staff and family who will feed the patient:

- Position the patient in an upright position with supports as needed.
- Face the patient while feeding.
- Make eye contact.
- Use a gentle tone of voice.
- Feed small amounts at a slow, consistent rate.
- Provide verbal encouragement and/or prompts.
- Check that the patient has swallowed before offering another bite or sip.
- Watch the patient closely for cues that he or she is having difficulty (DiBartolo, 2006).

TIPS FOR CAREGIVERS FOR FEEDING A LOVED ONE

Family members in particular need to be educated on nurturing without making their loved one feel pressured to eat:

- Prepare small portions of foods the patient usually enjoys.
- Offer snack-sized meals throughout the day instead of the traditional three meals a day.
- Be encouraging and accepting of amount of food patient feels like eating.
- You can still make every calorie count:
  - Snacks that are high in calories and nutrition (e.g., ice cream, puddings, milkshakes)
  - Discuss options with dietitian

COMFORT FEEDING ONLY

Palecek et al. (2010) suggest using the term *comfort feeding only* (CFO), with the goal of providing new language to describe how eating problems in patients with advanced dementia would be managed. *Comfort*, in CFO, has a twofold meaning:

- Refers to a stopping point in feeding, emphasizing that the patient will be fed only as long as it is not distressing.
- Refers to the goals of the feedings. The feedings are comfort oriented in that they are the least invasive and potentially most satisfying way of attempting to maintain nutrition through careful hand feeding.

Palecek et al. (2010) offer helpful information about comfort feeding only, including an example dialogue between physician and family member concerning end of life and eating. This term is preferable to *pleasure feeding*, which is sometimes used.

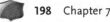

EDUCATING NURSES ON ASSESSING FEEDING: USING THE EDFED-Q

The Edinburgh Feeding Evaluation in Dementia Questionnaire (EdFED-Q) (Watson & Dreary, 1997) is an instrument designed to be used by nurses to determine the help patients with dementia need at mealtimes. This 11-item instrument helps nurses identify behaviors (e.g., turning away, spilling food) and develop a plan for each resident. It takes about 10 minutes to administer. It can be administered by watching a patient eat or by asking the caregiver questions.

Because eating is one of the last activities of daily living to be lost in dementia, identifying the best ways to help patients in end-stage dementia is beneficial not only to nursing staff but also to families. If appropriate ways to help the patient can be identified, families can stay engaged with the patient at mealtimes (Stockdell & Amella, 2008).

Helping Families Make Decisions

Caregivers of patients in advanced stages of dementia have likely faced many tough decisions over the progression of their loved one's disease, such as when to take over managing the finances, when to make the patient stop driving, or when to start going with their loved one to medical appointments. However, there is probably no harder decision than determining what to do when the patient loses interest in eating. Despite clear clinical evidence that placement of a feeding tube will neither prolong life nor enhance quality of life, families often feel that refusing a PEG means they are starving their loved one to death.

The SLP should seek out advice from the other members of the palliative care or hospice team in these instances. They can help guide the patient and family through the decision-making process regarding eating and drinking and the approach that will be taken should the patient develop pneumonia.

The SLP should also become familiar with articles that discuss issues of ethics related to feeding. It seems that U.S. law increasingly supports the position that food and liquid be considered like any other medical treatment that can be refused by a competent patient or by a family member or surrogate on behalf of the patient. As one of the members of the health-care team providing the most information about a patient's ability to eat and prognosis for recovery and rate of continued decline, the SLP may be asked by family members to help them make a decision.

SLPs help a family make decisions regarding a loved one's care by meeting with the family members and any other individuals involved in the patient's care, such as the following:

- The patient (when appropriate)
- The primary physician
- Nurses
- The social worker
- Spiritual, ethical, and/or legal advisers
- Representatives of the institutions involved

Decision Aids

Another way to help families facing decisions about tube feeding is to provide information about decision aids. One study analyzed the use of a decision aid by families and found that a decision aid improves the decision-making process for long-term tube feeding in older patients with cognitive impairments. It does this by decreasing decisional conflict and by promoting decisions that are informed and consistent with personal values (Mitchell, Tetroe, & O'Connor, 2001).

In a randomized trial of 256 residents in nursing homes and their surrogate decision makers, the use of a decision aid improved knowledge scores. After 3 months, intervention surrogates had lower Decisional Conflict Scale scores than controls and more often discussed feeding options with a health-care provider. Residents in the intervention group were more likely to receive a dysphagia diet and showed a trend toward increased eating assistance from staff. Tube feeding was rare in both groups even after 9 months (Hanson, Carey, et al., 2011). Another study found that patients with declared DNR/AND status had lower rates of tube placement (Teno et al., 2010).

Another study examined a video-based decision-aid about goals of care (GOC) that addressed more than just feeding. The GOC decision aid intervention was effective in improving end-of-life communication for nursing home residents with advanced dementia and enhanced palliative care plans while reducing hospital transfers (Brady, 2007).

A decision aid for advanced dementia and decisions about feeding that can be very helpful to families is Improving Decision-Making Feeding Decisions About Dysphagia in Dementia (n.d.). This is from the University of North Carolina School of Medicine and is available in PDF or video format. Another useful tool is "Making Choices: Feeding Options for Patients with Dementia" (n.d.).

Case Examples: Decision Making in Palliative and Hospice Care

The following eight case examples present some ethical dilemmas and challenging case management decisions.

Case 1: "I know it takes a long time to feed her, but Mom really enjoys eating."

The patient is a 75-year-old with advanced dementia. Her daughter says that she believes that the patient still understands everything going on around her and has chosen not to talk.

The daughter tells you the patient always loved to eat. The patient will not routinely open her mouth for the spoon. Food has to be forced between her lips, and it is almost impossible to tell when the patient has swallowed. In an hour and a half, the patient may take 15 bites and a few sips. She has had a modified barium swallow that was fairly inconclusive because of this behavior, but she did not show any aspiration on the few swallows of liquid poured into her mouth.

1. **The physician talks to you because she is concerned that the patient is losing weight and experiencing some skin breakdown related to poor nutrition. She wants to place a feeding tube and asks for your recommendation.**

   Discuss with the physician your impression that the patient's daughter thinks it is still a pleasurable event for her mother to eat but that, in your observation, this is not the case. Ask if the patient had ever expressed her wishes regarding whether she would like to have a feeding tube. A referral to palliative care or hospice might be appropriate. Discuss the risks of aspiration with a feeding tube.

2. **The physician wants you to observe the daughter feed the patient a meal and then discuss your observations with the daughter. What will you say to the daughter?**

   Try to help the daughter understand that feeding was a pleasurable event for her mother in the past, but having food forced between her lips for an hour and a half three times a day is probably not a pleasurable experience anymore. Help the daughter find a few things the patient can take without being force-fed.

3. **In the course of the discussion, the daughter asks, "If it were your mother, what would you do?" What do you say?**

   Try to guide the conversation back to the fact that the daughter has to make the decision about her mother. You might tell her that if you were in this position, you would want to consider all the information available, consider your mother's wishes, and determine what provides the patient with the most comfort at this time. You might provide a decision aid to the daughter.

Case 2: "I have to ask for a modified barium swallow order from Dr. Idon'tthinkso."

You completed a clinical swallow evaluation on a patient who showed several clinical signs of aspiration, including coughing immediately after thin, nectar-thick, and honey-thick liquids with wet vocal quality. The patient did not show clinical signs of aspiration with pudding-thick liquids. Dr. Idon'tthinkso notoriously refuses requests for modified barium swallows, saying they are a waste of money.

1. **How do you make your request to Dr. Idon'tthinkso?**

   It might be best to sit down with Dr. Idon'tthinkso and discuss the actual cost of a modified barium swallow study compared to the cost of treating aspiration pneumonia. Perhaps a radiologist who performs modified barium swallow studies or another specialist who frequently refers for these studies can help you with the discussion. You may even want to have a physician who is your ally talk with Dr. Idon'tthinkso, as physicians often listen to one another more readily than they do other professionals. A handout in the Supplemental Materials also provides useful information (see Education Materials, Staff/Physician, Instrumental Examination of Swallowing).

2. **Should you try to find another physician who treats this patient to get the order without consulting Dr. Idon'tthinkso?**

   Every facility and physician is different in terms of who will order special studies. Most often, unless the physician is the attending physician, he or she will not order any special studies without consulting the attending physician.

3. **Do you tell the family that it is not safe to feed the patient without the modified barium swallow study and ask them to talk to Dr. Idon'tthinkso?**

   It is very appropriate to share the results of your evaluation, including your diagnosis and prognosis, with the patient and his family. You can even share with them the fact that you are recommending a modified barium swallow study. However, if you are trying to build a working relationship with the physician, it probably would be better to work through the problem with the physician directly rather than indirectly through the family.

Case 3: "Does the doctor think I have X-ray vision?"

You have recommended a modified barium swallow study on a patient with a new onset of dysphagia after a bedside evaluation and have also recommended that the patient be made NPO until the study is completed. You have established a few oral-phase goals but cannot determine what the pharyngeal deficits are or which treatment techniques are indicated. However, Dr. Goaheadandfeed refuses the modified and writes the order: "SLP to feed whatever diet seems easiest and safest for this patient."

1. **Do you include presentation of any PO during your treatment sessions?**

   It is presumed that if you made a recommendation for NPO, you were unable to find any textures the patient appeared to eat safely or any positions or compensatory techniques that would allow the patient to eat safely. If that is the case, it would not make sense to include trial feedings during your therapy sessions. However, if you found one texture that the patient seemed to swallow safely, such as pudding-thick materials, you might use that consistency as needed when using treatment techniques.

2. **If you decide not to use food during the therapy sessions, what do you say to the doctor?**

   Either in person or in writing, communicate to the physician that you do not think it is safe for the patient to eat any textures and that no compensatory techniques are effective in eliminating what you consider significant clinical signs of aspiration. Indicate that you will begin therapy for the identified oral deficits, but you are declining to participate in presenting food to the patient. You can instruct nursing staff of safe feeding practices that might help reduce the risk of aspiration. Remind the physician that an instrumental study will help you plan appropriate treatment for the pharyngeal phase.

3. If you decide not to present food to the patient, what do you say to the patient and/or family?

This communication must be worded carefully. You definitely do not want to complain about the physician. If you had already counseled the patient and family about the results of the evaluation, you might tell them that the physician has decided that she does not want the patient to have the special X-ray study and wants the patient to eat.

Suggest some techniques that could reduce, but not totally eliminate, the risk of aspiration. For instance, show them how to position the patient at 90°, and discuss other positioning or compensatory techniques. Be sure the family understands why you are uncomfortable participating in therapeutic feeding.

4. If you decide not to feed the patient, what do you say to the staff?

Explain that you do not think there are any textures the patient can safely take and that your involvement would not be therapeutic at this time. Convey to the staff your concern about the risk for aspiration and ask that they carefully observe the patient for any further clinical signs of aspiration. Explain that without the instrumental study, you will not be able to develop a treatment plan.

Case 4: "But he never wanted a tube . . ."

An 87-year-old patient with advanced dementia and frail health has returned from a stay in an acute-care facility for aspiration pneumonia. While there, a modified barium swallow study demonstrated frank aspiration of all textures. No compensatory techniques were found to reduce or eliminate the aspiration.

The patient's family states that years ago the patient expressed that he "never wanted to have to eat my food through a tube in my nose." The patient cries, "I want water!" throughout the day. The doctor and family have decided against a tube, and the doctor writes an order for pureed diet and thick liquids. Staff wants you to feed the patient because "you will know how to do it."

1. Do you agree to feed the patient?

Consider whether feeding the patient at this point would be a skilled treatment service. It most likely is not, but you might decide to feed the patient for a short period to complete patient and family education about techniques that might reduce the risk of aspiration.

2. If you decide to feed the patient, how will you reduce the risk of aspiration?

Be sure to position the patient at 90° and use other general precautions, such as aggressive oral care, having the patient take small bites and sips, and making sure the patient's mouth is empty before presenting the next bite or sip.

3. Why might you decide not to feed the patient?

You may choose not to become involved if you decide the assessment completed at the acute-care facility contains all the information needed for staff to begin feeding the patient.

4. What will you tell the doctor and the family?

Communicate to the doctor that the assessment completed at the acute-care facility provides all necessary information for staff to feed the patient and that there is no need for skilled services at this time.

Discuss with the family that you understand their careful consideration of the issues and respect their decision to feed the patient. In this type of case, it seems that the physician and family have carefully considered the prognosis for this patient and are respecting the wishes of a statement the patient made at a time when he was able to make such decisions.

Explain that you will be happy to show them positioning techniques that might help, but you will not be involved further because they will be able to feed the patient, based on your recommendations.

5. Do you or the family give the patient sips of water per the patient's request?

You definitely do *not* want to give the patient sips of water since the order by the physician is for pureed diet and thick liquids. The family might decide to give water to the patient, but you should remind them that this is not the diet ordered.

You may want to discuss with the physician the fact that free water between meals is used with some patients with dysphagia in some facilities.

Many patients state that thickened liquids do not satisfy their feelings of being thirsty. This issue becomes a consideration of patient comfort because if the patient is taking enough thickened liquids, he or she is getting enough hydration.

6. What other considerations should be discussed?

It is likely this patient will continue to develop aspiration pneumonia. The physician and family should discuss whether to treat the aspiration pneumonia or whether referral to hospice is indicated.

Case 5: "What is it like to starve to death?"

The patient is an 80-year-old female who is in declining physical health (chronic obstructive pulmonary disease, diabetes mellitus, and heart failure) but cognitively alert. She had a recent brainstem stroke with resultant profound pharyngeal dysphagia and is aspirating everything. You have mentioned aspiration pneumonia to her as a probable consequence of eating. She asks you to sit down to discuss her options.

1. She asks what it is like to die of aspiration pneumonia and what it is like to starve to death. What do you tell her?

Explain to the patient that these questions are probably premature since her dysphagia is the result of an acute event and that you expect some recovery. Suggest that she try some alternatives, such as therapy and nonoral feedings. Mention that she could choose a time-limited trial of tube feeding and could decide at any point in the future to have the tube removed.

2. She wants to continue to eat and work with you on "exercises to improve my throat." Do you agree to treat her?

If you have every reasonable expectation that she can achieve some significant improvement in function, you might agree to work with her on exercises, but you probably would not want to present food to her.

3. The patient's son asks you to talk his mother into a feeding tube. What do you say to him?

Invite him to sit down and discuss the situation with the patient, the physician, and any other applicable individuals. Based on the information provided, a short trial of the feeding tube is probably the most appropriate treatment at this time.

Case 6: "What's the rush?"

You are called in to consult on a patient in acute care in the hospital who is two days post a right-hemisphere CVA and has an NG tube in place. The patient is believed to have aspiration pneumonia. The physician states she wants to change the NG tube to a G-tube to prevent further development of the aspiration pneumonia.

1. What do you say to the physician about the patient's risk of aspiration pneumonia?

Discuss that complete bedside and instrumental swallow assessments should give you enough information to make a prognosis for the length of time it might take the patient to return to full PO. If it is a short period, keeping the NG tube in place might be a better alternative. Also mention to the physician that many studies indicate that aspiration pneumonia occurs just as frequently with the G-tube and even the J-tube. Also discuss whether the aspiration could have occurred at the time of the CVA versus aspiration from the tube feeding.

Case 7: "My facility won't let me ask the doctor for an order for an instrumental exam."

You provide services in a long-term-care facility. The administrator has told you that sending patients out for instrumental assessment of swallowing is too costly and that you will need to plan dysphagia management without any instrumental exams.

1. What can you say to the administrator to convince her that this is not a good decision, in terms of either patient care or fiscal management?

Discuss which clinical swallow evaluations can and cannot tell you about the pharyngeal phase of the swallow. Share statistics about silent aspiration and the risk of aspiration pneumonia associated with patients who aspirate. Volunteer to find out what it costs to treat the patient if pneumonia develops. Even if patients are sent to a hospital, when they return, there will likely be costly medication that needs to continue. And with changes in reimbursement methodologies, the facility may even be responsible for some of the costs of the hospital stay. You may find some useful information in the handout in the Supplemental Materials. (See Education Materials Staff/Physician, Instrumental Examination of Swallowing.) Discuss the facility's legal liability if it does not provide all the care a patient needs and the patient ends up getting sick because of the facility's policy.

2. How can you show that you are not overreferring for instrumental exams?

Review your records and show the administrator how many clinical evaluations you have performed and how many times you have asked for instrumental exams in the past (e.g., 6 months, 1 year). If you have a protocol for determining which risk factors indicate the need for an instrumental exam, share those too.

Case 8: "My boss wants me to teach the OT how to treat dysphagia."

You work 3 days a week in a small rural hospital. The rehab director wants you to teach the OT on staff (who is there daily and has extra time) how to perform clinical dysphagia evaluations and modified barium swallow studies as well as explain how to treat dysphagia.

1. How do you prepare for the meeting you have requested to discuss this with the rehab director?

Prepare for the meeting by obtaining a copy of your state licensure law with your scope of practice and the OT law and their scope. See whether anything in the OT scope mentions pharyngeal phase of swallowing. Many OT laws describe self-feeding or oral motor skills but do not mention pharyngeal-phase skills. Also obtain a copy of your transcripts from graduate school showing your dysphagia classwork and related classwork, such as anatomy and physiology of the respiratory system, head, and neck, as well as documentation of continuing education in the area of dysphagia.

Review your Code of Ethics, specifically Principle of Ethics I, Rule E, concerning delegating provision of clinical services only to individuals who are qualified. Review the latest information from ASHA's National Outcomes Measurement System (NOMS) to see how much progress patients with dysphagia make when service is provided by a certified SLP (although this is not a comparison of the progress patients make when seen by an SLP vs. an OT, OT has no similar national data to combat your outcomes statement). Better yet, if your facility participates in NOMS, you will have your own data to share.

The ASHA website provides helpful information to demonstrate why speech–language pathologists are the preferred providers of dysphagia services at http://www.asha.org/SLP/clinical/Speech-language-Pathologists-as-the-Preferred-Providers-for-Dysphagia-Services/.

2. What do you say to the rehab director?

Begin by acknowledging that it is problematic that there is not daily coverage for patients with dysphagia. Suggest an arrangement whereby you (or another SLP) can be on call on the days you are not working at the facility. Most facilities have an already established "on call" rate that will cover the several hours or day the on-call staff must be ready to come into the hospital if called. Perhaps some of the OT "extra" hours could be reduced to pay for the needed SLP hours. If this alternative is not immediately acceptable, review the documents you have brought with you, which clearly indicate that while your education and training prepare you to work with patients with dysphagia, the OT's may not, particularly in the area of pharyngeal dysphagia. Explain why a team approach, with each professional evaluating and treating different components of the patient's problem, would yield the very best care for the patient. Summarize that your Code of Ethics prohibits you from delegating the provision of clinical services to persons who are not qualified.

3. What if the rehab director is not swayed by any of these arguments?

Then you must decide whether you can ethically agree to her demands.

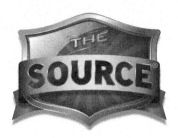

Chapter 8
Education and Advocacy

This chapter highlights the importance of providing education to a variety of audiences. Closely tied to education is advocacy, or taking action to solve a problem. The scope of practice in speech–language pathology comprises five domains of professional practice and eight domains of service delivery. Two of the domains of professional practice are advocacy and outreach, and education (Scope of Practice, 2016). Throughout this chapter there are references to related materials that can be found with the Supplemental Materials. The comprehensive list of Supplemental Materials is in the front of the book, following the Table of Contents. These materials include fact sheets about specific topics and example PowerPoint presentations that can be used when educating staff. Of course, information that can be used to educate various audiences is also found in chapters throughout the book.

Whom Do SLPs Educate?

Education has always been an important part of the services provided by speech–language pathologists (SLPs). SLPs educate patients and significant others whenever presented with an opportunity to interact with them. SLPs educate staff and physicians when sharing information about specific patients, and they use that information to plan the patient's care. Two other audiences are in need of education about dysphagia services and the value of these services: administrators and payers. It is critical that information be shared with administrators about the value that dysphagia services add to the care of the patient. It is also important to share information about how dysphagia care can reduce the overall cost of treating patients (for more information, see Chapter 10). Third-party payers are also very interested in the cost of the care provided as well as the results of that care. Payers need education to help them understand the importance of dysphagia management.

Educating Patients and Caregivers

Why is it important to educate a patient's family about feeding precautions and compensatory techniques? The speech–language pathologist cannot be with a patient every time the patient is being given something to eat or drink. If family members understand why these recommendations were made and how they are related to the patient's care, they may participate more actively in the patient's care. If a patient is a silent aspirator, it will not be easy for the family to understand why the patient's diet has been changed or why the family needs to employ certain strategies, for instance. However, showing family members a recording of the patient's instrumental study or a sample instrumental depicting aspiration may make it easier for them to understand. If education is begun with the family before the evaluation, and findings are discussed throughout, it is likely that the caregivers will be better allies in carrying out the recommendations.

Educating the Patient and Family About the CSE

BEFORE THE CLINICAL SWALLOW EVALUATION

If the family will be present at the evaluation, the speech–language pathologist should explain to the patient and caregivers in detail what they are going to do in the evaluation and what they will be looking for during the assessment. A handout in the Supplemental Materials will help you explain the purpose of the clinical swallow evaluation. It also explains the difference between this procedure and instrumental procedures that may be recommended (see Education Materials Patient/Family, Clinical or Bedside Swallowing Evaluation Information). The time before the evaluation is used to obtain information from the patient and family. The speech–language pathologist may be the first staff member who has spent a considerable amount of time listening to the family's questions and concerns about the patient's swallowing skills. They family may be able to report things about how the patient has swallowed in the past and how long the problem has been present. More detailed information may be gained from the patient or family than from the patient's medical record.

DURING THE CLINICAL SWALLOW EVALUATION

If the caregivers are observing the CSE, this is the opportunity for the speech–language pathologist to point out what is observed. For instance, if a patient is having trouble masticating a bolus and has a lot of pocketing in her cheek, the SLP can point this out to the family. If a patient is losing liquids out the front of her mouth when trying to drink from a cup, a compensatory technique could be demonstrated. Any explanation of observations should be shared with the patient as well. Discussing observations throughout the evaluation helps keep the care patient focused and prepares the patient to take responsibility for managing the disorder.

AFTER THE BEDSIDE OR CLINICAL EVALUATION

After the evaluation, the speech–language pathologist discusses findings and recommendations. Depending on the patient's physician(s), the speech–language pathologist may need to explain that recommendations will be suggested to the physician, who will make the final determination about the need for other evaluations, such as a VFSS or FEES study, or a consultation with another medical specialist. In many facilities, however, the speech–language pathologist has been granted the privilege to write these recommendations as orders to be later cosigned by the physician.

Educating the Patient and Family About the Videofluoroscopic Swallowing Study

BEFORE THE VFSS/MBS

When the study is scheduled, the patient may be given a handout found in the Supplemental Materials (see Education Materials Patient/Family, Modified Barium Swallow/VFSS FAQs). To point out the basic features of anatomy and what the speech–language pathologist will be carefully analyzing, the patient and her family can also be provided with the diagrams included in the Supplemental Materials (see Education Materials Patient/Family, Modified Barium Swallow/VFSS Information, and Phases of Swallow).

DURING THE VFSS/MBS

Letting family members observe the modified barium swallow study helps them understand the problem. Families are often surprised that they will be allowed to watch the study and will be told the results immediately. As with the CSE, discussing observations during the study and explaining any compensatory techniques help family members understand challenges the patient is facing.

AFTER THE VFSS/MBS
Similar to the recommendations made after a CSE, the speech–language pathologist has to phrase the information shared with the patient and family about the results of the study based on facility practice and the physician on the case. In some settings the physician may understand that the speech–language pathologist will make diet and compensatory recommendations without consulting the physician. For example, in some facilities the SLP department has advocated for more independent practice and can write diet orders without contacting the physician for a separate order. However, if the recommendation is for the patient to be NPO, this will need to be discussed with the physician. The recording of the study may be reviewed with the patient and family members after the study to point out the findings and explain the patient's response to any treatment techniques attempted. Patients and families may have a particularly difficult time understanding silent aspiration. If the patient "looks" all right when swallowing, it is puzzling to hear that food or liquid is entering the airway. Information included with the Supplemental Materials may be helpful in this situation. (See Education Materials Staff/Physician, Aspiration and Aspiration Pneumonia FAQs.)

Educating the Patient and Family About the Fiberoptic Endoscopic Evaluation of Swallowing

BEFORE THE PROCEDURE
The diagram in the Supplemental Materials showing pictures of FEES can be given to the patient and his or her family (see Education Materials Patient/Family, Fiberoptic Endoscopic Evaluation of Swallowing [FEES] Information). Because this procedure for inpatients is done at bedside, it provides an excellent opportunity for the speech–language pathologist to describe what is being done and what is observed during the procedure.

DURING THE FEES
The family will be able to watch the monitor and the speech–language pathologist can explain what they are seeing. The monitor can often be positioned so that the patient can see it. This is an especially powerful education and biofeedback opportunity. Some family members may decline the offer to observe the study, perhaps because they are uncomfortable with medical procedures.

AFTER THE FEES
If the family was present during the procedure, much will have already been explained to them. If not, the recording can be reviewed with them and the patient so they can see the problems. If aspiration was observed, there is helpful information in a handout in the Supplemental Materials. (See Education Materials Staff/Physician, Aspiration and Aspiration Pneumonia FAQs.)

Educating the Patient and Family About Therapeutic Feeding Treatment and Exercises

THERAPEUTIC FEEDING
If the patient is going to eat by mouth, it is very important to educate the patient and family on all the precautions and compensatory techniques they will need to know in order to help the patient eat safely. If the speech–language pathologist conducts therapeutic feeding sessions, the techniques being used should be explained.

Having the family observe the speech–language pathologist using specific techniques with the patient is useful. Having them then try the techniques while the speech–language pathologist observes is an effective teaching strategy. For example, it is an effective teaching technique for family members to actually try to position the patient in bed at 90°. Postural changes and compensatory techniques may be second nature to the SLP, but they are new to the family and patient. Opportunities to practice these techniques will help family members become more efficient and effective.

EXERCISES

Patients need to take responsibility for actively practicing the necessary swallowing exercises. Working with the speech–language pathologist even on a daily basis is not enough to achieve a change in swallowing physiology. The patient needs to practice the exercises the prescribed number of times per day and will likely need the support and encouragement of family. One of the best resources for educating patients and families is the website of the National Foundation on Swallowing Disorders (http://www.swallowingdisorderfoundation.com). This consumer-based advocacy group website has a handout describing common exercises as well as movies demonstrating how to perform many exercises.

The Supplemental Materials include two handouts for the patient in the Education Materials Patient/Family section. One is the list Swallowing Exercises and the other is the descriptive Swallowing Exercises Instructions.

Educating the Patient and Family About Oral Hygiene

Chapter 2 contains background information on the importance of oral hygiene and its relationship to oral health and overall health. Two common misperceptions of patients and families about oral hygiene are the following:

The patient is NPO, so why would he need to brush his teeth?

The patient does not have any teeth to brush.

Whether or not the patient is taking anything by mouth, it is still important to keep the oral cavity clean. And even with no teeth, the other surfaces of the mouth (gums, cheeks, tongue, roof of mouth) harbor bacteria and should be scrubbed. Two handouts in the Supplemental Materials may be useful (Oral Care Handout and a specific page for patients who cannot take thin liquids [see Education Materials Patient/Family, Oral Care Guidelines for Patients Who Cannot Have Thin Liquids]).

Documenting Family Progress on Goals

As with all services, documenting what was done is as important as doing it. Particularly for patients who are not independent with practicing rehabilitation techniques or are not independent with compensatory strategies at meals, the speech–language pathologist may want to devise specific goals for the family. An example is included with the Supplemental Materials (see Education Materials Patient/Family, Safe Feeding Goals for Family, as well as Safe Feeding Instructions for Family). In the acute-care setting, patient and family education is critical because the average length of stay has significantly decreased. In skilled nursing facilities, the speech–language pathologist may see families less frequently, thus making it challenging to provide teaching. In home health, the speech–language pathologist usually has good access to families and caregivers. Each of these settings may have different requirements for documentation.

Educating the Patient and Families About Dementia

Chapter 7 includes information about palliative and hospice care, including the effects of using a decision aid. Included with the Supplemental Materials is a handout explaining what families can expect about the patient's eating and swallowing at different stages of the disease. (See Education Materials Patient/Family, Dementia: Stages and Eating).

Web-Based Resources for Patients and Families

There are many resources available on the web for patients and families. A few suggested sites are the following:

- National Foundation on Swallowing Disorders (NFOSD) (https://www .swallowingdisorderfoundation.com). This organization was described above.

- American Board of Swallowing and Swallowing Disorders (AB-SSD) (http:// www.swallowingdisorders.org). This is the board that certifies SLPs as specialists in swallowing. The website has a long list of other consumer sites, with links to the sites.

Educating Patients and Families About Other Related Topics

Other patient and family education materials have been referenced in other chapters. For example, Lifestyle Modifications for Patients with Gastroesophageal Reflux Disease (GERD) is described in Chapter 1.

Educating Staff

Patient-Specific Education

The most frequent, and likely most effective, type of staff training is patient-specific education. It would be ideal if nursing staff and even physicians could observe diagnostic and therapy sessions. It is unlikely, however, that a staff member will have enough time to observe the modified barium swallow study and participate fully during a therapeutic treatment at mealtime as a family member might. One benefit of the FEES is that it is performed at bedside and the nursing assistant or nurse can be present for at least part of the study.

If nursing staff will be expected to follow through with dysphagia precautions, it is just as important that the techniques be demonstrated to the nursing staff. It should not be assumed that a nurse knows as much about swallowing as a speech–language pathologist. Recommendations should be very specific. For instance, if a patient is not allowed to have thin liquids, the speech–language pathologist should explain that this applies to cups of ice chips as well. If a patient needs to be upright when eating and drinking, the nurse needs to know this applies to the patient taking medications. This type of education typically occurs at bedside with the patient. This affords the staff the opportunity for hands-on practice, such as practice positioning the patient or cueing the patient to remember compensatory strategies.

Case Conferences

In facility settings some very specific recommendations for treatment of a patient's dysphagia may be discussed during a case conference. This is a wonderful opportunity to make sure that all staff involved with the patient hear the recommendations. It is not only nursing staff who have the opportunity to provide food or liquid to the patient; patients may ask the respiratory therapist, physical therapist, or occupational therapist to give them a drink of water. All staff in contact with the patient must be aware of any precautions.

General In-Services

It is often challenging to get nursing staff or nursing assistants to attend a general in-service. Working with the manager, the speech–language pathologist can determine the best time to offer in-services. Using a break room close to the nursing station may boost attendance. Offering the in-service at different times of the day to make it available to all shifts is important. The turnover of staff in many health-care facilities may be fairly high, so it is important to repeat these in-services at periodic intervals. The following are included with the Supplemental Materials and may help in planning and giving such in-services. When presented in slide format with notes, readers are encouraged to modify the content to customize it to their facility. See the following training materials:

Dysphagia In-Service (PowerPoint)—Designed to be 15–20 minutes.

Dysphagia In-Service (Supplemental Materials)—Use the outline to help supplement information on the slides.

Dysphagia In-Service Pre- and Posttest

Swallowing Guidelines Signs—Staff can be shown the signs they may see posted in patient rooms.

Managing Dysphagia: Role of Food Service Staff (PowerPoint)—10 minutes. Designed to help food service staff understand their important role in preparing dysphagia diets correctly. There is also a Dysphagia In-Service Pre- and Posttest that could be used with either of these in-services.

Oral Hygiene Importance (PowerPoint)—15 minutes. For nursing and nurse assistants. Designed to help them understand the importance of oral hygiene, a task nursing staff acknowledge as important but typically rate as a low priority to complete.

Oral Care Validation Tool—Competency validation tool.

Dysphagia and Palliative Care (PowerPoint)—30 minutes. Designed for professional staff (nursing, nurse assistants).

Helping the Patient With Dementia Eat (PowerPoint)—10 minutes. Designed for any staff member who interacts with patients with dementia at mealtime.

Educating Physicians

Educating physicians is a challenging proposition. Such education is typically patient specific and usually occurs slowly as rapport is built with the physicians. Sometimes the speech–language pathologist will have the opportunity to respond to a specific question from a physician. Two sample letters in the Supplemental Materials may be helpful if physicians raise specific questions about the cost and purpose of clinical swallow evaluations and instrumental examinations (see Education Materials Staff/Physician, Letter to Physician Samples).

Physicians may also have questions about the predicted outcome of dysphagia intervention and the relationship of the outcome to the cost of the service. Chapter 10 provides detailed information about outcomes. These particular handouts may be helpful when addressing specific questions raised by physicians. (See Education Materials Staff/Physician, Instrumental Examination of Swallowing; Dysphagia FAQs; Aspiration and Aspiration Pneumonia Q&A.) The speech–language pathologist should update and add recent references to support the claims made in the handouts. As research in the area of dysphagia continues, some conclusions and practice patterns change as well.

Educating Administrators and Payers

The questions raised by administrators and payers typically concern the cost of service, the predicted length of treatment, the projected functional outcome, and the cost–benefit ratio. It is important to explain how dysphagia services can reduce the risk of medical complications and save money for the facility or payer. For help describing the benefits of specific procedures (e.g., instrumental examinations) and explaining the role the examination plays in a comprehensive dysphagia management program, refer to the handout with the Supplemental Materials (see Education Materials Staff/Physician, Instrumental Examination of Swallowing). Chapter 10 provides more information on outcomes and efficacy that will help you prepare materials for education.

Advocacy

Advocacy means taking action to solve a problem, and it can occur at multiple levels, from advocating for a particular patient to get what he or she needs to facility-level advocacy, and even advocacy at the state and federal government levels.

At the patient level, for example, SLPs might advocate for the patient to be positioned appropriately for presentation of medications. SLPs advocate at the facility level by working to train all nursing and nursing assistant staff in appropriate ways to feed patients at risk of dysphagia. Many SLPs also become involved in advocacy efforts at the state or federal level. These efforts usually involve reimbursement or coverage issues.

Education and advocacy go hand in hand. Many of the education opportunities described above also involve advocacy. In educating staff about how to feed patients with dementia, the speech–language pathologist is also advocating for the patient to preserve his or her dignity and to optimize nutritional status. In educating administrators about the cost of services, one is advocating for the SLP program.

The most successful advocacy efforts utilize data to support statements. Many different types of data are available to clinicians. Data are likely available from the department (e.g., What percentage of instrumental studies result in the patient returning to a PO diet?). Comparing facility-specific data against national benchmark data, such as ASHA NOMS, is even more powerful. Perhaps the administrator of a facility views speech–language pathology as an expense only and does not see any cost benefit to the services. NOMS data can document how many patients who received swallowing treatment are able to discontinue tube feeding. The amount of money saved on tube feeding and nursing care related to the tube feeding can be compared to the cost of the speech–language pathology services rendered, demonstrating a clear cost savings.

Here are just a few examples of other problems SLPs encounter and suggestions for the type of data used to address each problem:

1. Development of a clinical pathway: If the facility is developing a clinical pathway for stroke patients that indicates when speech–language pathology will be called on to see the patient regarding dysphagia, the following can be utilized:

   - Information about decreased length of stay for CVA patients when a dysphagia management program is in place

   - Cost data comparing cost of tube feeding with cost of SLP services

2. Refusal to allow referral for instrumental assessments: If the skilled nursing facility refuses to allow the speech–language pathologist to request instrumental assessments because it does not want to pay for the exam, what data might be needed?

   - Data about aspiration pneumonia rates and the relationship between aspiration and development of pneumonia

   - Cost data regarding treating the pneumonia (when the patient returns from acute care after a hospital stay for the pneumonia)

- Data about cost of tube feeding compared to oral feeding plus therapy (noting that therapy cannot be planned without instrumental exam)

- Data about how many patients can resume oral feeding as a result of instrumental exam

3. Family needs information: The family of a patient with a new CVA wants to know whether their father will be able to go home after rehabilitation and eat food without supervision. What information is needed to counsel the family?

  - Outcomes data from a national database, as well as specific information from the facility about similar patients, will allow the SLP to give an informed answer about prognosis.

For real change to take place, SLPs must be advocates as well as clinicians. Successful advocates are ones who have data to back their arguments. The following examples of advocacy are actions that every SLP who works with patients with dysphagia should take:

- Be in regular contact with representatives in Congress to let them know of the negative effects reimbursement changes have had on patient care.

- Use information from a variety of sources when counseling patients and families about the patient's disorder and prognosis.

- Use research data to supplement discussions with physicians concerning the value of dysphagia services.

- Use data to talk with administrators about the value and cost–benefit ratio of dysphagia services.

- Sign up to collect outcomes data for the national database ASHA NOMS.

- Contact a researcher and volunteer to help with a research project on dysphagia, or better yet, suggest the topic for such a study and help identify the patients.

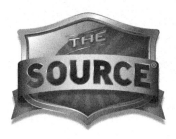

Chapter 9

Reimbursement: Coding and Documenting Dysphagia Services

Many patients with dysphagia are elderly and therefore have Medicare as their payment source. Being familiar with Medicare guidelines is important for that reason, but also because many other payers, such as Medicaid and private insurance companies, adopt and follow Medicare guidelines. Patients with dysphagia are seen in every health-care setting, including acute care, inpatient rehabilitation facilities, skilled nursing facilities, home health, and outpatient. Depending on the setting, the services for patients with Medicare may be covered by Medicare Part A or Part B. It is beyond the scope of this chapter to describe reimbursement requirements for each setting related to Part A services. Readers are referred to Documentation and Reimbursement for SLPs: Principles and Practice (Swigert, 2018), and to the ASHA Reimbursement website.

Medicare Definition of Dysphagia

The Medicare definition of *dysphagia* is found in the Medicare National Coverage Determination for Speech–Language Pathology Services for Treatment of Dysphagia (170.3).

> Dysphagia is a swallowing disorder that may be due to various neurological, structural and cognitive deficits. Dysphagia may be the result of head trauma, cerebrovascular accident, neuromuscular degenerative diseases, head and neck cancer, or encephalopathies. While dysphagia can afflict any age group, it most often appears among the elderly. Speech–language pathology services are covered under Medicare for the treatment of dysphagia, regardless of the presence of a communication disability.
>
> Patients who are motivated, moderately alert and have some degree of deglutition and swallowing functions are appropriate candidates for dysphagia therapy. Elements of the therapy program can include thermal stimulation to heighten the sensitivity of the swallowing response, exercises to improve oral-motor control, training in laryngeal adduction, compensatory swallowing techniques, and positioning and dietary modifications. Design all programs to ensure swallowing safety of the patient during oral feedings and to maintain adequate nutrition. (National Coverage Determinations Alphabetical Index, 2016).

Medicare Regulations

Specific Medicare regulations are written for Part B services but may be used by auditors and reviewers to determine appropriateness of services provided under Part A.

Medicare Benefit Policy Manual

Many of the regulations regarding dysphagia services are found in the *Medicare Benefit Policy Manual: Therapy Policies*. The manual itself can be found on the official CMS website (http://www .cms.hhs.gov) by searching for "paper or internet manual." Therapy services are also mentioned in other manuals:

- 100-04 *Medicare Claims Processing Manual*
- 00-08 *Program Integrity Manual*

Local Coverage Determinations

In addition to these national guidelines, some regulations are written by regional insurance companies contracted by CMS to administer the Medicare program. These contractors are called Medicare Administrative Contractors (MACs) and typically cover a multistate area (Medicare Administrative Contractors, 2016).

These guidelines are found in documents called local coverage determinations (LCDs). Most MACs write an LCD for speech-language services and a separate one for dysphagia services. The LCDs contain information about the type of service that is reimbursable, definitions of services, and typically a list of diagnostic and procedure codes covered by Medicare. Determine who at your facility receives the updates to the LCDs and ask that they share them with you.

Definitions Found in Medicare Benefits Policy Manual

Some definitions found in the national *Medicare Benefits Policy Manual* are important concepts related to funding and reimbursement.

UNDER THE CARE OF A PHYSICIAN

For Medicare to pay for the therapy service, the client must be under the care of a physician.

MEDICALLY NECESSARY

Services are medically necessary if the documentation indicates they meet the requirements for medical necessity, including that they are skilled, rehabilitative services, provided by clinicians with the approval of a physician or NPP, safe, and effective (i.e., progress indicates that the care is effective in rehabilitation of function).

REASONABLE AND NECESSARY

It should be expected that the individual's rehabilitation potential is significant in relation to the extent and duration of therapy services. If it is not, the services are not considered reasonable and necessary.

SKILLED SERVICE

Skilled services are those furnished by a certified, licensed speech–language pathologist and cannot be safely and effectively furnished by someone less skilled. For example, practicing an effortful swallow to clear residue throughout a meal is not considered skilled. However, that same activity, when first introduced to the patient, with the SLP providing cues, changing the difficulty of the task based on the analysis of the client's performance, providing reinforcement, and so on indicates a level of skill that could not be provided by a caregiver or family member (*Medicare Benefit Policy Manual*, 2016). Much more information about documenting skilled service can be found in Chapter 5, Documenting Treatment.

EXPECTATION OF IMPROVEMENT

Historically, Medicare reimbursed for services only if the client was expected to make improvements, even with a chronic, progressive, degenerative, or terminal illness. If no improvement was expected, then a maintenance program could be established but therapy was not likely to be covered. In 2013, in a case called *Jimmo v. Sebelius*, a court determined that Medicare may not deny speech–language pathology services simply because the beneficiary shows no functional progress, such as those individuals with degenerative and progressive diseases (e.g., multiple sclerosis, Parkinson's disease, amyotrophic lateral sclerosis). Rather, Medicare must cover skilled services that prevent deterioration and maintain functional levels (*Jimmo v. Sebelius Settlement Agreement Fact Sheet*, 2014).

Medicare Requirements for Part B Services

The following are important considerations when you provide services to Medicare patients covered by Part B. This is most often in outpatient settings, but some patients in inpatient facilities may be covered by Part B. This may happen, for example, if the patient has exhausted Part A coverage or does not qualify for Part A. This information is found in the *Medicare Benefit Policy Manual*.

Order Not Required Before Services in Outpatient Settings

When a patient covered by Medicare presents without an order, a plan may be established and treatment begun with the expectation that there is a physician or nonphysician practicioner (NPP) who will certify the plan and provide treatment to the patient. NPPs are physician assistants, advanced practice registered nurses (APRNs), certified nurse-practitioners, and clinical nurse specialists. Payment will be denied if the plan is not approved.

Plan of Care

For dysphagia services to be covered in the outpatient setting, the services need to be considered reasonable and necessary. A plan of care (treatment plan) has to be established by the physician or NPP, or the therapist, and is periodically reviewed by the physician or NPP. The plan must be established before treatment begins. It may be written on the same day as evaluation and initial treatment. If the plan is established by the speech–language pathologist providing the treatment, treatment may begin before the plan is written, but the plan must be established by the close of business (COB) the next day. This policy allows you to evaluate a patient and begin treatment that day before you have actually written the plan. The plan of care should contain at least the following:

- Diagnoses
- Long-term treatment goals
- Type, amount, duration, and frequency of therapy services
- Signature, date, and professional identity of the person who established the plan

The plan should be modified for significant changes in condition. A change in long-term goals would be a significant change. An insignificant alteration in the plan would be a decrease in the frequency or duration due to the patient's illness or a modification of short-term goals to adjust for improvements made toward the same long-term goals. If a patient has achieved a goal and/or has had no response to a treatment that is part of the plan, the therapist may delete a specific intervention from the plan of care before physician or NPP approval. This deletion should be reported to the physician or NPP responsible for the patient's treatment before the next certification.

Assessment Versus Evaluation Versus Reevaluation

Evaluation is a separately billable, comprehensive service that requires professional skills to make clinical judgments about dysphagia, based on objective measurements and subjective evaluations of patient performance and functional abilities. Evaluation is warranted, for example, for a new diagnosis or when a condition is treated in a new setting. These evaluative judgments are essential to development of the plan of care, including goals and the selection of interventions. *Assessment* is included in the course of therapy services and is not separately billable. Assessment requires data collection through observation and patient inquiry and may include limited objective testing and measurement to make clinical judgments regarding the patient's condition(s). Assessment determines, for example, changes in the patient's status since the last visit and whether the planned procedure or service should be modified. Based on these assessment data, you may make a judgment about progress toward goals and/or determine that a more complete reevaluation is indicated.

Reevaluation is billable separately and is periodically indicated when your assessment indicates a significant improvement or decline in the patient's condition or functional status. Some regulations and state practice acts require reevaluation at specific intervals. Reevaluation may also be appropriate at a planned discharge. A reevaluation assesses progress toward current goals and includes decisions about continuing care, modifying goals and/or treatment, or terminating services. Reevaluation requires the same professional skills as evaluation. Current procedural terminology (CPT) does not define a reevaluation code for speech–language pathology; use the evaluation code.

When More Than One Profession Is Involved

Although Medicare guidelines do not distinguish between SLPs, OTs, and PTs regarding dysphagia services, the guidelines do state that swallowing assessment and rehabilitation are highly specialized services. In addition, speech–language pathology is often referred to directly. The professional rendering care must have education, experience, and demonstrated competencies. Competencies include, but are not limited to, identifying abnormal upper aerodigestive tract structure and function; conducting an oral, pharyngeal, laryngeal, and respiratory function examination as it relates to the functional assessment of swallowing; recommending methods of oral intake and risk precautions; and developing a treatment plan employing appropriate compensations and therapy techniques.

Occupational therapists and physical therapists often provide service with SLPs, but these services must not duplicate one another. If you are involved in a team approach in which two or more of these professions are providing intervention for a patient with dysphagia, the notes documented by each must reflect the different areas addressed.

EXAMPLE NOTES WHEN MORE THAN ONE PROFESSION IS TREATING

When a patient is seen for dysphagia by two different professions, each writes a note reflecting the skilled care provided:

Speech—"Patient able to close lips around spoon with tactile assistance on 8 of 10 trials during therapeutic feeding at lunch. Analysis of patient's ability to actively close lips around spoon revealed patient unable to do so without the tactile stimulation. If support is not provided to the right lower corner of the lip, patient has anterior loss with thin liquids. Patient able to manipulate bolus of pureed consistency from front to back of mouth with minimal oral residue on 10 of 10 trials. Patient used chin-down position for thin liquids without cues 100% of the time when small sips were presented from a straw."

An occupational therapist providing treatment during a meal would certainly follow all the precautions described above, but their treatment might be documented as follows:

"Patient positioned at upright at the beginning of meal with extra pillow placed behind her head. Patient able to maintain head at midline for approximately 3 minutes at a time. Patient could reposition head at midline with tactile cues in 6/7 trials. Patient able to locate items on tray when cued to look to the left. Patient showed adequate sensation to wipe residue from right side of face without cues. Patient using weighted handle spoon for presentation of pureed foods."

Skilled Level of Care

Skilled therapy may be needed, and improvement in a patient's condition may occur, even where a chronic or terminal condition exists. For example, a terminally ill patient may begin to exhibit self-care, mobility, and/or safety dependence requiring skilled therapy services. The fact that full or partial recovery is not possible does not necessarily mean that skilled therapy is not needed to improve the patient's condition. In the case of a progressive, degenerative disease, for example, service may be intermittently necessary to determine the need for assistive equipment and establish a program to maximize function. The deciding factors for care are always whether the services are considered reasonable, effective treatments for the patient's condition and require the skills of a therapist or whether the services can be safely and effectively carried out by others, such as family members, friends, and nursing assistants, without the supervision of qualified professionals. (See Table 5.5 for examples.)

If an individual's expected rehabilitation potential would be insignificant in relation to the extent and duration of therapy services required to achieve such potential, therapy would not be covered because it would not be considered rehabilitative or reasonable and necessary.

Services are not considered rehabilitative if they can be delivered safely and effectively by non-skilled personnel without the supervision of qualified professionals. If at any point in the treatment of an illness it is determined that the treatment is not rehabilitative, or does not legitimately require the services of a qualified professional for management of a maintenance program as described below, the services will no longer be considered reasonable and necessary. Services that are not reasonable and necessary should be excluded from coverage.

Remember that if all you are doing is routine, repetitive observation or standby cueing, it is probably not going to be viewed as skilled rehabilitation. The services of a certified and licensed SLP are needed because you are able to observe and analyze what the patient is doing and make changes based on your observations. These changes may be in treatment techniques, positioning techniques, and diet. However, a note such as the one below would probably indicate that the services being provided are not skilled. There is nothing in the note that indicates a nursing assistant or family member could not do the same thing:

"Watched patient at lunchtime. Fed patient pureed diet by spoon and thin liquids from cut-out cup. Patient consumed 80% of pureed foods and 100% of liquids."

During the last visits for dysphagia therapy, the speech–language pathologist may develop a maintenance program. The goals of a maintenance program would be, for example, to maintain functional status or to prevent a decline in function. The specialized knowledge and judgment of a qualified therapist would be required. Services are covered to design or establish a plan; ensure patient safety; train the patient, family members, and/or unskilled personnel; and make infrequent, but periodic, reevaluations of the plan.

The services of a qualified professional are not necessary to carry out a maintenance program and are not covered under ordinary circumstances. The patient may perform such a program independently or with the assistance of unskilled personnel or family members.

Instrumental Examinations

The SLP performs clinical and instrumental assessments and analyzes and integrates the diagnostic information to determine candidacy for intervention as well as appropriate compensations and rehabilitative therapy techniques.

The equipment used in the examination may be fixed, mobile, or portable. Professional guidelines recommend that the service be provided in a team setting with a physician or NPP who provides supervision of the radiological examination and interpretation of medical conditions revealed in it.

Coding for Diagnosis and Treatment Procedures

Coding systems were designed to collect data for research and health statistics and to aid in the payment of claims. There are two coding systems used in health care. The coding system used to describe the reason the client is being seen is the *International Classification of Diseases–10th Edition* (ICD-10-CM). Codes to describe the service provided are called Current Procedural Terminology (CPT) codes. The Current Procedural Terminology (CPT) process is owned and managed by the American Medical Association (AMA) (CPT Current Procedural Terminology, 2017).

ICD-10-CM

This coding system is used to assign codes to diagnoses, or the reason the patient is being seen. The ICD-10 is owned by the World Health Organization, but the National Center for Health Statistics (NCHS) and the Centers for Medicare and Medicaid Services (CMS) are the U.S. governmental agencies responsible for overseeing all changes and modifications to the ICD-10-CM. The "CM" means clinical modification and is the U.S. modification of ICD-10.

USES FOR ICD-10

These diagnostic codes have many other uses besides coding for reimbursement. ICD is used around the world to identify health trends and to gather statistics. Internationally it is the standard for reporting diseases and health conditions. ICD is the standard for research purposes. Because it is a standardized system, it allows for the following:

- An easy way to store, retrieve and analyze health information so that evidence-based decisions can be made

- A way for health-care facilities, regions, and countries to share and compare health data

- A location to compare data over a period of time (e.g., reporting an increase or decrease in a specific disease, such as an increase in diabetes in a region over time)

- A standardized way to describe a disease or disorder on a health-care claim

ICD-10 uses a seven-character alphanumeric system. The first character is alphabetical, the second is numeric, and the third through seventh characters are either alphabetical or numeric. ICD-10 has about 68,000 codes available.

RULES FOR DIAGNOSTIC CODING OF THERAPY SERVICES

ICD-10 code should support procedure code. For therapy services to be reimbursed, the client must have a diagnosis that supports the need for services of a speech–language pathologist. For example, it is logical that a client might need an evaluation by a speech–language pathologist if the client has a diagnosis of stroke, Parkinson's disease, multiple sclerosis, or other similar illnesses. However, if the only diagnosis on a client's bill was something like broken hip or hypertension, services of a speech–language pathologist would not seem to be indicated. It is important that all appropriate diagnoses be listed. For example, a client might have suffered a broken hip, a code that does not warrant SLP services, but the patient might also have dementia. If the dementia is not coded on the bill along with broken hip, then the charge for speech-language services would likely be denied. Medicare probably has the most stringent guidelines about which diagnostic codes it considers as supporting the need for speech–language services.

Physician codes medical problem. The physician is responsible for determining the code for the medical problem (e.g., stroke), and the speech–language pathologist can apply the code or codes to describe the swallowing problem for which the client is being treated. When submitting a claim, the primary diagnosis is the condition (disease, symptom, injury) that is chiefly responsible for the visit or the reason for the encounter. This primary code is listed on the first line of the list of diagnoses. Secondary diagnoses, which are then listed below the primary diagnosis, are coexisting conditions or symptoms, or things discovered after the evaluation. Sometimes there is an obvious medical disorder (e.g., stroke, ALS, dementia) causing the dysphagia. When there is not, dysphagia might be the only medical diagnosis listed. In that case, the physician might use R13.10 Dysphagia Unspecified.

SLP codes phase of dysphagia. The speech–language pathologist can then add the more specific code when the phase(s) involved have been determined, which adheres to the guidance is that you should always code to the highest degree of specificity. That means, if there is a code with three characters and one with four characters that could describe the disorder, choose the one with four characters. If there is a four-character code and a five-character code and either describes the disorder, but the code with five characters more specifically describes the problem, then choose the code with five characters. Some ICD-10 codes use the terms *not otherwise specified* (NOS) and *not elsewhere classified* (NEC). These codes are not very specific and seem to indicate that the clinician does not really know what is wrong with the client. Avoid using these codes when possible. ICD-10-CM guidelines indicate that clinicians should not use terms like *rule out* or *probable*, *likely*, *suspected*, and *questionable*. Instead, the report should indicate the reason for which the patient was referred. For example, if a patient is referred for signs of pharyngeal dysphagia, but the instrumental assessment reveals no deficits, the code should be for pharyngeal dysphagia and the report should explain that the findings were within normal limits.

There are many more codes for dysphagia than those listed in Table 9.1 that describe dysphagia by the phase(s) affected. For example, in the "I" series of codes, dysphagia is associated with a number of stroke-related neurological causes. Dysphagia following non-traumatic intracerebral hemorrhage; or I69.291 Dysphagia following other nontraumatic intracranial hemorrhage). These would need to be applied by the physician ("2018 ICD-10-CM Diagnosis Codes Related to Speech, Language and Swallowing Disorders," 2017).

Current Procedural Terminology Codes (CPTs)

In addition to coding the diagnosis, the reason the client is being seen, the clinician also uses codes to describe what procedure(s) were performed. These procedural codes are the Current Procedural Terminology Codes. Unlike the ICD-10-CM process, which is managed by government agencies, the CPT process is owned and maintained by the American Medical Association (AMA), which has copyright protection of the codes (CPT Current Procedural Terminology, 2017).

There are CPT codes that apply to dysphagia evaluation and treatment. The best place to locate information about the codes is on the ASHA website (http://www.asha.org/practice/reimbursement/medicare/SLP_coding_rules/). Read the descriptions of each code and choose one that accurately describes what you have done with the patient. Note that Medicare has indicated that regardless of the modality used (e.g., electrical stimulation), the treatment code 92526 is to be used.

CPT codes are used to bill outpatient therapy services. Speech–language pathologists working in inpatient settings may be asked to use CPT codes, but this is for internal tracking and productivity purposes. Since all inpatient settings under Medicare are paid through prospective payment systems, it is irrelevant how many and which CPT codes were used.

Table 9.1
ICD-10-CM Codes for Phases of Dysphagia

R13.1 Note: Code first, if applicable, dysphagia following cerebrovascular disease (I69. with final characters 91) Excludes 1: psychogenic dysphagia (F45.8)

Code	Description
R13.10	Dysphagia, unspecified
	Difficulty in swallowing NOS
R13.11	Dysphagia, oral phase
R13.12	Dysphagia, oropharyngeal phase
R13.13	Dysphagia, pharyngeal phase
R13.14	Dysphagia, pharyngoesophageal phase
R13.19	Other dysphagia
	Cervical dysphagia
	Neurogenic dysphagia

Note. From *ICD-10-CM Tabular List of Diseases and Injuries* (2010), retrieved from https://www.cms.gov/medicare/coding/icd10/downloads/6_i10tab2010.pdf.

The facility then attaches a discipline-specific modifier that indicates which rehabilitation professional rendered the service. These modifiers are very important, as more than one discipline may be billing the same CPT code on the same day. The modifier for SLP services is GN; for OT, GO; and for PT, GP.

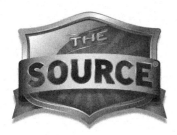

Chapter 10

Practicing From an Evidence Base

As a scientific profession, speech–language pathologists (SLPs) have long been expected to use evidence and data to manage decisions about treating patients with dysphagia. However, external demands for data have accelerated our interest in the topic. Health-care reimbursement rules and methodologies are ever-changing, but the one constant is an increasing demand to demonstrate value. *Value* is defined as outcome over expense. Are the services adding value without costing too much money? Is the desired outcome being achieved, and in particular, is it the functional outcome desired by the patient and caregivers? SLPs are being asked by a variety of audiences to demonstrate the value of dysphagia treatment as well as how involvement with patients with dysphagia is going to make a difference. Who are the people making these demands?

Third-party payers want to know about the bang for their buck. If they pay for the service, what will the outcome be? For example, will the patient still need to be on tube feeding? Consumers and their family members want to know whether the patient will be able to eat a regular, unrestricted diet. Referring physicians may ask whether the patient's swallowing skills will improve more rapidly with treatment than without. Savvy consumers and payers also ask similar questions about specific techniques and modalities.

Demands such as these make it important for clinicians to understand the kinds of data and evidence available, as well as ways to use the information to provide better services. A profession must also be aware of the kinds of data that are lacking, and sorely needed, to answer questions that will be faced in the future about dysphagia services. It is expected that health care providers will continue to receive more questions about outcomes from a variety of sources and that those questions will become more rigorous.

Types of Data

Three broad types of data are available to clinicians when operating from an evidence base: outcomes data, outcomes research, and treatment research (Table 10.1). Each type contributes to the clinician's knowledge base and guides decision-making for individual clients. In this chapter a subtle distinction is made between outcomes data *collection* and outcomes *research,* which are described below. For a more comprehensive resource on outcomes data collection, outcomes research, and models of treatment research, readers are referred to *Outcomes in Speech–Language Pathology* (Golper & Frattali, 2013).

Outcomes Data Collection

Clinicians are used to collecting data on the patient level. Data are collected on objective evaluation measures, on patient performance in treatment and status at discharge. The data collected are used to develop a treatment plan, select long- and short-term goals, and establish treatment objectives to meet those goals. In this way, clinicians are able to demonstrate a patient's progress

Table 10.1

Types of Data Available to Clinicians

Type of data	What it is	What it can do	What it cannot do	Examples
Outcomes				
Outcomes data collection	Data collected in clinical situations without rigorous controls, typically using a rating scale.	Provide data about what happens in real-world situations.	Cannot "prove" that the change demonstrated by the patient was attributable to the treatment.	ASHA NOMS Functional Independence Measure (FIM™)
Research				
Outcomes research Designs include experimental and nonexperimental (e.g., data synthesis, observational)	Likely uses rating scales like outcomes data collection but applied in a more controlled situation than data collection. Typically focuses on patient-centered and policy-relevant outcomes.	Serve as a bridge between data collection and rigorous treatment efficacy research. Causal interpretations must still be qualified because the research is done in less controlled atmosphere.	Typically does not answer questions about changes in physiology.	Measuring outcomes like: physiologic changes function health status patient satisfaction quality of life
Treatment research	Evaluates effectiveness (efficacy) of a clinical approach (e.g., clinical swallow evaluation, specific technique).	Answer specific questions about whether an approach is effective in doing what it purports to do.	Address policy-relevant outcomes.	See citations in Chapters 2, 3, and 4.

Note. Adapted from Golper and Frattali (2013); Rubenfeld et al. (1999).

from session to session as well as from the beginning to the end of treatment. However, if the only data available are on an individual patient's performance, then clinicians will not be able to answer questions such as the following:

- How many sessions does it typically take before a patient no longer needs tube feeding and can eat by mouth?

- What is the likelihood a patient's swallowing will improve during a short stay in acute care?

- In general, does more therapy yield more significant improvement in similar patients?

For answers to questions such as these, outcomes data is needed on a large number of similar patients. Outcomes data describe what a patient was like at the end of a period of treatment. One cannot necessarily attribute any change that took place over the course of treatment to the treatment itself. (For that kind of data, see the discussion of efficacy later in this chapter.) Any such interpretation of cause must be qualified due to the many unrelated and uncontrolled factors, but can lend support to experimental evidence of efficacy. Outcomes data simply state that at the end of the period of treatment, this is what the patient was like compared to what she was like at the beginning of treatment. When outcomes data are collected on a large number of patients and submitted to a data collection system, the data can be analyzed and used in patient and program management. For example, data from an aggregated source can be used to benchmark an individual patient's performance against other similar patients in similar situations or a facility's program against similar programs.

National Outcomes Data Collection Systems for Benchmarking

National systems allow for benchmarking, which is a more powerful tool in several ways. Comparing an individual patient's progress to that of a group of patients with similar deficits provides the basis for an informed prognosis. Benchmarking meets the demands of accrediting agencies that want programs to compare themselves to a standard and set goals to improve the program's performance. Information from a national system can form the basis for quality improvement and program management activities. In addition, national data can stimulate change in practice patterns.

FUNCTIONAL INDEPENDENCE MEASURES (FIM)

Such national data may be embedded in a comprehensive assessment instrument, such as the Functional Independence Measure (FIM) developed by the Uniform Data System for Medical Rehabilitation (UDS) in 1995. The FIM was designed to measure a level of independence in areas such as locomotion, sphincter control, transfers, self-care, and communication. Each variable within those categories is scored on a 7-point scale. The drawback to use of the FIM to show functional change in swallowing is that it is rated on a self-care scale called *eating*. The eating scale focuses not just on the ability to eat or swallow but also on self-feeding skills like bringing a utensil to the mouth. Clinicians report it is not specific enough to measure change in swallowing. In addition, the eating scale does not have to be scored by an SLP (Kidd et al., 1995).

ASHA NATIONAL OUTCOMES MEASUREMENT SYSTEM (NOMS)

To meet the demands on SLPs for data to demonstrate the value of services, ASHA developed the National Outcomes Measurement System. NOMS was launched in 1998, but the new, enhanced NOMS was released in September of 2013. The new NOMS has simplified data collection forms with optional interim reporting and a new goal-setting feature with access to real-time national benchmarking data.

The registered user (an SLP) rates the patient's functional level on admit, at other points within the period of care, and at the end of therapy. (See description below of the functional communication measures.) These ratings, along with demographic information, diagnostic codes, treatment setting, and amount of treatment, are submitted to ASHA.

ASHA compiles the data that have been submitted and prepares a national report card to answer questions like these:

- How many treatment units does it take for a patient with a CVA to move from Level 3 to Level 5 on the swallowing FCM?

- Do patients receive more or fewer treatment units in skilled nursing facilities compared to home health agencies, and is their amount of change affected by the amount of service?

- Do patients make more or less progress when seen in group treatment?

Such national data provide important information to the profession and to consumers and payers. For facilities that participate and contribute data to the national database, the data are available in real time to be used in performance improvement and quality initiatives and also to help determine a prognosis for an individual patient. There is no cost to ASHA members to participate in NOMS. For information, contact ASHA via the website http://www.asha.org/NOMS.

Rating Scales of Functional Outcomes

Outcomes data collection and outcomes research typically involve the use of a rating scale or other measurement tool that can be used before and after treatment to show that change has occurred. Some scales combine some functional ratings with physiological ratings, while others focus just on changes in function. Some scales are rated by the clinician, while others are based on patient self-report. Other scales focus on physiologic changes rather than changes in function.

Rating scales that describe functional outcomes differ from physiological rating scales that describe an outcome as a change in some aspect of the complex physical act of swallowing (e.g., better tongue movement, increased laryngeal elevation). Functional outcomes describe change in a way that is meaningful to someone other than an SLP, and is particularly important to the patient. Functional change implies a change in an applied aspect of the skill. That is, because the underlying physiology has improved, the result is a practical change.

ASHA NOMS FUNCTIONAL COMMUNICATION MEASURES (FCMs)

The NOMS measures change in a variety of areas through the use of 7-point rating scales called Functional Communication Measures (FCMs). These FCMs have been developed for 15 areas including, of interest here, swallowing

The swallowing FCM takes into account several factors that contribute to a change in functional ability to eat, such as kinds of solid foods the patient can eat, kinds of liquids the patient can swallow safely, amount of cueing needed, and which of the patient's nutritional needs are met by mouth. For example, Level 1 indicates that the patient has no functional swallow and receives all nutrition and hydration by nonoral means. Level 3 indicates that an alternative method of feeding is still required, as the individual takes less than 50% of nutrition and hydration by mouth, and/or swallowing is safe with consistent use of moderate cues to use compensatory strategies, and/or patient requires maximum diet restrictions. At Level 7, the patient's ability to eat independently is not limited by swallow function, and swallowing is considered safe and efficient for all consistencies. Compensatory strategies are effectively used when needed.

THE DYSPHAGIA OUTCOME AND SEVERITY SCALE (DOSS)

The DOSS is a scale that allows clinicians to make recommendations about diet, independence, and type of nutrition. Examining one of its seven levels demonstrates how physiology and function are combined on the same scale. For example, Level 3: Moderate Dysphagia is described as "total assist, supervision or strategies; two or more diet consistencies restricted." The scale then lists symptoms that may be exhibited, such as moderate retention in the pharynx or oral cavity and airway penetration. Combining severity of physiological deficits and functional skills on one scale makes the scale less meaningful to payers, although the authors state that the tool lends some objective measurement to the functional description (O'Neil, Purdy, Falk, & Gallo, 1999, p. 142).

THE FUNCTIONAL ORAL INTAKE SCALE (FOIS)
Similar to the DOSS and to the ASHA FCM, the FOIS is a 7-point scale developed to document clinical change in oral intake in patients after stroke (Crary et al., 2005).

Patient-Reported Outcomes (PROs) Tools

Patient-reported outcomes (PROs) have been defined as "any report of the status of a patient's health condition that comes directly from the patient, without interpretation of the patient's response by a clinician or anyone else" ("Patient Reported Outcomes," n.d.). PROs tools measure what patients are able to do and how they feel by asking questions. These tools enable assessment of patient-reported health status for physical, mental, and social well-being (Cella et al., 2010).

Several examples of PROs in dysphagia are SWAL-QOL, SWAL-CARE, MDADI, and EAT10. Initially, the SWAL-QOL was a 93-item quality-of-life and quality-of-care outcomes tool for dysphagia researchers and clinicians. Because its length made it impractical for clinical use, the researchers used psychometric techniques to reduce the 93-item instrument into two patient-centered outcomes tools: the SWAL-QOL, a 44-item tool that assesses 10 quality-of-life concepts, and the SWAL-CARE, a 15-item tool that assesses quality of care and patient satisfaction. The scales have been shown to have good internal-consistency reliability and short-term reproducibility. The scales differentiate normal swallowers from patients with oropharyngeal dysphagia and are sensitive to differences in the severity of dysphagia as clinically defined (McHorney et al., 2002).

The Eating Assessment Tool is a self-administered, symptom-specific outcome instrument for dysphagia. The researchers concluded that the EAT-10 has good internal consistency, test–retest reproducibility, and criterion-based validity. The normative data suggest that an EAT-10 score of 3 or higher is abnormal. The instrument may be utilized to document the initial dysphagia severity and monitor progress in treatment (Belafsky et al., 2008).

The MDADI, MD Anderson Dysphagia Inventory, was the first validated and reliable self-administered questionnaire designed specifically for evaluating the impact of dysphagia on the QOL of patients with head and neck cancer. The MDADI is a 20-item 5-point Likert questionnaire that assesses dysphagia in three domains (functional, emotional, physical) (Chen et al., 2001).

Physiological Scales

Some scales used in research studies do not address function as much as they measure change in a physiologic parameter. Using ICF terminology, scales such as these focus on disability rather than function. Examples of physiologic rating scales are seen in Table 10.2. The 8-point Penetration–Aspiration Scale measures biomechanical action during swallowing. It can be used to objectify what is observed during videofluoroscopic studies. It measures the depth of penetration of the bolus and effectiveness in attempts to clear the material (Rosenbek, Robbins, Roecker, Coyle, & Wood, 1996). The scale can also be used to establish pre- and post- ratings of physiological skills to demonstrate change that has taken place between the initial fluoroscopic study and any repeat studies. The PAS has also been used during FEES (Colodny, 2002).

Steele and Grace-Martin (2017) proposed a reorganization of the 8-point scale into a four-level categorical penetration–aspiration scale, with increasing levels of physiological severity. This categorization describes Levels 1 and 2 as normal function and Level 4 as a healthy response to penetration. Levels 3, 5, and 6 reflect failure of closure at the entrance to the airway in which

Table 10.2
Examples of Physiologic Rating Scales

Rating scale	Reference	What it does
Penetration-Aspiration Scale (Pen-Asp)	Rosenbek, Robbins, Roecker, Coyle, & Wood, 1996; Steele & Grace-Martin, 2017	Used during instrumental studies to describe depth of penetration of material into airway, patient response, and effectiveness of response
Secretion Rating Scale	Murray, Langmore, Ginsberg, & Dostie, 1996	Rates amount and location of secretions viewed endoscopically and predicts likelihood of aspiration
Yale Pharyngeal Residue Scale	Neubauer, Rademaker, & Leder, 2015	5-point scale of residue location and amount on FEES
Normalized Residue Ratio Scale (NRRS)	Pearson, Molfenter, Smith, & Steele, 2013	Measurement that incorporates the ratio of residue relative to the available pharyngeal space and the residue proportionate to the size of the individual

Note. Steele and Grace-Martin (2017).

material remains in the vestibule after the swallow. Levels 7 and 8 reflect aspiration with either an effective response or no response.

Murray and colleagues developed a rating scale from 0 to 3 to describe the amount and location of secretions on the FEES. This rating was used to predict the likelihood of aspiration but could also be used in repeat studies to demonstrate change (Murray, Langmore, Ginsberg, & Dostie, 1996).

Two scales measure the amount of residue on FEES and on VFSS. The Yale Pharyngeal Residue Scale is a 5-point ordinal rating scale based on residue location (vallecular and pyriform sinus) and amount (none, trace, mild, moderate, and severe) viewed on a FEES exam. The article contains color images for each of the ratings in the valleculae and pyriform sinuses (Neubauer, Rademaker, & Leder, 2015). The Normalized Residue Ration Scale (NRRS) is a continuous measurement that incorporates both the ratio of residue relative to the available pharyngeal space and the residue proportionate to the size of the individual. However, this scale requires use of open-source software and spreadsheets and therefore is not likely to be used clinically on a routine basis (Pearson, Molfenter, Smith, & Steele, 2013).

Outcomes Research

Outcomes research encompasses the features described above concerning outcomes data collection but typically in a more controlled fashion. The results of the research can be found published in journals, whereas the information from a data collection system like NOMS or FIM is generally contained in reports, often available only to subscribers. Outcomes research typically focuses on patient-centered and policy-relevant outcomes and considers the effects of treatment on endpoints important to patients and society (Rubenfeld et al., 1999). Outcomes research is also sometimes referred to as treatment effectiveness research and is suited to making statements about trends, associations, and estimates (Golper & Frattali, 2013).

Categories of Functional Change

Functional outcomes research in dysphagia is generally grouped into measuring the following categories of functional change. Consider how each might be patient-centered and/or policy-relevant.

ABILITY TO EAT

As reflected in some of the scales described above, the outcome is measured related to the types of food and liquids the patient can consume, number of compensatory strategies needed, level of independence in eating, length of time it takes to eat, and other variables. This kind of outcome would be particularly relevant to the patient.

HEALTH STATUS

Some studies compare the results of dysphagia management to the patient's health status. Certain chemical and physiologic measures (e.g., body weight, serum albumin levels) and overall health status (e.g., pneumonia, readmission to the hospital) measures are used to determine if the intervention was successful. These results are patient centered and policy relevant; the latter because patients with a poor health status outcome cause increased cost to the health-care system.

PATIENT AND CAREGIVER SATISFACTION

The clinician's view of a successful outcome may be very different from the patient's and caregiver's views. For example, the clinician may be pleased to have advanced the patient from NPO status to eating a pureed diet with mildly thick liquids with only a few compensatory strategies. This may not be deemed a success from the patient or caregiver perspective.

QUALITY OF LIFE

Quality of life is also from the patient and/or caregiver's perspective and can encompass many different factors. These might include the factors described above related to the ability to eat, but could also include measures of how confident the patient is when eating in front of others or how much the patient is able to participate in family meals. This is very patient-centered research.

Treatment Research

Outcomes measurement tools, data collection, and outcomes research can yield important information about change in patient status over time. As described, these outcomes range from change in physiology to change in quality of life. Outcomes data can answer many questions, as stated previously. Outcomes data cannot, however, answer questions such as these:

- Do patients get better as a result of the treatment provided?
- Do patients with impaired swallow improve more quickly as a result of treatment Technique A or B?

For the answers to such questions, we need efficacy data.

Efficacy and Effectiveness

Studies that SLPs read in refereed journals that seek to answer such questions are generally considered studies of efficacy or effectiveness. Rosenbek (1995, p. 263) states that efficacy is "improvement resulting from treatment applied in a rigidly controlled design when treatment and no-treatment conditions are compared. A comparison of two treatments of unproven efficacy is not an efficacy study."

Using Rosenbek's definition, the first question listed above (Do patients get better as a result of the treatment provided?) would be part of an efficacy study if a treatment and no-treatment design were applied. For the second question (Do patients with impaired swallow improve more quickly as a result of treatment Technique A or B?) to be part of an efficacy study, both treatments A and B would have to have undergone the rigorous treatment and no-treatment design and been shown to be efficacious.

Clinicians might look to the literature for evidence of the following:

- Efficacy of a particular therapy approach

- Efficacy of clinical swallow evaluations

- Efficacy of instrumental exams

Examples of efficacy literature have been included throughout *The Source* related to these and other areas of practice.

As clinicians, it is important that we become sophisticated users of the research literature. We must not simply read the description of the study and the conclusions and then apply the technique to our patients. We must also analyze the methods used, population selected, dependent variables chosen, and the like. In short, we must read every study the way we were taught in our research design course in graduate school. As critical consumers of research, we can decide when the information reported will be helpful to us and our patients.

How to Obtain Research Findings

Practicing clinicians face significant productivity demands at work and many other demands on their time away from work, both of which make it challenging to find time to search for, read, interpret, and apply research findings to their day-to-day work with patients. How can the practicing clinician stay current on research findings? Some suggested resources are listed in Table 10.3.

CONFERENCES

Attending conferences presented by SLPs who endorse evidence-based practice and share up-to-date findings is one effective way to stay current. When considering which conferences or web-based training to take, consider the presenter's credentials. If the course is on a particular evaluation or treatment approach, first review the literature to make sure the topic has been addressed in the research literature. Be aware that ASHA CE sponsors who put on programs do not have to get approval from ASHA for the content or the presenter. They are, however, supposed to vet both topic and presenter to determine that EBP principles will be followed. One might be wary of a particular CE provider who offers only courses on one particular topic or with one constant speaker. The ASHA website is a good place to find a listing of live and web-based events and training that are provided by various ASHA CE sponsors (Continuing Education, 2017).

Table 10.3
Finding and Using Evidence

Sources for evidence	Notes
ASHA-CE–approved courses from presenters who endorse EBP	https://www.asha.org/ce/
Journals (various)	Google Scholar Search Engine
Dysphagia Journal	https://link.springer.com/journal/
ASHA Practice Portal	https://www.asha.org/practice-portal/
ASHA Evidence-Based Maps	https://www.asha.org/Practice-Portal/Clinical-Topics/Adult-Dysphagia/
Perspectives of Division 13	https://www.asha.org/SIG/13/
Ask a Colleague: ASHA Community Page	Must belong to SIG 13 to access https://www.asha.org/SIG/

JOURNALS

Research on swallowing and swallowing disorders can be found in many different types of journals, including ASHA journals. An example of a journal focused solely on dysphagia research is *Dysphagia*, the journal of the Dysphagia Research Society (https://link.springer.com/journal/). One does not have to work at a large hospital to have access to many journals. Using a search engine like Google Scholar can help the clinician find many pertinent references, and often the articles are in the public domain and do not require a subscription to a particular journal.

ASHA PRACTICE PORTAL

This section of the ASHA web page is designed to help audiologists and speech–language pathologists by providing the best available evidence and expertise in patient care, identifying resources vetted for relevance and credibility, and increasing practice efficiency. It comprises Clinical Topics, Professional Issues, Client/Patient Handouts, and Tools & Templates.

ASHA EVIDENCE-BASED MAPS

An especially relevant part of the portal to the discussion about evidence-based practice is evidence-based maps. After development of an initial outline, and vetting by subject-matter experts, ASHA's National Center for Evidence-Based Practice (N-CEP) develops an evidence map for the topic. The resources identified in the maps—including systematic reviews, guidelines, and patient perspectives, as well as ASHA policy documents and resources—provide the basis for the initial content on the page.

The articles included on the evidence map are organized to provide:

- Citation
- Link to article
- Article quality ratings
- Article details
- Conclusions

It is the easiest place for a clinician to start to find journal articles on a particular topic (Evidence Maps, 2017).

ASHA *PERSPECTIVES ON SWALLOWING AND SWALLOWING DISORDERS*

Special Interest Group 13 (Swallowing and Swallowing Disorders) produces *Perspectives*, a peer-reviewed "newsletter" that is more like a minijournal. Members of any of the 19 special interest groups of ASHA can access the Perspectives of any of the groups. These publications usually have a theme for an issue so that all the articles in that issue are on a related topic.

ASHA SIG 13 COMMUNITY PAGE

Members of SIG 13 also have access to a web-based "chat" area where questions can be posted to seek input from colleagues. The replies shared are not necessarily evidence based, however, and may just be the opinion of the writer. Clinicians should first seek evidence-based information from one of the other sources listed above.

Treatment Techniques or Protocols With No Published Efficacy Data

In the area of dysphagia, perhaps more so than in other areas of speech–language pathology, clinicians seem willing to apply a technique or approach to their patients when no published proof exists. To a certain extent, that is a natural progression in a clinical field. If we waited until every technique had undergone careful treatment and no-treatment design studies, we would have few techniques at our disposal. However, we need to recognize the difference between published data and to a presenter's claiming, "This has worked with 90% of my patients!" When the results of a study are submitted to a scientific journal, the article is subject to critical analysis and review by respected peers. Any faults in the design of the study or in the interpretation of the results will be pointed out. Serious design flaws or misinterpretation of the data can keep the study from being published at all. This process used by scientific journals affords the readers some assurances that the study is scientifically sound.

Here are some questions you should ask yourself before beginning to use a technique you learned at a conference or heard about from a colleague if there is no published research to support it.

DOES THE TECHNIQUE MAKE SENSE, GIVEN WHAT YOU KNOW ABOUT THE PHYSIOLOGY OF THE SWALLOW?

For example, if a presenter told you that having the patient forcefully open and close the jaw would reduce pyriform sinus residue, you would quickly argue that jaw movement has nothing to do with laryngeal movement (which is largely responsible for reducing pyriform sinus residue).

IS THERE A POSSIBILITY OF HARM TO THE PATIENT?

Will the technique cause the patient any undo discomfort? For example, would a technique utilizing hot-pepper sauce increase saliva flow and increase risk of aspirating bacteria-laden secretions?

IF THERE IS NO EFFICACY DATA PUBLISHED, WHY NOT?

Just having a presenter or colleague tell you that a technique works does not mean you should try it. Our Code of Ethics (Principle I, Rule J) states that "individuals shall accurately represent the intended purpose of a service, product, or research endeavor and shall abide by established guidelines for clinical practice and the responsible conduct of research" (ASHA Code of Ethics, 2016). If the researcher or clinician has been using the technique or protocol and is so confident of its efficacy that he or she is willing to teach others how to do it, then that individual has an obligation to submit the data for critical peer review.

IF IT SEEMS TO WORK FOR YOUR PATIENTS, IS THAT ENOUGH PROOF FOR YOU?

Remember the placebo effect. If you are excited about a new technique and tell the patient how wonderful it is and how well it will work, that alone can have an effect on the patient. In addition to the placebo effect, just judging efficacy by how well it works for several patients does not help you determine what other variables you have failed to control that might be accounting for the change.

ARE YOU TAKING TIME AWAY FROM TREATMENT WITH A MORE TRADITIONAL TECHNIQUE THAT HAS BEEN SHOWN TO BE EFFECTIVE?

If you spend time in therapy having the patient hold a bag of ice because you believe increasing sensitivity in the hand increases the speed of onset of the swallow, are you not taking time away from use of thermal-tactile stimulation, which has some support in the literature?

WHAT DO YOU TELL A PATIENT WHEN YOU DECIDE TO USE WHAT MUST BE CONSIDERED AN EXPERIMENTAL APPROACH?

You should disclose to the patient that the technique you are using does not yet have any published efficacy data to support it. The Code of Ethics again provides guidance to us in Principle III:

A. "Individuals' statements to the public shall provide accurate and complete information about the nature and management of communication disorders, about the professions, about professional services, about products for sale, and about research and scholarly activities.

B. Individuals' statements to the public shall adhere to prevailing professional norms and shall not contain misrepresentations when advertising, announcing, and promoting their professional services and products and when reporting research results" (p. 7).

Abbreviations

ABG	Arterial blood gas
AB-SSD	American Board of Swallowing and Swallowing Disorders
AND	Allow natural death
ANH	Artificial nutrition and hydration
APM	Alternative payment models
APRN	Advanced practice registered nurse
ARDS	Acute respiratory distress syndrome
BiPAP	Bilevel positive airway pressure
BID	Bis in die, meaning twice a day
BJH-SDS	Barnes-Jewish Hospital–Stroke Dysphagia Screening
BOT	Base of tongue
BPM	Breaths per minute
CCI	Correct Coding Initiative
CFO	Comfort feeding only
CMS	Centers for Medicare and Medicaid Services
COPD	Chronic, obstructive pulmonary disease
CP	Cricopharyngeus
CPAP	Continuous positive airway pressure
CPT®	Current Procedural Terminology
CSE	Clinical Swallow Exam
CTAR	Chin tuck against resistance
CVA	Cerebrovascular accident (i.e., stroke)
DNR	Do not resuscitate
DNI	Do not intubate
DRG	Diagnostic-related group
EAT-10	Patient Reported Outcome Tool: Eating Assessment Tool
EGD	Esophagogastroduodonoscopy
EHR	Electronic health record
EMR	Electronic medical record
EMST	Expiratory Muscle Strength Trainer
EPAP	End positive airway pressure
EPG	Effortful pitch glide
ETT	Endotracheal tube
FCM	Functional Communication Measure (part of ASHA NOMS)
FEES	Fiberoptic Endoscopic Evaluation of Swallowing
FEES®	FEES following Langmore's protocol
FEEST	Fiberoptic Endoscopic Evaluation of Swallowing with Sensory Testing
FIO2	Fraction of inhaled oxygen
FFWP	Frazier Free Water Protocol
GERD	Gastroesophageal reflux
GI	Gastrointestinal
HFNC	High-flow nasal cannula
HPV	Human papilloma virus
HRM	High-resolution manometry
HTN	Hypertension
ICF	International Classification of Function, Disability, and Health
ICU	Intensive care unit
IOPI	Iowa Oral Performance Instrument

IP	Inpatient
IPAP	Inspiratory Peak Airway Pressure
JOAR	Jaw opening against resistance
LCD	Local Coverage Determination
LES	Lower esophageal sphincter
LPR	Laryngopharyngeal reflux
LTG	Long-term goal
MAC	Medicare Administrative Contractor
MDADI	MD Anderson Dysphagia Index
MEBDT	Modified Evans Blue Dye Test
MIPS	Merit-based incentive payment system
MTD	Muscle tension dysphagia
NEC	Not elsewhere classified
NFOSD	National Foundation on Swallowing Disorders
NG	Nasogastric
NJ	Nasojejunal
NMES	Neuromuscular electrical stimulation
NOMS	National Outcomes Measurement System (ASHA)
NOS	Not otherwise specified
NPO	Nil per os
NPP	Nonphysician practitioner
NSAID	Nonsteroidal, anti-inflammatory drugs
OCE	Outpatient coding editor
OP	Outpatient
PA	Physician assistant
PAS	Penetration-Aspiration Scale
PD	Parkinson's disease
PEEP	Positive End Expiratory Pressure
PEG	Percutaneous endoscopic gastrostomy
PEJ	Percutaneous endoscopic jejunostomy
PES	Pharyngo-esophageal segment
PPI	Proton pump inhibitors
PPS	Prospective payment system
PRN	Pro re nata, meaning "as necessary"
PRO	Patient-reported outcomes
PWD	Person with Parkinson's disease
QOL	Quality of life
RAD	Radiation-associated dysphagia
ROM	Range of motion
SCSE	Source Clinical Swallow Evaluation
sEMG	Surface electromyography
SIMV	Synchronized intermittent ventilation
STG	Short-term goal
SWAL-CARE	Patient reported outcome tool: Swallow CARE
SWAL-QOL	Patient reported outcome tool: Swallow Quality of Life
TOR-BST	Toronto Bedside Swallowing Screening
TPN	Total parenteral nutrition
UES	Upper esophageal sphincter
UGI	Upper gastrointestinal
VAP	Ventilator-associated pneumonia
Vt	Tidal volume

Glossary

achalasia	failure of the smooth muscle fibers to relax at the top of the stomach, resulting in the backup of food
adjunctive	describes an additional therapy used for increasing the efficacy or safety of the primary therapy or for facilitating its performance
advance directive	a legal document that allows a patient to state wishes about the use of life-support machines and medical treatment; also used to name someone else who can make medical choices for the patient
adventitious	abnormal breath sounds
agnosia	inability to interpret sensations
albumin	a protein found in the blood; known as serum albumin
allow natural death	term used to indicate that individual does not want any extraordinary life-extending efforts; comfort measures only
anticholinergics	blocking the passage of impulses through the parasympathetic nerves
antidepressants	medicines effective against depressive illness
antihistamines	substances capable of counteracting the effects of histamine
antihypertensives	agents that prevent or relieve high blood pressure
arrhythmia	a variation from the normal heartbeat
atelectasis	incomplete expansion or collapse of pulmonary alveoli or of a segment or lobe(s) of the lung
beneficence	performing kind acts (principle of ethics)
bolus tube feeding	tube feeding given in a concentrated dose rather than spread out on a slower drip over time
bradykinesia	atypically slow movements
BUN (blood urea nitrogen)/ creatinine ratio	the ratio of urea nitrogen to creatinine found in the blood; the ratio provides a rough estimate of kidney function; an extremely high ratio of BUN to creatinine may indicate dehydration
cervical auscultation	in swallowing, generally describes listening with a stethoscope over the larynx for breath sounds during swallowing
cervical osteophyte	a bony growth on the anterior part of the cervical spine that protrudes into the esophagus
chronic obstructive	a general term describing any obstructive breathing problem
clostridium difficile	bacterium that causes severe intestinal symptoms
cuffed trach tube	a tracheostomy tube with a cuff that can be inflated; the cuff rests below the vocal folds and serves as an anchor in the trachea
Current Procedural Terminology (CPT)	billing codes approved by the American Medical Association
deglutition	the oral and pharyngeal phases of swallowing
dehydration	a condition in which a patient is not getting enough fluids to keep cells hydrated
dentifrice	paste or powder for cleaning teeth and/or dentures
diuretics	medicines that stimulate the flow of urine

duodenum	the first part of the small intestine
dysgeusia	altered sense of smell
dyspnea	shortness of breath
edema	swelling caused by an abnormal accumulation of fluid in the intercellular spaces
edentulous	without teeth
endoscope	a tubular instrument that usually has a light source that can be inserted into a body cavity to permit visualizing the interior
erythrocytes	mature red blood cells
esophageal reflux	as opposed to gastroesophageal reflux, in which the contents of the stomach move up into the esophagus, esophageal reflux generally means that food remains in the esophagus and then moves back up toward the proximal esophagus
Fiberoptic Endoscopic Evaluation of Swallowing (FEES®)	a procedure in which an endoscope is passed transnasally into the pharynx for assessment of swallowing
fistula	abnormal or surgically made opening in the body
gastroesophageal reflux	movement of the contents of the stomach up and out of the stomach into the esophagus
GER or GERD	gastroesophageal reflux or gastroesophageal reflux disease
GI	gastrointestinal; pertaining to the stomach and intestines
globus	a feeling of fullness or sensation of a lump in the throat
gram negative bacilli	a type of bacteria found in the mouth
hematocrit	a lab value that reflects the amount of erythrocytes in a given volume of blood
hemodynamic	related to the flow of blood in organs and tissues of the body
hyolaryngeal complex	the hyoid bone and larynx considered as a unit
hypoxemia	low arterial oxygen supply
idiopathic	a disease or condition that comes about spontaneously, with unknown cause
infiltrate (pulmonary infiltrates)	indicates that some substance has passed into the lungs and is viewed via X-ray; does not necessarily mean that it is an aspirated substance
intubation	the art of inserting a breathing tube through the larynx into the trachea to attach the patient to a ventilator
isometric	a sustained movement designed to strengthen without contracting the muscle
isotonic	a muscle movement with normal contraction
jejunum	the second part of the small intestine between the duodenum and the ilium
Likert scale	A scale that uses fixed-choice response formats, often used to measure attitudes or opinions
lymphedema	swelling caused by blockage of the lymphatic system
maleficence	harm or causing harm

malnutrition	a condition in which the patient is not getting enough food to maintain adequate health or the patient's body may not be able to absorb and distribute the nutrition the patient is receiving
meta-analysis	a type of review that combines qualitative and quantitative reviews to form a conclusion
nasal cannula	small tubing that carries oxygen directly into the nose
neoplasm	a tumor
neuroleptic drugs	drugs prescribed to treat psychotic behavior
nonmaleficence	do no harm to the patient (principle of ethics)
nonsteroidal, anti-inflammatory drugs	class of drugs that reduce chemicals that promote pain and inflammation
nosocomial pneumonia	pneumonia acquired in a health-care facility
NPO	nil per os, which means "nothing by mouth"
odynophagia	pain or a feeling of obstruction on swallowing
orthostatic blood pressure	blood pressure taken in an upright position
ostomy	artificial opening in the body
parenteral	any feeding route other than the digestive tract; can be used to describe routes that are intravenous, subcutaneous, intramuscular, or mucosal
parenteral nutrition	a patient's total caloric needs are being met by intravenous route (a deep line is surgically placed into the subclavian artery and nutrition in a clear solution is delivered directly into a chamber of the heart; sometimes called total parenteral nutrition [TPN] or parenteral hyperlimantation)
paternalism	a mode by which a person in authority makes decisions for others, presumably in their best interest
patulous	distended
peristalsis	a wavelike progression of contraction and relaxation of muscle fibers in the esophagus
Physician extender	physician's assistant or advanced practice registered nurse
protein-calorie malnutrition	a condition in which the patient is malnourished in both calories and protein
rale	an abnormal respiratory sound
reflux	see gastroesophageal reflux
rhonchi	coarse, dry rales in the bronchial tubes
sensitivity	accuracy identifying patients who have a particular characteristic
serum osmolality	a measure of particle concentration in the blood; a high osmolality may indicate dehydration
specificity	accuracy ruling out patients who do not have a particular characteristic
tardive dyskinesia	a form of hyperkinetic dysarthria that may develop after prolonged use of neuroleptic drugs
thrush	disease caused by the fungus *Candida albicans*, which results in white patches on the mouth, throat, and tongue, usually accompanied by pain and fever

total parenteral nutrition (TPN)	delivers nutrients intravenously; often used when the gut is not working
trismus	fibrosis of the muscles of mastication
UGI (upper GI)	a videofluoroscopic study of the lower (distal) esophagus, the stomach and the stomach emptying into the small intestine
upper esophageal sphincter (UES)	the sphincter at the top of the esophagus formed by the cricopharyngeus
vallecula	a depression created between base of tongue and epiglottis
Valsalva maneuver	trying to exhale forcefully while tightly closing the glottis; increases intrathoracic pressure
vasoconstrictor	drugs that cause constriction of small blood vessels and reduce swelling
wheeze	a whistling respiratory sound
xerostomia	dry mouth